A Comprehensive Approach to

Stereotactic Breast Biopsy

Contributors

Andrea Dawson, M.D. — Department of Pathology, University of Rochester Medical Center, Rochester, New York.

Gia A. DeAngelis, M.D. — Assistant Professor of Radiology, University of Virginia Health Sciences Center, Charlottesville, Virginia.

W. Phil Evans, M.D. — Susan G. Komen Breast Center, Baylor University Medical Center, Dallas, Texas.

Laurie L. Fajardo, M.D. — Vice Chairman of Research and Professor of Radiology, University of Virginia Health Sciences Center, Charlottesville, Virginia.

Paul R. Fisher, M.D. — Director of Breast Imaging, Breast Care Center, Portsmouth, Virginia; Adjunct Professor of Radiology, University of Virginia Health Sciences Center, Charlottesville, Virginia.

Jennifer A. Harvey, M.D. — Assistant Professor of Radiology, University of Virginia Health Sciences Center, Charlottesville, Virginia.

Roy A. Jensen, M.D. — Department of Pathology, Vanderbilt University Medical Center, Nashville, Tennessee.

Shahla Masood, M.D. — Professor and Associate Chair, Department of Pathology, University of Florida Health Science Center; Chief of Pathology, University Medical Center, Jacksonville, Florida.

Gillian M. Newstead, M.D. — Faculty Practice Radiology, Breast Imaging Center, New York, New York.

David L. Page, M.D. — Department of Pathology, Vanderbilt University Medical Center, Nashville, Tennessee.

Robert J. Pizzutiello, M.S., F.A.C.M.P. — President, Upstate Medical Physics, Inc., Victor, New York.

Debra S. Saunders — Manager, Clinical Applications, LORAD®, a division of Trex Medical Corporation, a Thermo Electron Company, Danbury, Connecticut.

Richard Van Metter, Ph.D. — Research Physicist, Eastman Kodak Company, Rochester, New York.

Mark B. Williams, Ph.D. — Assistant Professor of Radiology, Division of Radiology Research, University of Virginia Health Sciences Center, Charlottesville, Virginia.

Kathleen M. Willison, R.T. (R)(M) — The Elizabeth Wende Breast Clinic, Rochester, New York.

A Comprehensive Approach to

Stereotactic Breast Biopsy

Edited by

Laurie L. Fajardo, M.D.

Kathleen M. Willison

Robert J. Pizzutiello

This book was made possible by an educational grant from LORAD®, a division of Trex Medical Corporation, a Thermo Electron Company.

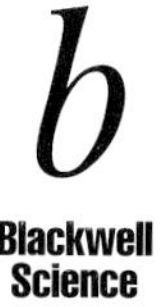

Berlin • Boston • Edinburgh • London • Melbourne • Oxford • Paris • Tokyo • Vienna

Blackwell Science
Editorial offices:
238 Main Street, Cambridge, Massachusetts 02142, USA
Osney Mead, Oxford OX2 0EL, England
25 John Street, London WC1N 2BL, England
23 Ainslie Place, Edinburgh EH3 6AJ, Scotland
54 University Street, Carlton, Victoria 3053, Australia
Arnette Blackwell SA, 1 rue de Lille, 75007 Paris, France
Blackwell Wissenschafts-Verlag GmbH
Kurfürstendamm 57, 10707 Berlin, Germany
Feldgasse 13, A-1238 Vienna, Austria

Distributors:
North America
Blackwell Science, Inc.
238 Main Street
Cambridge, Massachusetts 02142
(Telephone orders: 800-215-1000 or 617-876-7000)

Australia
Blackwell Science Pty Ltd
54 University Street
Carlton, Victoria 3053
(Telephone orders: 03-347-0300
fax: 03-349-3016)

Outside North America and Australia
Blackwell Science, Ltd.
c/o Marston Book Services, Ltd.
P.O. Box 87
Oxford OX2 0DT
England
(Telephone orders: 44-865-791155)

Typeset by: Pierce Brown Associates Inc.
Printed and bound by: Mercury Print Productions, Inc.
Rochester, New York

Printed in the United States of America
00 99 98 97 5 4 3 2 1

Notice: The indications and dosages of all drugs in this book have been recommended in the medical literature and conform to the practices of the general medical community. The medications described do not necessarily have specific approval by the Food and Drug Administration for use in the diseases and dosages for which they are recommended. The package insert for each drug should be consulted for use and dosage as approved by the FDA. Because standards of usage change, it is advisable to keep abreast of revised recommendations, particularly those concerning new drugs.

Library of Congress Cataloging-in-Publication Data
A comprehensive approach to stereotactic breast biopsy / edited by
Laurie L. Fajardo, Kathleen M. Willison, Robert J. Pizzutiello.
p. cm.
Includes bibliographical references and index.
ISBN 0-86542-467-5 (alk. paper). — ISBN 0-86542-467-5 (alk. paper)
1. Breast—Needle biopsy. 2. Stereotaxic techniques.
I. Fajardo, Laurie L. II. Willison, Kathleen M. III. Pizzutiello, Robert J., 1955-
[DNLM: 1. Biopsy, Needle—methods. 2. Stereotaxic Techniques.
3. Breast Diseases—pathology. 4. Breast Diseases—radiography.
WP 840 C737 1995]
RG493.5.B56C65 1995
618.1' 90758—dc20
DNLM/DLC 95-44397
for Library of Congress CIP

To Dr. Wende Logan-Young,
who fosters creative thought and intellectual growth
beyond what is merely conventional or expected.
All who are committed to the detection of early breast cancer
owe her an incalculable debt,
as a pioneer, a clinician, and as a superb interpreter
of the radiographic signs and clinical symptoms of breast disease.

Contents

Foreword

In the last quarter century, the diagnostic radiologist has gradually evolved from passive interpreter of the mammogram to the physician who is most capable of establishing the diagnosis of breast cancer. This evolution began with the expansion of the radiologist's role to include clinical breast examination, additional tailored mammographic views, ultrasonography, and fine needle aspiration cytology.

And now, finally, we have 14-gauge needle core biopsy, whose arrival could not be more timely. This accurate substitute for open-surgical biopsy arrives amidst the cost containment efforts of health maintenance organizations, industry, and government. Not only is 14-gauge needle biopsy an inexpensive method of diagnosing breast cancer, it is also amazingly well-tolerated by patients, who gratefully appreciate the quickness and ease of the procedure, the absence of scar tissue, and core biopsy's ready availability compared with the difficulty of scheduling operating room time.

Large-core gun biopsy offers other advantages as well. First, if the patient has an abnormality that is suggestive of carcinoma, a 14-gauge gun biopsy can establish the diagnosis without subjecting her to an additional surgical procedure. The patient much prefers undergoing an immediate 14-gauge gun biopsy to a surgical biopsy at some later date in a hospital setting. If the core biopsy diagnosis is carcinoma, the patient can forego the open-surgical biopsy and proceed directly to either a wedge resection and lymph node dissection, or a modified radical mastectomy.

Second, the increased utilization of mammography means the detection of increasing numbers of nonpalpable abnormalities. In addition to establishing the diagnosis of probable breast cancer, core biopsy also allows radiologists to investigate indeterminate abnormalities. In a perfect world, all radiologists would agree on which abnormalities require open-surgical biopsy and which need monitoring at short intervals. But in reality, radiologists often disagree in their interpretations and recommendations.

At one end of the spectrum are radiologists who advise as many as 10 women to undergo biopsy for every cancer that is surgically confirmed. These radiologists could perform core biopsies on the most benign-appearing of those abnormalities for which they would ordinarily recommend open-surgical biopsy. In other words, they would perform core biopsy on abnormalities just *above* their threshold for recommending open-surgical biopsy.

At the opposite end of the spectrum are radiologists, like those at our clinic, who advise only three women to undergo surgical biopsy for every two cancers verified. These radiologists could perform core biopsies on those patients whom they would not ordinarily send for surgical biopsy, but would instead monitor at short intervals. In other words, they would perform core biopsy on abnormalities that are just *below* their threshold for recommending open-surgical biopsy.

Thus, core biopsy will reduce the percentage of surgical biopsies recommended by the radiologist who has a high ratio of surgical biopsy to cancer. Core biopsy will also find more early cancers in women whose mammograms are assessed by the radiologist who has a low ratio of recommended surgical biopsy to cancer.

Only us "oldies" who, in the early 1970s, attempted to interpret mammograms with poor contrast (often with motion artifact), obtained with nondedicated equipment, can truly appreciate the miraculous improvements that have occurred in the last 25 years. Now, our task is to convince radiologists to assume an expanding role in diagnosing breast cancer. We must also convince health maintenance organizations, industry, and government that this is the best approach to diagnosing breast cancer. This excellent book will be extremely helpful for those learning to perform stereotactic biopsy—an integral and vital tool in the fight to reduce deaths due to breast cancer.

Wende W. Logan-Young, M.D.

The Elizabeth Wende Breast Clinic

Preface

To date, much of the educational literature focuses on the results and efficacy of stereotactic breast biopsy (SBB). Little is written that addresses the practical matters of the procedure. The goal of this text is to bridge the gap between theory, numbers, and practice.

The editors have put together a comprehensive text on SBB, endeavoring to keep the content to that of a practical nature. Although the procedural emphasis is on stereotactic large gauge automated biopsy (core biopsy), the contributing authors discuss stereotactic breast biopsy as one diagnostic element in a broad breast cancer detection program, having specific indications and contraindications. The text presents various disciplinary perspectives to assist the biopsy team in establishing and maintaining a successful breast needle biopsy (BNB) program.

The text meets the practical needs of the increasing number of clinicians and technologists performing stereotactic procedures. It will also be useful to medical physicists and administrators who, although at the periphery of the procedure, are involved in quality assurance issues, equipment purchase, and policy making. The text contains basic information for the novice but also provides useful methods and practices for more experienced users.

Digital imaging systems are in wide use for SBB procedures. In many cases, SBB will be the biopsy team's first encounter with a digital modality. Digital operation is sufficiently diverse from conventional imaging to warrant an entire chapter on the subject.

Kathleen M. Willison

The Elizabeth Wende Breast Clinic

Acknowledgments

The editors would like to thank several people who had a significant impact on the completion of this text. First and foremost, we thank all of the contributing authors who took the time to impart the specifics of their specialty to improve our understanding of BNB and to enhance the value of this text. A special thanks to Dr. Paul Fisher of the University of Virginia for his technical comments and encouragement. We also thank Dr. Richard Van Metter for entering midway though this project, despite a busy schedule. The chapter on digital imaging would not be complete without his significant contribution.

We are grateful to several people at The Elizabeth Wende Breast Clinic in Rochester, New York. A special thanks to Dr. Wende Logan-Young for providing teaching cases. To Dr. Stamatia Destounis for her encouragement and valuable insight. Thanks also go to Kathryn Barnsdale, L.R.T. and Judy Labella, R.T. (R)(M) for their suggestions and comments. The Clinic's technologists also were extremely helpful; we thank them for their assistance in compiling case studies for this text. We are also grateful to Nancy Wayne, Barbara Briody, and Jamie Egan at the Clinic, and Dave Mezzoprete (S & W X-Ray of Rochester, Rochester, New York) for their contributions to this project.

We would also like to thank Bronwyn Chaple, Manager, South Australian Breast X-Ray Service, Wayville, Australia for her comments and suggestions on chapter 2. Special recognition is also in order for Jeff Blackman for his expertise in clinical and medical photography.

A special thanks and appreciation go to the staff of Pierce Brown Associates Inc., Rochester, New York. As project manager and copy editor, Lorraine Trude provided a cohesive, readable presentation of the information and coordinated the layout of the text. We would also like to thank Joanne Farr, art director, who was responsible for graphic design, illustration, and typography. She provides the book with its superb aesthetic appearance. We also thank Donna Stubbings for compiling and proofreading the text, and Mike D'Alessandro, who established the print production quality of this book.

We extend our sincere appreciation to LORAD® for underwriting this project, in particular, we thank Hal Kirshner, President, who understands the value of practical techniques in the successful use of equipment. We offer our highest regard to Tony Pellegrino, CEO, for his ongoing commitment to provide equipment that is not only serviceable for the patient, but also addresses the needs of the user. Special thanks go to Kenneth DeFreitas for his technical assistance, time, and patience. We also thank Debra Saunders for her expertise and technical suggestions on the positioning chapter, and Alan Rigo, who made it technically possible for us to use LORAD digital images in the text. A very special thanks and recognition go to Anne Smith for coordinating the entire project.

We are especially grateful to the publisher, Blackwell Science, Inc. and Executive Editor, Christopher Davis for believing in the need for this text.

Finally, we would like to thank our families for their steadfast support and encouragement throughout this project.

Overview of Breast Needle Biopsy

Kathleen M. Willison

1

This chapter will familiarize the reader with current methods of the breast needle biopsy (BNB) procedure and introduce the practical aspects of implementing a breast needle biopsy program. A detailed discussion of techniques and how to establish a BNB program can be found in subsequent chapters.

Minimally invasive breast needle biopsy can replace surgical excisional biopsy for diagnosing most breast abnormalities. The two methods currently in use for BNB are fine needle aspiration cytology (FNAC, FNAB) and large-core automated needle biopsy (core biopsy). The main distinction between these two methods is the ease with which clinicians can obtain, preserve, and interpret a sample. Core biopsy yields a large core of tissue (histologic material), whereas FNAC provides a sampling of cells (cytologic material). Because of the small sample extracted with FNAC, it is more difficult to become proficient in obtaining an adequate sample, compared with core biopsy. The preparation and interpretation of the cytological sample also demands meticulous technique and, most important, a pathologist trained in cytopathology of the breast. In most cases, core biopsy also offers a more definitive diagnosis when compared with FNAC[1-6].

Biopsy Methods

FNAC is performed with a 20 to 23-gauge needle attached to a syringe directly, or with connective tubing. A variety of needle types are in use, however, chiba or spinal needles are the most common. Needle length varies depending on the depth of the abnormality in the breast and the biopsy modality. Once the needle is introduced into the abnormality, negative pressure is applied by pulling back on the syringe, allowing the aspiration of material for sampling. The cytologic or cellular material is preserved on slides for interpretation by a cytopathologist. Depending on the modality used for biopsy, FNAC can be accomplished in a relatively short period of time, 3 to 30 minutes.

Core biopsy is performed with a specially designed 14 to 18-gauge needle (14-gauge is most popular) that is placed in a rapid-fire automated biopsy instrument, commonly called a biopsy gun. Once the needle is placed at the appropriate depth, the spring-loaded, double-action gun rapidly advances the two-stage needle, taking a core of tissue during its excursion. Histological or tissue samples procured with core biopsy are preserved in formalin for interpretation by a histopathologist. Depending on the modality used, the core biopsy procedure requires 20 minutes to one hour or more to perform.

Biopsy Modalities

Breast needle biopsy can be performed with either *clinical guidance* or one of three *image guidance* modalities. Imaging methods for biopsy include the grid coordinate system, ultrasound, and stereotactic breast biopsy. These methods require varying degrees of training, experience, procedure time and equipment, and each provides a different degree of accuracy.

Clinical Guidance—Clinically guided BNB can be accomplished on palpable abnormalities that may or may not be mammographically and sonographically occult. The clinician places the needle by hand, relying on palpation of the breast abnormality. The abnormality is subject to movement because the breast is not fixed in position.

Clinically guided biopsy is primarily employed with FNAC. Clinically guided core biopsy requires greater skill and experience than clinically guided FNAC due to the difficulty of maneuvering the heavier biopsy instrument, and the excursion and speed of the biopsy needle in the unfixed breast. Care must be taken to maintain the needle in a position parallel to the chest wall. These factors can compromise accuracy, sterility and safety, further emphasizing the need for a skilled clinician.

One major disadvantage of clinically guided BNB is that no systematic method exists to document accurate needle placement. Therefore, depending on the initial level of clinical concern, *negative* results may pose a dilemma for the clinician. The clinician is often faced with the choice of open excisional biopsy or follow-up interval mammography, based on how the abnormality felt. However, if needle biopsy is *positive*, the patient can avoid excisional biopsy and make appropriate choices regarding definitive treatment.

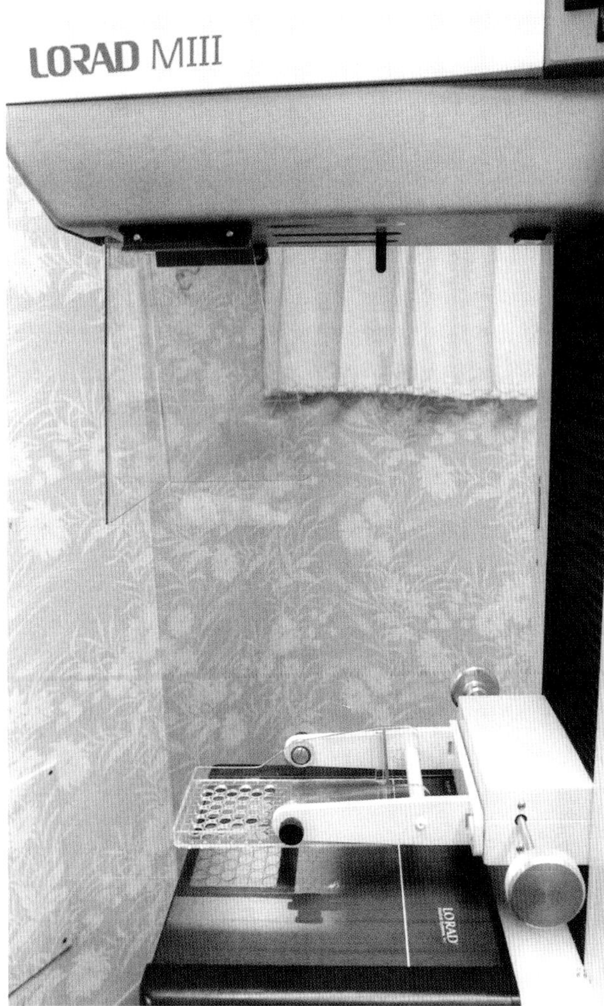

Figure 1.1. Grid Coordinate System.

Grid Coordinate System—The grid coordinate system utilizes dedicated mammography equipment and a needle localization grid (**Figure 1.1**). The clinician uses the localization grid to locate the abnormality in *two dimensions*. Although relatively inexpensive and a sound method for needle localization, this method does not determine or guarantee access to the third dimension, that is, the correct *depth* of the abnormality. At best, the depth of the abnormality can only be estimated. Freehand-guidance of the needle further diminishes accuracy of needle placement.

Ultrasound-Guided Biopsy (Sonographic)—Sonographic biopsy has application for palpable or nonpalpable abnormalities. The same challenges exist in sonographic biopsy that exist in clinically guided biopsy. But unlike clinical guidance, real-time ultrasound enables monitoring of needle movement. This is especially true when performing FNAC, yielding exceptional accuracy in trained hands. However, the excursion of the biopsy needle during core biopsy is not as easily monitored, due to the rate of speed at which the needle moves.

In a recent study comparing ultrasound-guided biopsy with stereotactic-guided biopsy, it was reported that greater than 50% of all abnormalities and more than 60% of carcinomas *could not* be visualized with sonography[8]. Calcifications, architectural distortions, and small masses that measure 6 millimeters or less in size pose the greatest sonographic imaging difficulties[9].

Stereotactic Guidance—Stereotactic breast biopsy (SBB) requires specially designed equipment to calculate the location of an abnormality. This is accomplished by using two angled radiographs approximately 30° apart (+/-15° from center), and a coordinate system (see chapter 2). Studies have shown that the location of an abnormality is possible in three dimensions and is accurate to within 1 mm tolerances[10-12]. There are few exceptions to the types of abnormalities that can be biopsied using stereotactic guidance. Calcifications, masses, and architectural distortions are identifiable in most cases.

The stereotactic procedure is less dependent on clinician skills than are ultrasound or clinically guided methods because the breast is held immobile by a compression device. Consequently, the abnormality is less likely to move. In addition, the biopsy instrument is not handheld and manually guided — a guidance system holds the biopsy instrument as the needle is directed into the breast for sampling the abnormality. With most stereotactic equipment, orientation of the needle parallel to the chest wall eliminates the possibility of excursion beyond the limits of the breast into the chest wall or thorax.

The two types of stereotactic equipment in use today are upright add-on units and prone tables **(Figures 1.2 and 1.3)**. Add-on units require the patient to be upright in a sitting position during the procedure, and prone tables allow the patient to be recumbent.

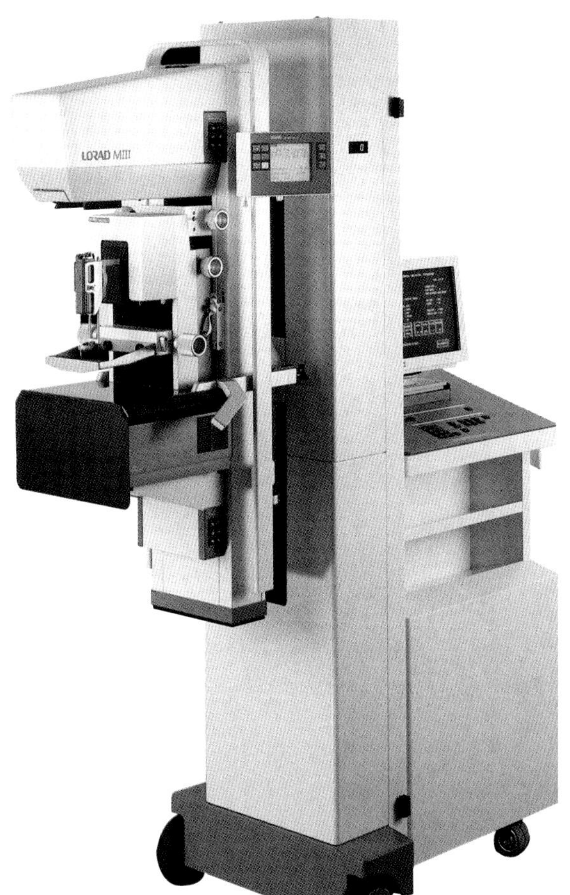

Figure 1.2. Add-On Unit (LORAD® MIII with StereoLoc®). Photo, courtesy of LORAD, a division of Trex Medical Corporation, a Thermo Electron Company.

Developing and Maintaining a Breast Needle Biopsy Program

Organization and planning are the first steps to creating a successful BNB program **(Figure 1.4)**. Determining the biopsy team, identifying methods and modalities, developing marketing strategies, organizing the biopsy suite, and defining patient care protocols are all matters for consideration.

The Biopsy Team

A dedicated, caring, and enthusiastic biopsy team is essential to the success of any BNB program. The biopsy team should consist of a clinician and one or two technologists, and a nurse, if desired. The number of clinicians and technologists trained in these procedures should be kept to a minimum. A small, dedicated team will develop greater proficiency with imaging guidance systems with exposure to a variety of patients and abnormalities than would a larger team, given a comparable case load.

The team clinician should be the person most closely associated with the breast diagnosis. The technologist should be a competent, experienced mammographer who welcomes new techniques. Knowledge and expertise in mammographic problem solving will aid in learning the techniques necessary to perform stereotactic procedures.

To encompass all aspects of patient care, an administrator, office staff, and medical physicist should also be members of the team. Each team member's area of expertise will affect the quality of the BNB program.

Providing education for the biopsy team can take many forms. Stereotactic equipment manufacturers provide training that focuses on the use of the equipment and imaging modalities. Tutorials and seminars on all modes of biopsy are available to provide the clinician and technologist with a comfortable level of confidence to perform their initial procedures.

Methods and Modalities

Selecting the appropriate methods and means of biopsy for the BNB program will depend on a variety of factors, which are discussed in chapters 7-10. The selection of stereotactic equipment usually involves the administrator, radiologist, technologist, and medical physicist (see chapter 4).

Marketing the BNB Program

A marketing strategy will help develop a referral base. Attention to this matter, during the equipment selection

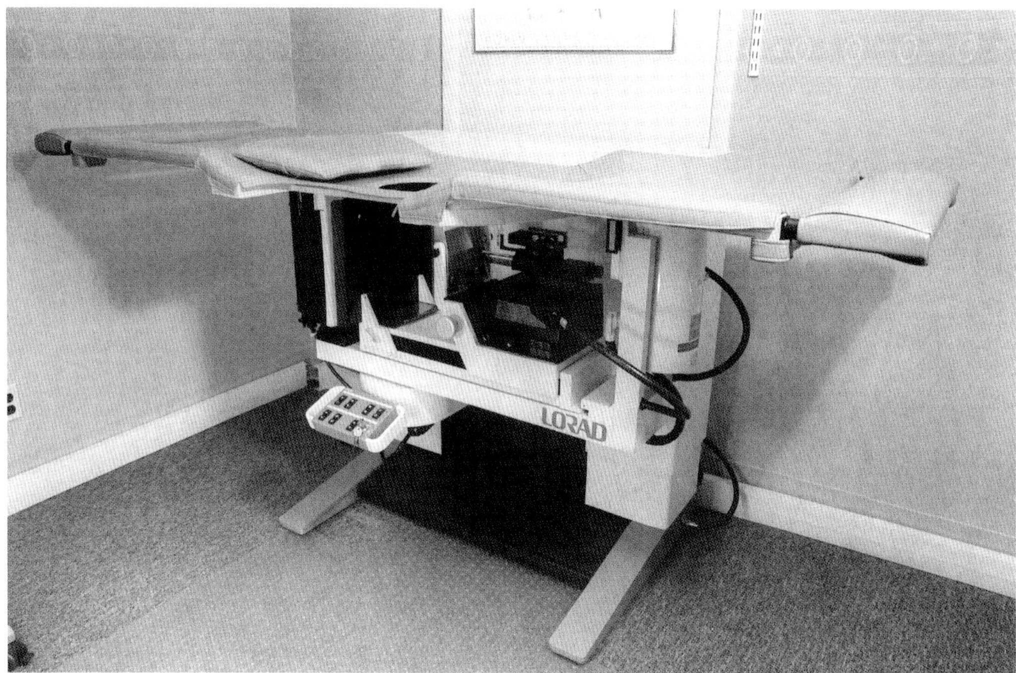

Figure 1.3. Prone Table. (LORAD® StereoGuide® prone breast biopsy system). Photo, courtesy of LORAD, a division of Trex Medical Corporation, a Thermo Electron Company.

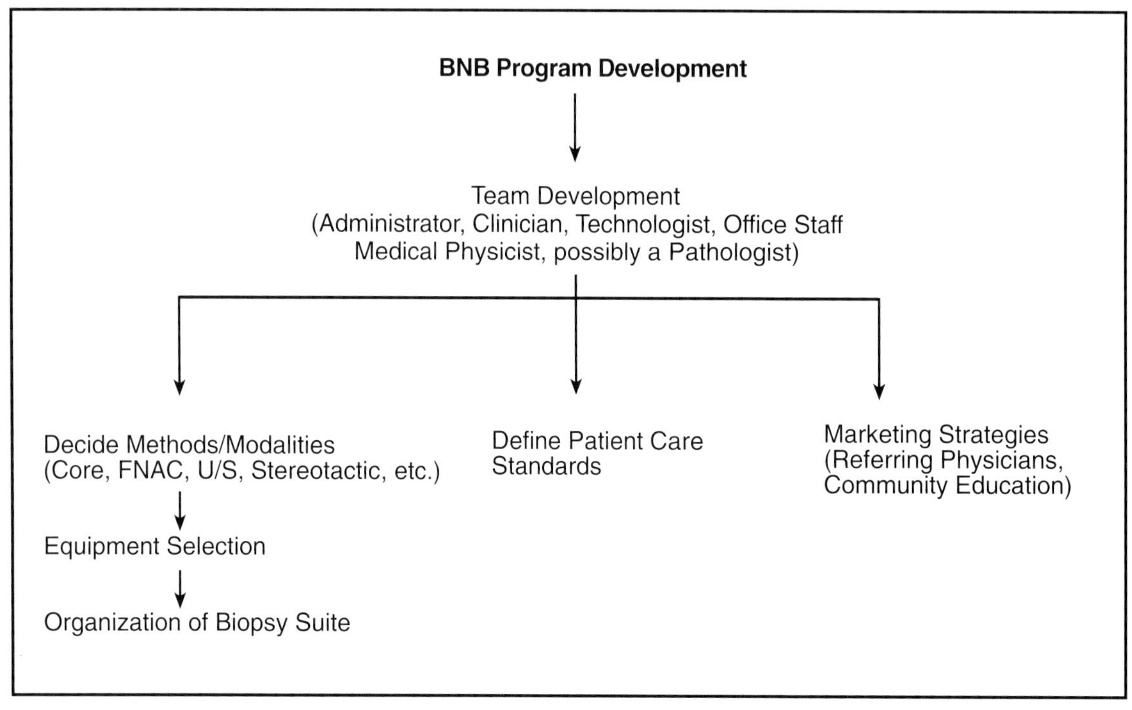

Figure 1.4. BNB Program Development.

process and while waiting for its arrival, eliminates the potential problem of having the team and equipment in place but no patients. Educational lectures for both referring physicians and the community can have a significant positive effect on a referral base (see chapter 7).

Organizing the Biopsy Suite

Organize the biopsy suite to maximize efficiency during the procedure (**Figure 1.5**). There should be adequate counter space to work on and storage space for supplies. A sink is a necessity in planning a biopsy suite. Installation of a radiographic viewbox provides the biopsy team with the ability to review mammograms during the biopsy procedure. Use space effectively, taking into account the total number of people that may be working at one time. The equipment manufacturer can help with the suite layout to ensure the correct placement of the stereotactic equipment. Identify and order supplies to stock the room and the sterile tray. Items necessary for the procedure are listed in appendix A.

Setting Patient Care Standards

Quality patient care should be the focus of the BNB program from the first contact with the patient, through the biopsy process, to interval or yearly follow-up. To ensure success, define all administrative and clinical aspects prior to the inception of the BNB program. Quality assurance standards should be available as detailed written protocols to provide a blueprint for the direction of the program (**Figure 1.6**). The written protocols aid in maintaining quality and consistency of patient care and the assignment of responsibilities. Appropriate members of the team should make protocol decisions and re-evaluate them periodically.

The following section describes clinical and administrative protocols. Although some of the same subjects fall under both categories, the tasks may vary.

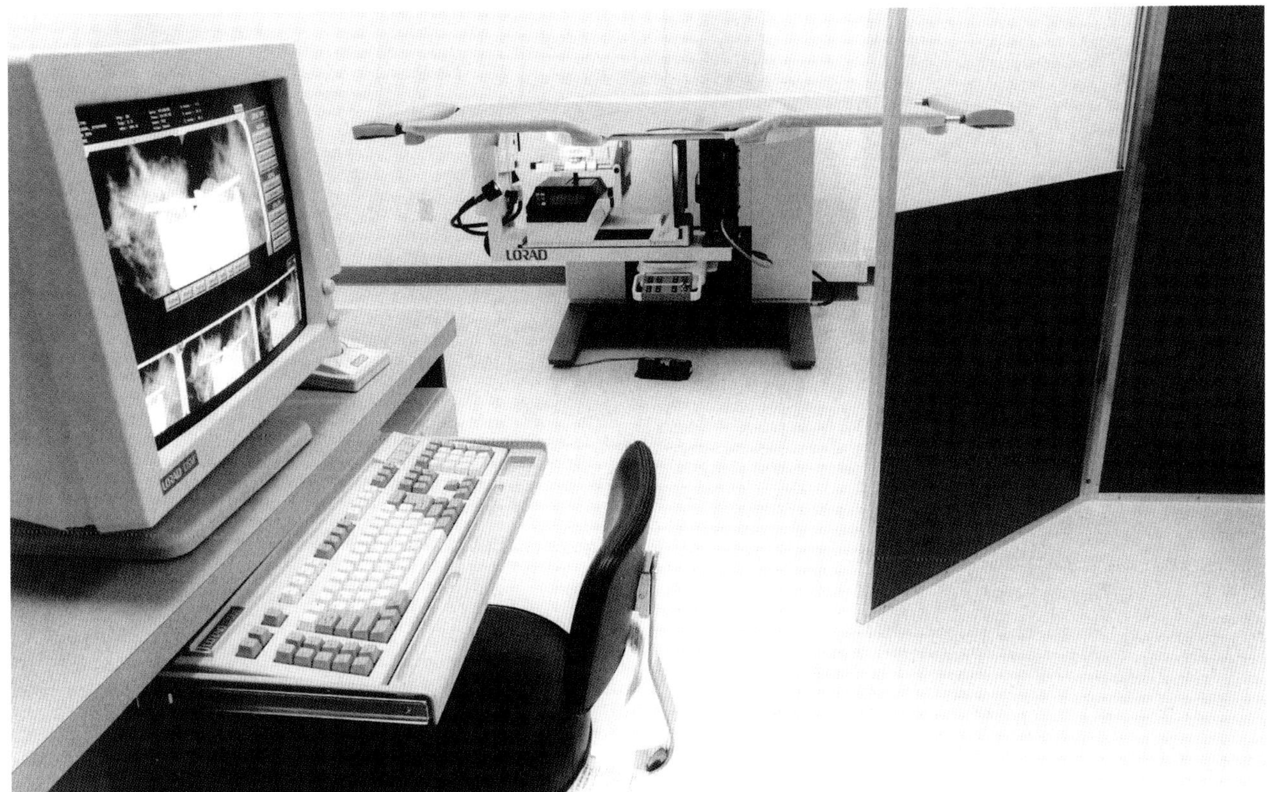

Figure 1.5. The Biopsy Suite.

Clinical and Administrative Protocols
Clinical
Patient selection
Abnormality selection
Correlative studies (FNAC vs. core vs. open biopsy)
Contact with Pathology Department
Procedure protocols for biopsy
Role of the clinician in patient care and follow-up
Follow-up of patients with benign results
Prebiopsy instructions
Immediate postbiopsy care
Next day follow-up care
Tracking pathological results (practice audit)
Administrative
Exposure control plan for blood borne pathogens
Appropriate literature, consent form, prebiopsy information/instructions, postbiopsy instructions
Protocols for patient scheduling
System to retrieve outside mammograms for review
Transporting samples to Pathology Department
Appropriate labeling and requisitions for samples
Record keeping
Quality assurance

Figure 1.6. Issues of Importance for Defining Clinical and Administrative Protocols.

Clinical Protocols

The clinician should define and establish a review process for the following protocols:

Patient Selection

Obtain the patient's medical history prior to the date of biopsy, especially for core biopsy candidates. It is best to see the patient and speak directly with her. Some restrictions may require preparation for biopsy, or a change in biopsy method.

Medications—If a patient is taking anticoagulants, she might not be a candidate for core biopsy; however, FNAC might be a viable choice. If core biopsy is desired, then her medication might be altered prior to and following biopsy. Instruct the patient to contact her physician regarding any change in medication. If the patient requires prophylactic antibiotics for dental work, she may also need them for core biopsy.

Patient Tolerance—Generally, BNB procedures are widely accepted by patients. However, severe back pain, neck pain, or injury might inhibit a patient's ability to remain immobile for stereotactic procedures, regardless of the equipment available. A patient's inability to be recumbent eliminates the possibility of using a prone table, whereas the use of upright equipment can eliminate those patients who cannot tolerate being immobile in an upright position for up to an hour or more.

Abnormality Selection

The types of abnormalities that are subject to biopsy, and the specific method applied, will depend on prevailing approaches to breast diagnosis and on the referring physician's acceptance of new modalities. The accepted list of abnormalities for biopsy will most likely expand as experience with BNB develops, and as referring physicians gain greater confidence in the procedure. Chapters 8-11 provide additional information to guide the physician in abnormality selection.

The clinician can define categories for mammographic abnormalities by utilizing a classification system, such as the American College of Radiology system. With this categorization, protocols for abnormality selection can be further defined for all BNB methods and modalities.

Establish Correlative Studies

Due to the political climate and despite evidence in the literature of the efficacy of BNB, it might be necessary to establish comparative studies of BNB with open biopsy. For this reason, establish protocols *prior to* the inception of a BNB program.

Review Process for Referred Patients

When patients are referred by an outside source, there must be a system to procure the patient's mammograms for review to determine the viability of biopsy. For these patients, it may be necessary to perform additional mammographic and sonographic work-up, in advance, or on the day of biopsy.

Define the Role of the Clinician

The clinician performing BNB must define his or her role in patient follow-up care. This includes reporting results and ensuring that patients return for interval mammography (see chapter 7).

Establish Contact with Pathology

Establish contact with the Pathology Department to determine appropriate sample preservation, enabling cytopathologists and histopathologists to correctly interpret the sample. Contact with Pathology is especially important in FNAC, where preservation of cellular material has a more critical effect on diagnosis.

Establish Procedural Protocols for Biopsy

To assure smooth performance, outline the steps of the procedure and delegate various tasks to team members. This allows each team member to anticipate the next task and ensures maximum team efficiency.

Postbiopsy Care

Patient care immediately after the core biopsy procedure may include:

1. Compression of the biopsy site until bleeding subsides.
2. Application of an antibiotic ointment.
3. Closure of the mammotomy site, using steristrips. Placing a pressure dressing over the biopsy site to prevent hematoma is optional.
4. Application of single-use ice packets to alleviate discomfort and reduce edema.

Fifteen minutes is usually sufficient to observe postprocedural complications.

The clinician should counsel the patient regarding postbiopsy care. Give the patient a written explanation of instructions (see *Administrative Protocols*).

Next Day Follow-Up

Patient morbidity related to BNB is low. It is best to contact the patient 24 hours following the procedure to determine if there are complications and to ensure that the patient is following instructions for postbiopsy care. The technologist usually contacts the patient by phone.

Tracking of Pathological Results

To develop confidence in the procedure and to instill confidence in the medical community, it is essential to track the results of the BNB program. Tracking results also enables the clinician to become more proficient at the procedure. Information can be gathered as to the types of abnormalities that are suitable for BNB. Tracking results can help further define methods and modalities appropriate for various abnormalities. Practice audits mandated by law will require this type of monitoring in the near future (see chapter 12). A *Patient Log for Breast Needle Biopsy,* shown in **Figure 1.7,** demonstrates the type of information needed to track results.

Administrative Protocols

Safety with Blood Borne Pathogens

All personnel involved in the biopsy procedure, including those who transport specimens to Pathology, must be trained

Patient Log for Breast Needle Biopsy

Patient ID	FNAC	Core	U/S	Clinical	Stereotactic	Mass	Ca++	Arch/dist	Mass/Ca ++	Size in mm, less than				Incomplete*					Results			
										5	10	15	20	1	2	3	4	5	B	M	Atyp	Other
Totals																						

*Code
1 = Patient could not tolerate
2 = Cyst/pseudo mass, procedure aborted
3 = Nonvisualization, radiographically
4 = Nonvisualization, positional
5 = Other

Figure 1.7 Sample Patient Log for Breast Needle Biopsy.

in *universal precautions* pertaining to the handling of blood and blood borne pathogens. Rules and regulations for the handling of blood, including specimen handling and transport, cleaning of equipment, and staff training are set forth by the Occupational Safety and Health Administration[13] (OSHA).

Develop Necessary Forms

The clinician and the administrator need to develop the following literature:

Consent Form— Consult appropriate personnel to develop an informed consent.

Instructions Prior to Core Biopsy—This brochure should inform and educate the patient about the procedure and any necessary preparation. Food and drink intake need not be restricted prior to core biopsy or FNAC. However, if the patient is to lie in a prone position for biopsy, suggest light meals prior to biopsy.

Postcore Instructions—The patient should restrain from strenuous activity for the remainder of the day, especially if an activity requires the use of the ipsilateral arm. Instruct the patient to take acetaminophen (such as Tylenol®) for discomfort. It is advisable to avoid aspirin or aspirin-containing products to prevent the possibility of bleeding. Bruising around the biopsy site is common with core biopsy. The patient should examine the site for hardness or a lump (indicating hematoma), and for heat or redness (indicating infection). Although complications are rare, include an emergency number on the instruction form. This form can also indicate when she can expect the results and who will contact her.

Scheduling

At the time of discovery of the abnormality, the clinic can perform BNB if it is prepared for immediate procedures. Otherwise, protocols for scheduling should consider the following:

1. Personnel to make the appointment.

2. Pertinent patient information, such as name, address, phone, etc.

3. Medical history, including current medications, physical limitations prohibiting the procedure (that is, weight or musculo-skeletal limitations), or a medical condition that may require prophylactic antibiotics, for example, mitral valve prolapse or diabetes.

4. Insurance review to determine if a referral is necessary.

5. Follow-up appointments after benign biopsy.

Scheduling is best made directly with the patient, especially for follow-up visits.

Labeling and Transport of Specimens

The Pathology Department requires specific labeling of the tissue sample, with appropriate requisitions. Decide how to and who will transport the samples. Request that the Pathology Department set timelines for reporting results, which is important information for the patient.

Outside Mammograms

Establish protocols to obtain outside mammograms prior to the date of biopsy. This allows the clinician to review images to determine the viability of biopsy.

Record Keeping

Develop a patient log to record breast needle biopsy activity to aid in proper follow-up and tracking of the patient. See Figure 1.7 for a sample patient log.

It is important to consider provisions for the archival and storage of patient images, including hard copy and digital media (such as optical disk). Develop appropriate folders and labels for all patient records.

Quality Assurance

It is important to include the necessary time and cost in the BNB program to perform ongoing quality control testing of the stereotactic biopsy unit. Although the Food and Drug Administration has not yet set quality assurance guidelines for SBB equipment, it is important to ensure that the unit functions properly. *In addition, poor equipment performance can result in greater patient rejection due to nonvisualization of the abnormality.* Acceptance testing and interval quality control testing by a medical physicist establishes a *performance standard* for the unit (see chapter 13). The technologist should then perform applicable tests from the American College of Radiology recommendations for mammography units[14]. Not all the recommended tests apply to the stereotactic unit. However, the following activities will ensure that the unit is functioning properly:

- Phantom imaging. Perform at least once a month.

• Quality control visual checklist. Perform quarterly. The technologist can establish a checklist specific to the SBB equipment. A sample visual checklist appears in appendix A.

• Technique chart. The technologist should develop a technique chart to set guidelines for technique selection.

• Repeat reject analysis. This will help the technologist to determine if she is improving at positioning and imaging abnormalities.

• Daily calibration checks for coordinate calculation of all SBB equipment (see chapter 2). The technologist will need additional time to complete this test.

The advent of digital imaging brings other issues of quality assurance to the forefront. At this time, quality assurance testing for the components of the digital system are in the research stage of development. Of particular importance is the proper setup and functioning of the monitor. Additional testing to determine the proper functioning of the coupling system and the digital camera (including the CCD, analog-to-digital converter, and cooling system) is also needed. Until standards and tests are determined and perfected, it is necessary to rely on the equipment manufacturer to perform tests and preventive maintenance. Without this testing, it is difficult to determine if the equipment is functioning properly. The ACR is currently developing a voluntary QA program for stereotactic systems.

Establishing a practice audit will provide valuable information for the clinician. See chapter 12 for a detailed discussion.

Maintaining Proficiency

In the early stages of a BNB program, the number of patients may be scarce. Practice, which can be accomplished with phantom work, is a prerequisite to increased proficiency and confidence. Use commercial or homemade phantoms to keep skills sharp (**Figure 1.8**). If the biopsy team performs less than two procedures a week, allow additional time for training and skill development.

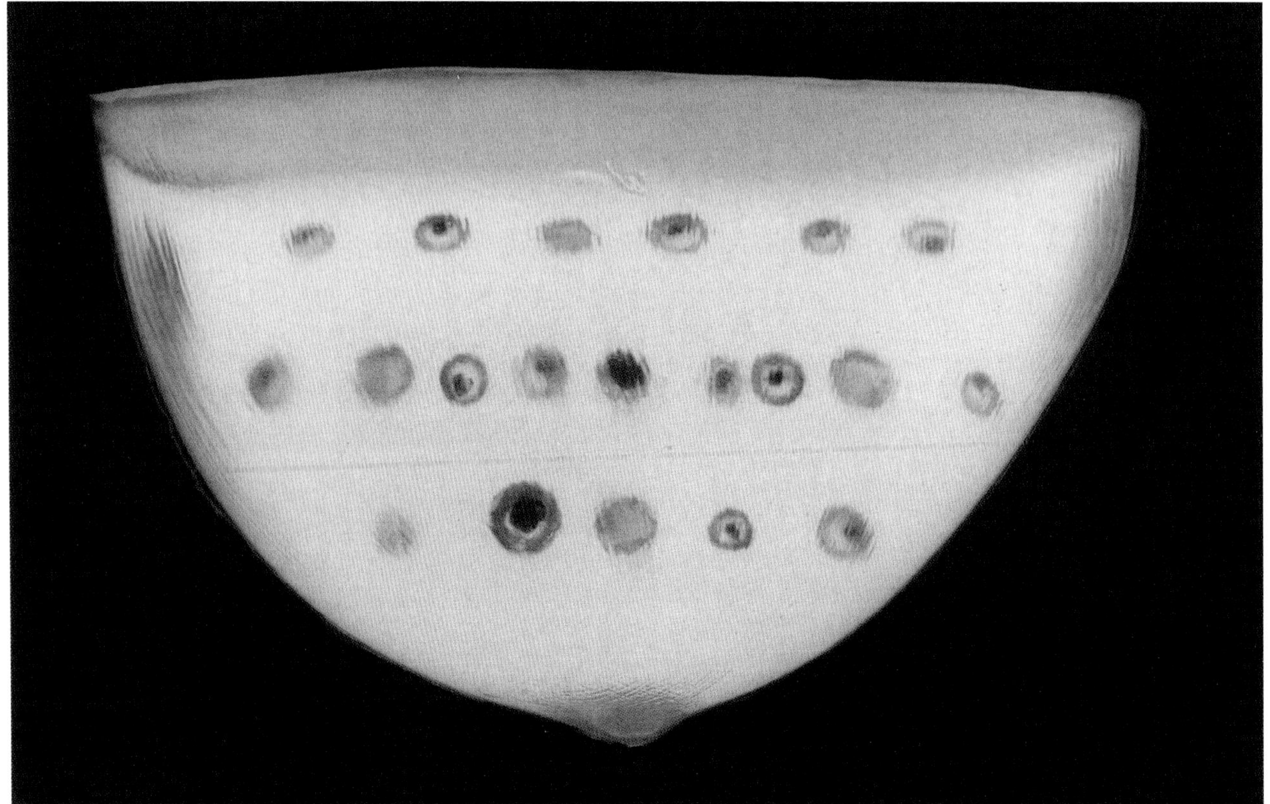

Figure 1.8. A Typical Commercial Practice Phantom. This phantom is a product of Nuclear Associates, Division of Victoreen, Inc.

References

1. Gent, H. J. 1986. Stereotaxic Needle Localization and Cytological Diagnosis of Occult Breast Lesions. *Annals of Surgery* 204:580-585.

2. Lofgren, M., Andersson, I., Bondeson, L., Lindholm, K. 1988. X-ray Guided Fine Needle Aspiration for the Cytologic Diagnosis of Non-palpable Breast Lesions. *Cancer* 61:1032-1037.

3. Azavedo, E., Svane, G., Auer, G. 1989. Stereotactic Fine Needle Biopsy in 2594 Mammographically Detected Non-palpable Lesions. *Lancet* 1:1033-1036.

4. Ciatto, S., Del Turco, Mr., Bravetti, B. 1989. Non-palpable Breast Lesions: Stereotaxic Fine Needle Aspiration Cytology. *Radiology* 173:57-59.

5. Parker, S.H., Lovin, J.D., Jobe, W.E., Luethke, J.M., Hopper, K.D., Yakes, W.F. 1991. Nonpalpable Breast Lesions: Stereotactic Automated Large Core Biopsies. *Radiology* [JC:qsh] 180 (August) (2):403-7.

6. Parker, S. H., Lovin, J.D., Jobe, W.E., Luethke, J.M., Hopper, K.D., Yakes, W.F., Burke, B.J. 1990. Stereotactic Breast Biopsy with a Biopsy Gun. *Radiology* 176 (September) (3):741-7.

7. Logan-Young, W. and Hoffman, N.Y. 1994. Breast Cancer: A Practical Guide to Diagnosis. Rochester: Mt. Hope Publishing Co., Inc., Vol. 1.

8. Elvecrog, E.L., Lechner, M.C., Nelson, M.T. 1993. Nonpalpable Breast Lesions: Correlation of Stereotaxtic Large-Core Needle Biopsy and Surgical Results. *Radiology* 188 (August) :453-455.

9. Fornage, B.D., Coan, J.D., David, C.L. 1992. Ultrasound-Guided Needle Biopsy of the Breast and Other Interventional Procedures. *Radiologic Clinics of North America* 30:167-185.

10. Bolmgren, J., Jacobson, B., Nordenström, B. 1977. Stereotaxic Instrument for the Needle Biopsy of the Mamma. *American Journal of Roentgenology* [JC:3ae] 129 (July) (1):121-5.

11. Nordenström, B. 1977. Stereotaxic Screw Needle Biopsy of Nonpalpable Breast Lesions In: *Breast Carcinoma: The Radiologists Expanded Role* edited by W.W. Young. New York: John Wiley & Sons, Inc.

12. Nordenström, B., Zajicek, J. 1977. Stereotaxic Needle Biopsy and Preoperative Indication of Non-Palpable Mammary Lesions. *Acta Cytologica* [JC:Oli] 21 (March-April) (2):350-1.

13. Federal Register, Part 1910.1030, Blood Borne Pathogens.

14. Technologists Manual–American College of Radiology Committee on Quality Assurance in Mammography. 1994. *American College of Radiology.*

Fundamentals of Stereotactic Breast Biopsy

Kathleen M. Willison

2

Introduction

The primary tasks of stereotactic breast biopsy (SBB) are positioning and imaging by the technologist, and targeting and sampling by the clinician. Developing expertise in these roles requires an understanding of stereotactic principles and the biopsy procedure.

The ability to mentally visualize the three-dimensional structure (clinician) and the position of an abnormality (technologist) in the breast from the two-view mammogram are invaluable skills. The clinician should understand the three-dimensional structure of the abnormality in terms of size, shape, and distribution. This awareness is essential for problem solving and significantly aids in appropriately targeting the abnormality. When the technologist and clinician are attentive to these and other visual cues, they can avoid incorrect sampling, faulty positioning, and procedural difficulties.

Although a computer performs the mathematics necessary to calculate localization, computations are based on the information provided by those performing the procedure. If the input information is inaccurate, errors will result. Faulty localization is rarely a malfunction of the stereotactic system or computer, but more often results from human error.

The purpose of this chapter is to describe the principles of stereotactic localization and stereotactic imaging, and the fundamentals of the core biopsy procedure. With this reserve of information, the biopsy team can prevent or recognize an error, preferably prior to needle insertion. This chapter also seeks to foster a thought process that aids the team in accomplishing safe, efficient, and successful biopsy.

Principles Of Stereotactic Localization

Stereology is the science of determining three-dimensional information about an object based on planar (two-dimensional) views. A familiar comparison, albeit oversimplified, is the stereoscopy the brain accomplishes through the human visual system. Each eye gives a different perspective of an object and the brain reconstructs the object three-dimensionally. This is simple to demonstrate — hold an object in front of the eyes and alternately close one eye and then the other, realizing the different perspective each eye is relaying to the brain. Take this one step further—alternately look at this object with one eye and then the other in *reference* to a more distant (or near) object. The distance of the apparent "shift" of the object in relation to the reference object is **parallax**. The brain solves the parallax problem (that is, the difference in relation to the reference) and accurately perceives the distance of the object. The resulting *depth perception* allows us to know how far to reach out to accurately touch the object. Depth perception is severely inhibited (in the absence of other visual or familiar clues) with loss of vision in one eye, or with only one perspective of the object. This problem is evident with the mammogram, where vertical and horizontal measurements are fairly easy to determine but the accurate measurement of depth is elusive.

Stereotactic breast localization involves the same visual principles that the brain and eyes use to accurately see a three-dimensional object. The object under consideration is the nonpalpable breast abnormality. For our purposes, the three-dimensional result is not reconstruction but accurate, quantitative computation of the location of the abnormality in the breast in three dimensions — horizontal, vertical, and depth. Accurate location of the abnormality is provided by: 1) the **stereo pair,** consisting of two planar images of the abnormality from different perspectives, 2) the **reference point** or points, providing the relative comparison of shift of the abnormality to determine depth and other coordinates, and 3) a **computer** that solves the mathematics of the parallax effect and determines location to within 1 mm.

Three-Dimensional Localization

The following provides an overview of three-dimensional localization/biopsy in the breast. A **scout image** properly demonstrating the abnormality in the biopsy window is a prerequisite. Two images, acquired with the x-ray tube at two different positions, are projected side by side on film or on another image receptor (monitor) to form the **stereo pair** (**Figure 2.1**). The clinician then targets the abnormality of interest. The computer determines location based on the abnormality's shift from the reference point. The computer also provides a **coordinate system** for translation of the results for practical use. After coordinate determination, a needle is placed in the breast for sampling, and a **confirmation (or prefire) stereo pair** is acquired. If the second stereo pair demonstrates accurate needle placement, then sampling of the abnormality is completed. Subsequent samples can be taken with or without other stereo images.

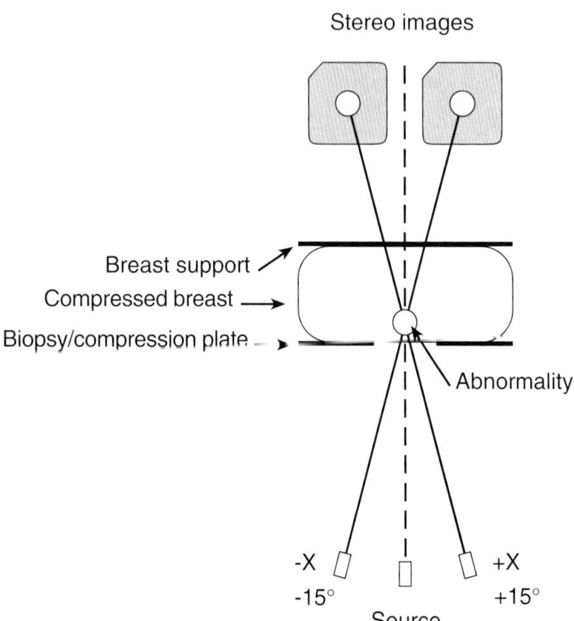

Figure 2.1. Three-Dimensional Localization. Acquisition of two planar images from different source positions provides the means for three-dimensional localization.

The following detailed discussion of three-dimensional localization will provide technical information and visual cues that are helpful during the procedure. Because variations among units are inevitable, each biopsy team should endeavor to discover each unit's unique characteristics.

Coordinate Systems

The primary purpose of a coordinate system is to identify a unique visual point in the breast that will be used as the target for the biopsy needle. The coordinate system, *regardless of type*, will give the location of the abnormality in three dimensions (**Figure 2.2**). The horizontal plane is expressed by *X* or *H*; the vertical plane by *Y* or *V*; and depth by *Z* or *D*.

There are two types of coordinate systems, Cartesian and polar. *A **Cartesian coordinate system** defines a point by distances from three axes that intersect at right angles.* The familiar X, Y, Z coordinates are the distances from the reference point in the X (left-right axis), Y (up-down axis), and Z (depth) directions (**Figure 2.3**). An example of abnormality location would be as follows: X = +4 mm, Y = 10 mm, Z = 22 mm. Perhaps the most obvious advantages of the Cartesian method are its familiarity and the intuitive ease with which most people adapt to its use. The simplicity of this coordinate system permits users to easily adjust needle position. For example, if analysis of the *prefire stereo pair* suggests that the needle is 5 mm too far to the left, it is easy to visualize repositioning the biopsy needle 5 mm to the right for correction. A Cartesian system also allows easier correlation with other aspects, such as *scale* and *reference*, which are described below.

*A **polar coordinate system** defines a target by the distances from a fixed point, and the angular distances from a reference line* (**Figure 2.4**). Coordinates are most often given as H, V, D. Horizontal and vertical coordinates are given in angles rather than millimeters. While this system is accurate, it is more difficult for the user to recognize errors, unless gross in nature. Correcting an error requires trigonometric calculations too complex to be practical during a procedure. Because the needle travels on an arc, a correction of H, V, or D may change the accuracy of the other coordinates. Thus, acquiring a new stereo pair and retargeting the abnormality would be the most effective method to correct an error.

Scale

Although the coordinate system is not visible on the biopsy

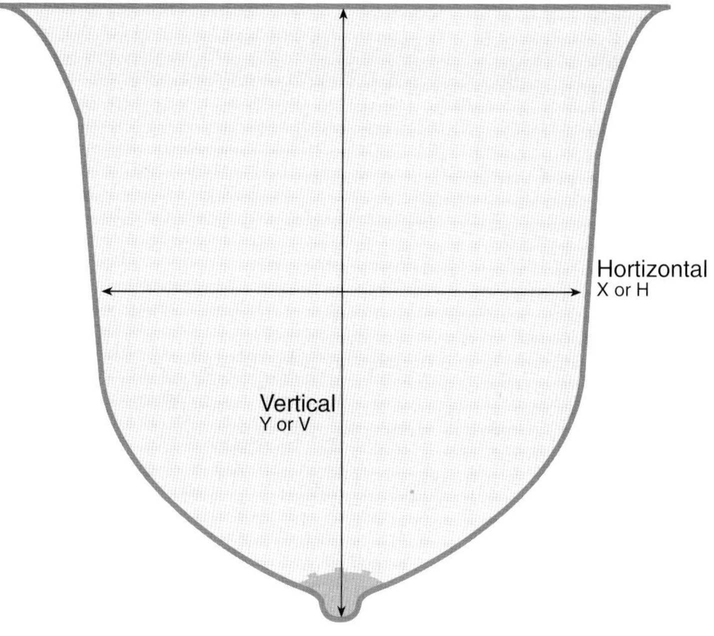

Frontal or Superior View
(prone unit) (upright unit)

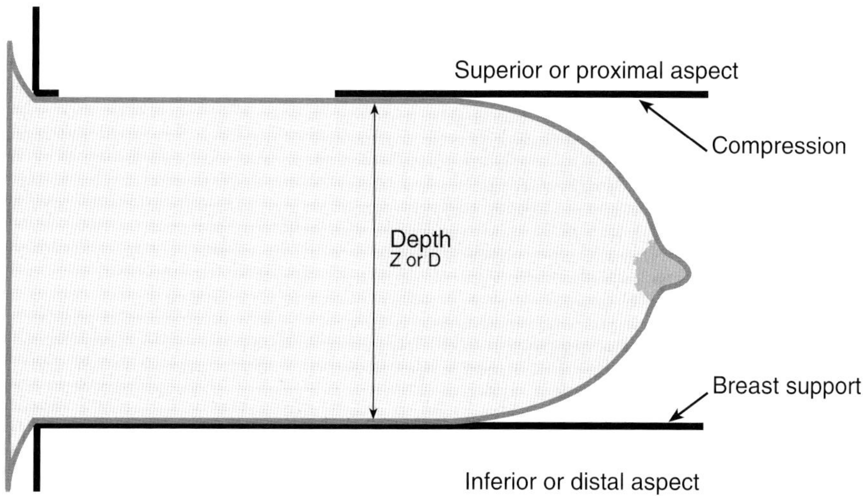

Lateral View

Figure 2.2. Three-Dimensional Coordinates. A coordinate system gives the location of the abnormality in three dimensions: X or H represents the horizontal plane, Y or V, the vertical, and Z or D, the depth.

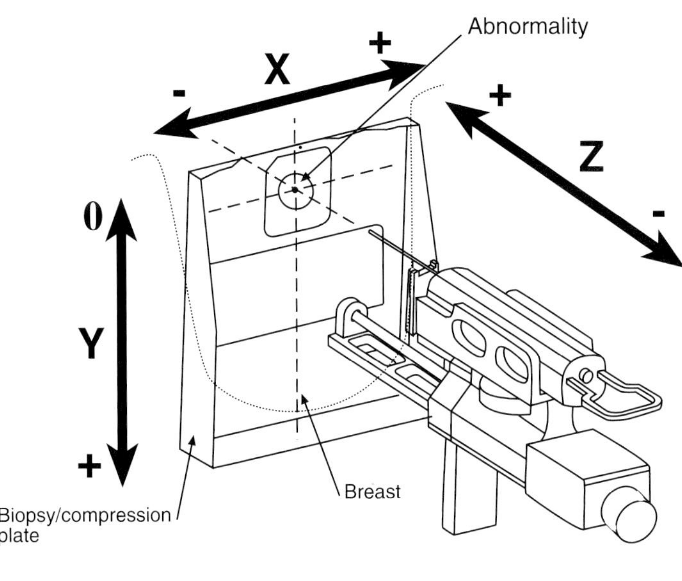

Figure 2.3. Cartesian Coordinates. A Cartesian system identifies the location of a unique point by three axes intersecting at right angles.

window, an applicable scale exists for the horizontal, vertical, and depth axes. The coordinate scale, usually expressed in millimeters, defines the location of point 0 for the vertical and hortizontal axes, and divides the biopsy window into positive and negative halves, or quadrants. **Figure 2.5a** demonstrates the biopsy window from two different stereotactic units. Although both use Cartesian systems, point 0 is in a different location for each unit. This information is useful in checking calculated coordinates against the scout image. The scout image demonstrates an abnormality at a specific point on the scale of the biopsy window; coordinate calculation should match this position. If abnormality location is in a negative quadrant, coordinates should be negative, etc. (**Figure 2.6**).

Correlation of coordinates and scout position may be difficult with the scale of a polar system, as the angles that define target location are not easily related to its position on the scout image. However, the biopsy window is divided into negative and positive halves. The clinician can detect an error prior to needle insertion, when the set position of the biopsy needle is contrary to the position of the target on the scout image.

The scale also defines point 0 for the depth axis. **Figure 2.5b** illustrates 0 (or the zero plane) for the depth axis at either the distal or proximal surface of the breast. The depth

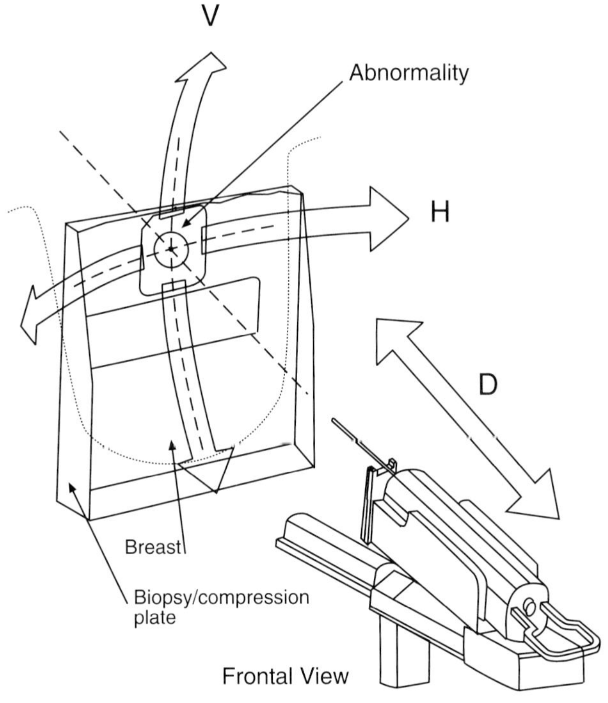

Figure 2.4. Polar Coordinates. A polar system identifies the location of a unique point by the distances from a fixed point and the angular distances from a reference line.

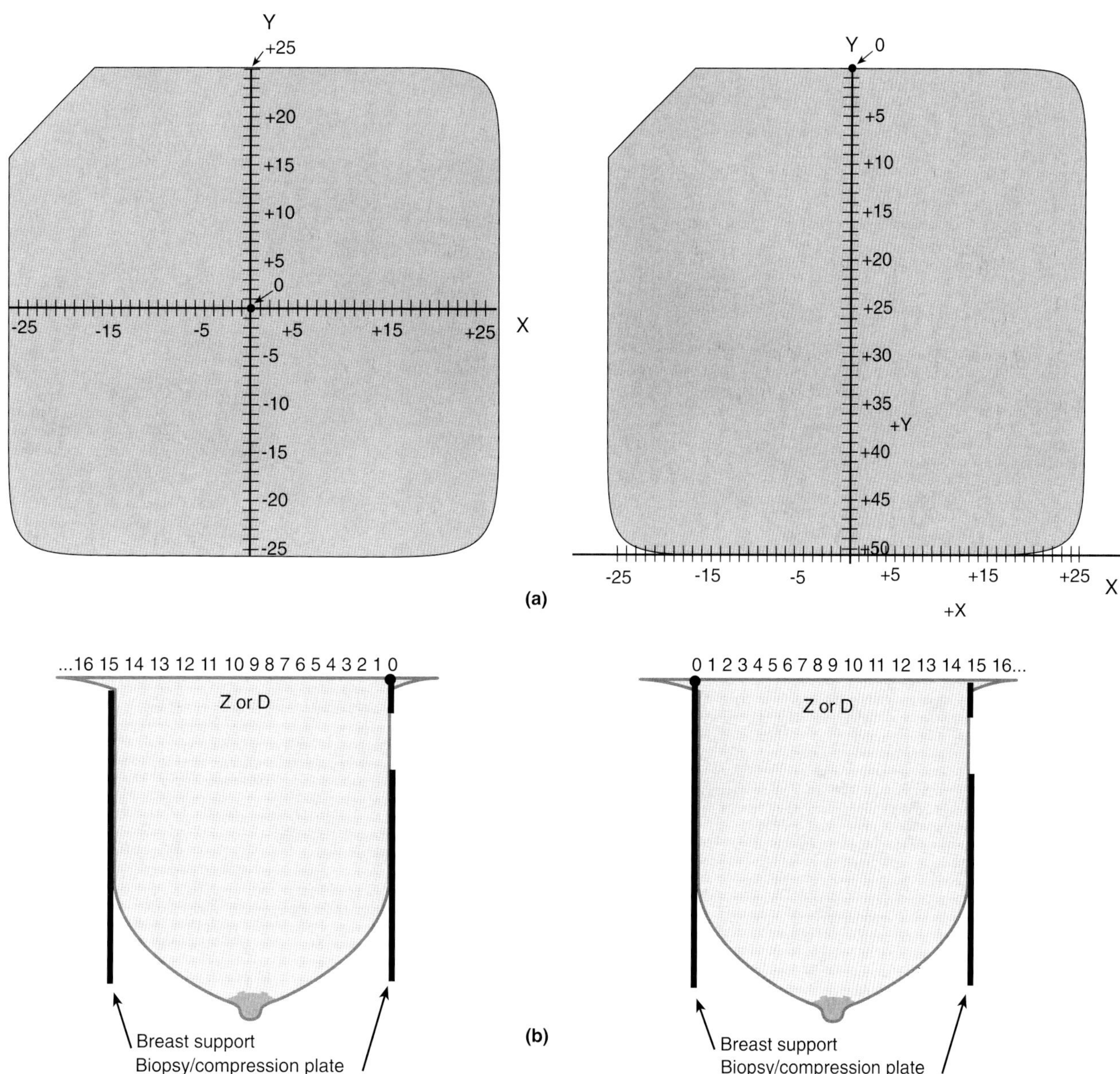

Figure 2.5 a and b. This figure demonstrates how scale is applied to the biopsy windows of two different SBB systems. The scale divides the biopsy window into negative and positive halves or quadrants **(a)**. Note that *0* has a different location for each biopsy window. Scale is also applied to depth **(b)**. Note that *0* is at the breast support for one system and at the biopsy/compression plate for the other system.

coordinate of an abnormality is expressed in millimeters from 0 to the abnormality. This number can be correlated with the expected depth in the breast based on the two-view mammogram. A depth coordinate that differs greatly from the expected depth should raise concern for the clinician. With at least one stereotactic unit, an arbitrary scale defines the depth coordinate. This scale does not directly relate to the distance of the abnormality from either the proximal or distal skin surface. With an arbitrary scale, the clinician has no correlative data to assure that the depth coordinate is accurate. In fact, no direct visible information exists to correlate coordinate depth with expected abnormality depth,

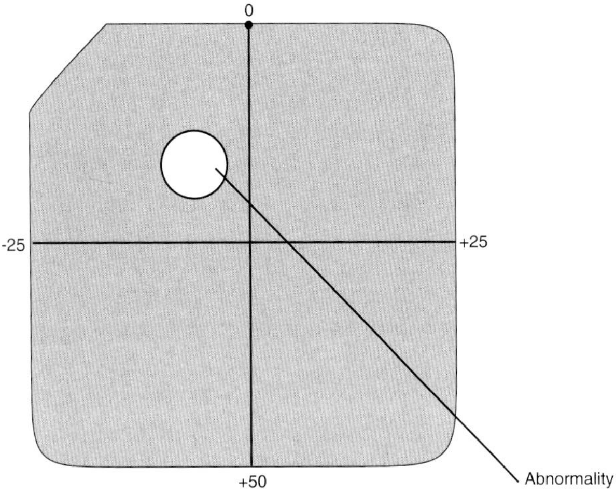

Figure 2.6. Applying the Scale. Coordinate calculation should match the position of the abnormality on the scale of the biopsy window. This is a good visual check to assure proper targeting and procedural tasks. In the case above, the horizontal coordinate should be a negative number of approximately 10 mm; the vertical coordinate should be a positive number, about 18 mm. Obvious differences in polarity or measurement would signal an error.

prior to needle insertion. However, during needle insertion, the clinician can correlate centimeter markings on the needle with the expected depth of the abnormality.

The Reference

All coordinates are determined from measurements based on a reference point or points. The shift of a targeted abnormality on the stereo pair, in relation to this established recognized reference, provides for the exact three-dimensional position to within 1 mm.

Location of the Reference—The location of the reference point(s) is determined by the equipment manufacturer. For some units, the established reference is located on the *biopsy/compression plate* between the compressed breast and the x-ray tube. Because the biopsy/compression plate is removable, it is critical to place it on the unit accurately. If the centering of the biopsy/compression plate is in error, reference placement and coordinate determination will be in error. Other manufacturers locate the reference point(s) on the *breast support*, between the compressed breast and the image receptor.

Visualization of the reference on the resultant image is a very useful visual aid, allowing coordinate calculation with actual abnormality position.

Proximal vs. Distal Reference Location—Units that provide a reference point on the biopsy/compression plate determine the depth coordinate from the *proximal aspect* of the breast, along the pathway the biopsy needle will travel. The depth coordinate has a direct relationship to the depth of the abnormality, relative to the skin surface **(Figure 2.7a)**. Because of this relationship the clinician can check the depth coordinate against information available from the mammogram. A depth coordinate significantly different from what is expected, or a negative coordinate, should raise concern that the abnormality was not properly localized.

Checking the depth coordinate is more difficult with those units employing a distal reference **(Figure 2.7b)**, which determines the depth coordinate from the breast support. To correlate the depth coordinate, the clinician must subtract the depth from the compression thickness to determine the depth of the abnormality from the proximal skin surface.

Principles of Stereotactic Imaging

The Scout and Stereo Pair

Acquiring a scout image of the abnormality is the first step in obtaining the stereo pair. The x-ray tube is positioned perpendicular to the breast support with left to right centering of the abnormality in the imaging field. Although the scout image is necessary for postioning, it is not a part of the localization algorithm.

It is useful to have the scout image available during the procedure. The scout provides a reference for many visual cues that can facilitate the biopsy process.

After proper scouting of the targeted abnormality, the next step is acquisition of the two planar images that form the stereo pair. Moving the x-ray tube in the horizontal plane to different source positions, usually +/- 15° from the perpendicular, provides two separate fields of view **(Figure 2.8)**. For screen-film acquisition, the stereo images are recorded adjacent to each other on the same film; with digital imaging, the image pair is juxtaposed on the monitor. With the use of a screen-film image receptor, the cassette will also be moved between acquisitions to prevent superimposition of the two planar images **(Figure 2.9)**. With a digital receptor, the computer prevents the overlap of images.

Proper ***display*** *of the planar images and apparent* ***shift*** *of the abnormality within the planar images provide the basis*

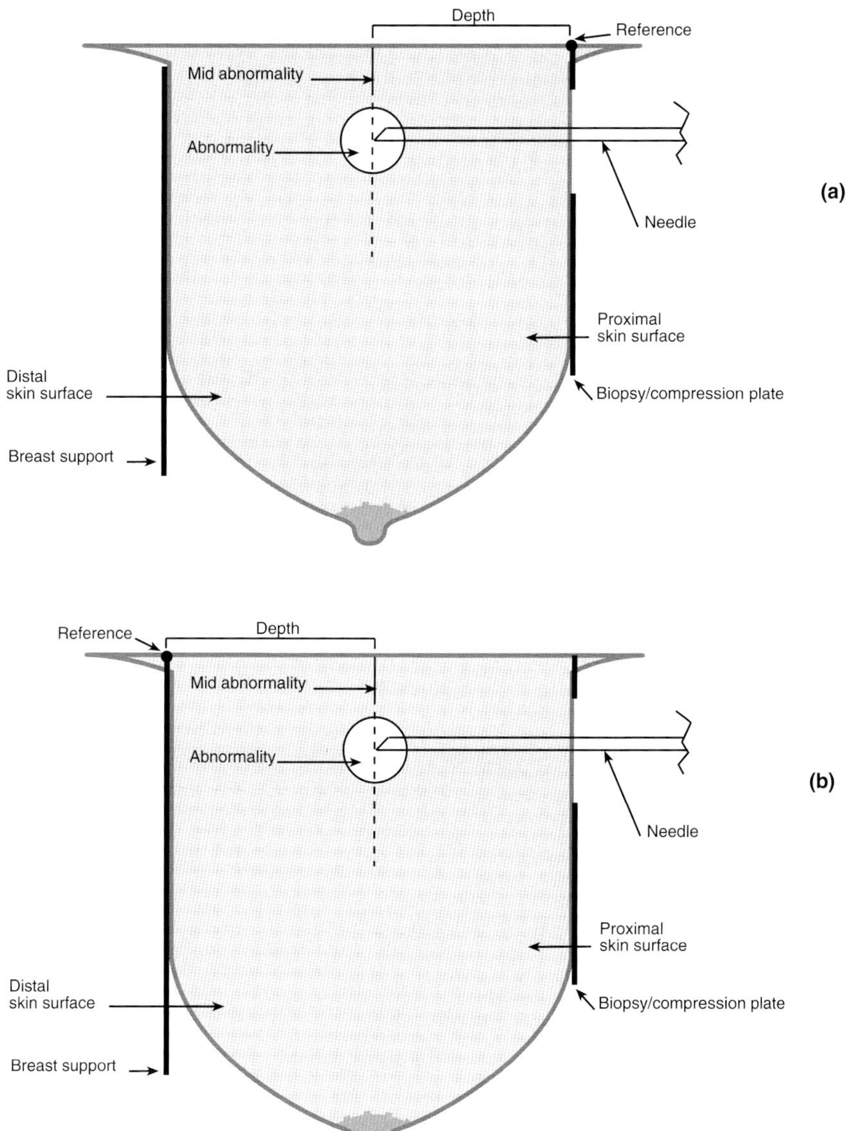

Figure 2.7 a and b. Proximal vs. Distal Reference Location. An SBB system with a proximal reference **(a)** determines the depth coordinate from the proximal skin surface, allowing the clinician direct correlation of this coordinate with expected depth relative to skin surface, based on the two-view mammogram. To correlate the depth coordinate using a distal reference **(b)** requires the clinician to subtract the depth from the compression thickness to determine the depth of the abnormality from the proximal skin surface.

for determining target coordinates. In addition to providing the means for accurate localization, abnormality shift and display of the planar images provide useful information for both the clinician and the technologist performing the procedure (discussed in greater detail below).

Acquisition and Display of the Planar Images

The programmed mathematical algorithm for coordinate determination requires the correct display of the +/- planar images for accurate localization. Recording of the stereo pair on the image receptor is specific and must remain consistent. The positive-angled image should always be placed to one

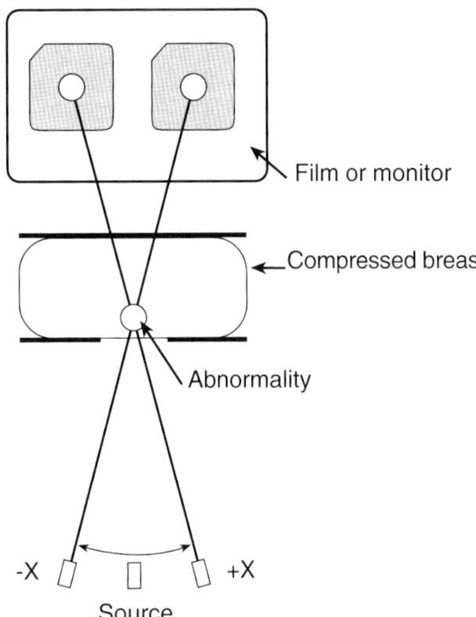

Figure 2.8. Stereo Pair. Acquisition of the stereo pair requires two projections with the x-ray tube moved horizontally to different source positions, usually +/- 15° from center. These projections are placed side by side on a monitor or on the same film.

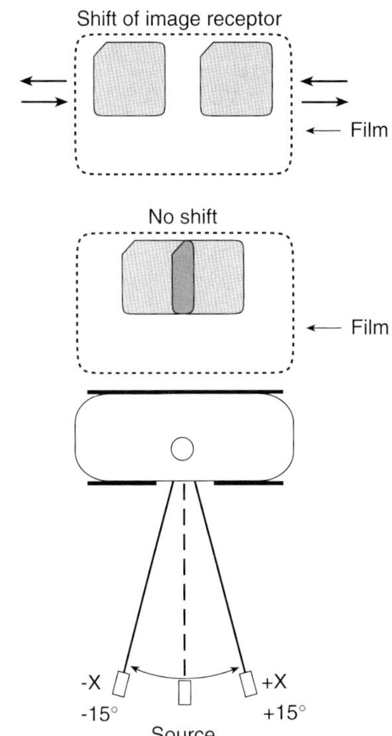

Figure 2.9. Screen-Film Image Receptor Shift. With a screen-film system, shift of the image receptor with x-ray tube movement is necessary to prevent superimposition of the planar images.

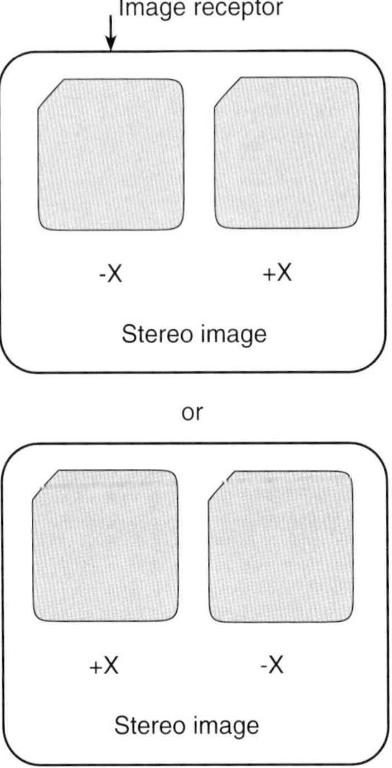

Figure 2.10. Recording and Display. Recording and display of the +/- planar images are specific to each manufacturer and imaging modality. The positive image should be displayed to the right (or left) of the image receptor and the negative image on the opposite side.

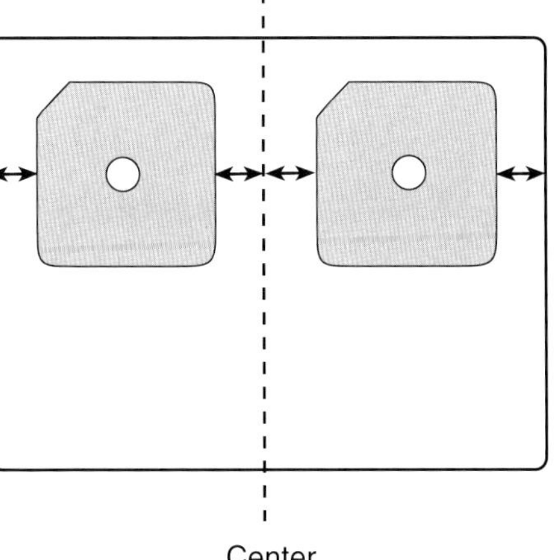

Figure 2.11. Display Characteristics. The display of the planar images includes visual characteristics that inform the team that acquisition is correct. In the above example, the planar images should always appear equidistant from the center of the film and each edge of the film.

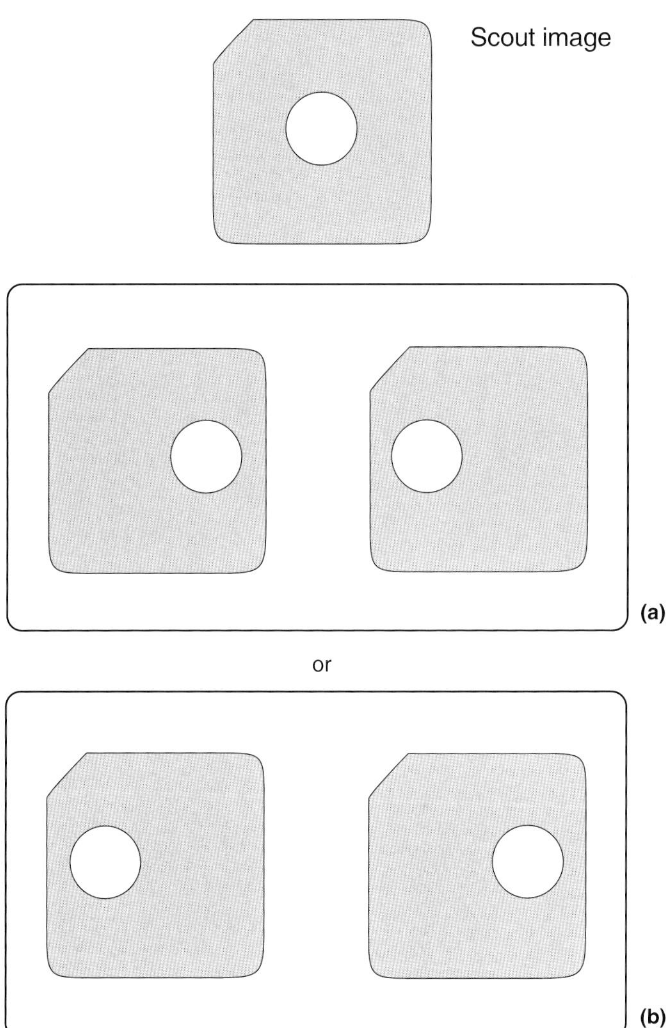

Figure 2.12 a and b. Direction of Abnormality Shift. The display of the planar images determines the direction of shift of the abnormality. Viewing the stereo pair appropriately, the projected image of the abnormalities will appear to move toward **(a)** or away from **(b)** one another.

side of the film or monitor (that is, left or right) and the negative-angled image should always be placed on the opposing side **(Figure 2.10)**. This requires appropriate movement of the x-ray tube and, with some systems, the image receptor, as specified by each manufacturer. Display of the stereo pair may depict other visual characteristics (specific to the unit) to inform the technologist and clinician of correct acquisition **(Figure 2.11)**. Misalignment is a visual cue of faulty tube and/or image receptor movement. Image placement characteristics can be learned through applications and phantom work.

Order of Acquisition — The order of acquisition of the +/- planar images is arbitrary with screen-film combinations because *specific movements* of the tube and image receptor will place images in a consistent manner. However, with a digital receptor, the stereo images must be taken in *specific order*. The computer cannot recognize the difference between the +/- projections, and can make accurate calculations only for the preprogrammed order of image acquisition. One way to determine appropriate acquisition of the stereo images is to recognize the direction of abnormality shift.

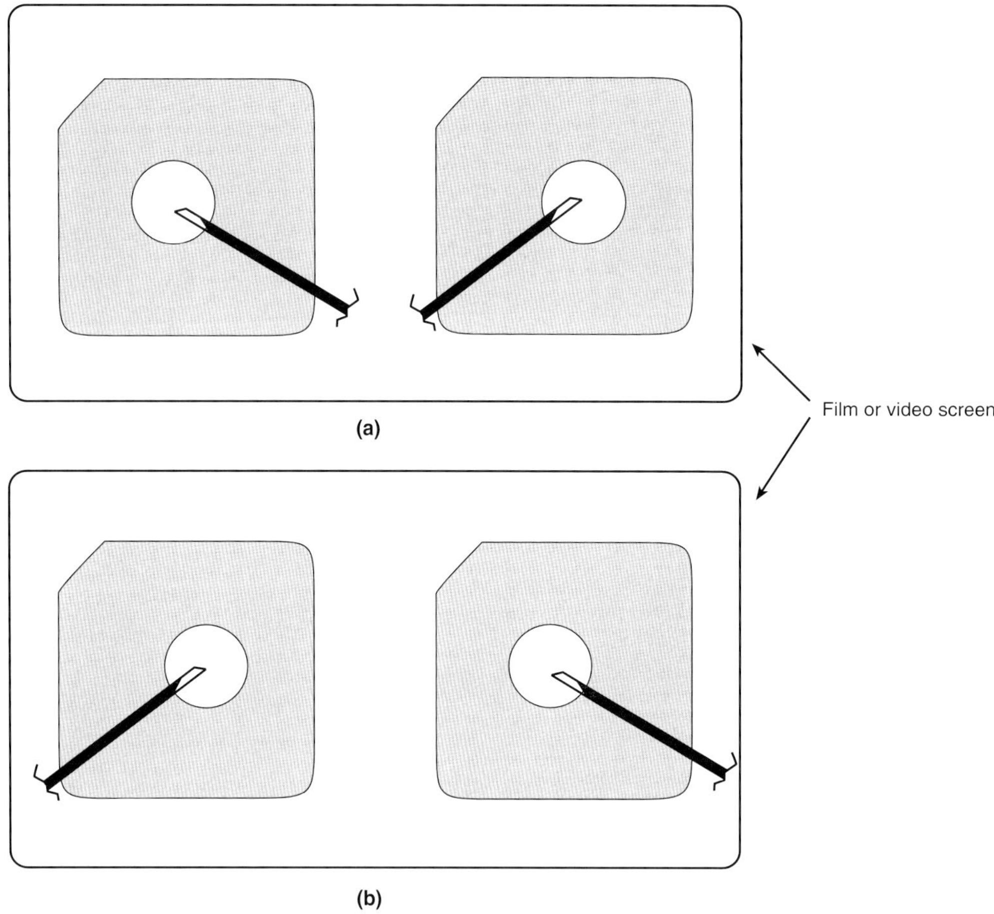

Figure 2.13 a and b. Needle Direction. The display of the planar images determines needle direction. The needles will be oriented toward **(a)** or away from **(b)** one another.

Shift of the Abnormality within the Stereo Image

Direction of Shift —Within each +/- planar image, the projected abnormality will shift in the horizontal plane relative to its original position on the scout image, and on some units, relative to the reference point(s). The direction of shift is determined by the manufacturer and the display of the planar images. Viewing the stereo pair appropriately (as recommended by manufacturer), the projected image of the abnormalities will move either toward or away from one another in the horizontal plane only (**Figure 2.12**). This directional shift will remain constant for a specific unit and image receptor. The display of the planar images also determines the appearance of the biopsy needle after it is positioned in the breast; the needle tips will be directed toward one another, or away from one another (**Figure 2.13**).

The technologist and clinician should be familiar with the circumstances of placement and directional shift as this offers correlative visual assistance. For example, visual clues such as errant directional shift or misdirected needle tips indicate mistakes early in the procedure. X-ray tube or image receptor movement and acquisition order are all possible errors. If the mistake is undetected, then coordinate calculations will be in error (**Figure 2.14**).

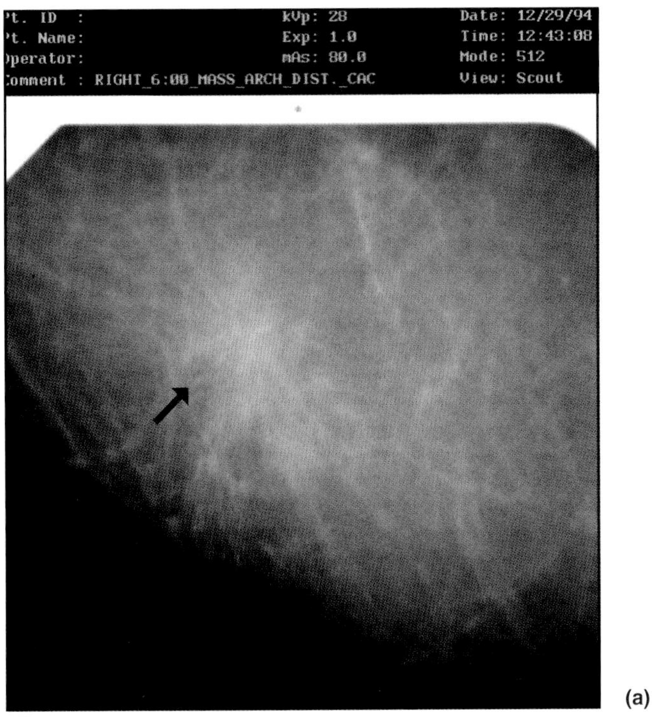

(a)

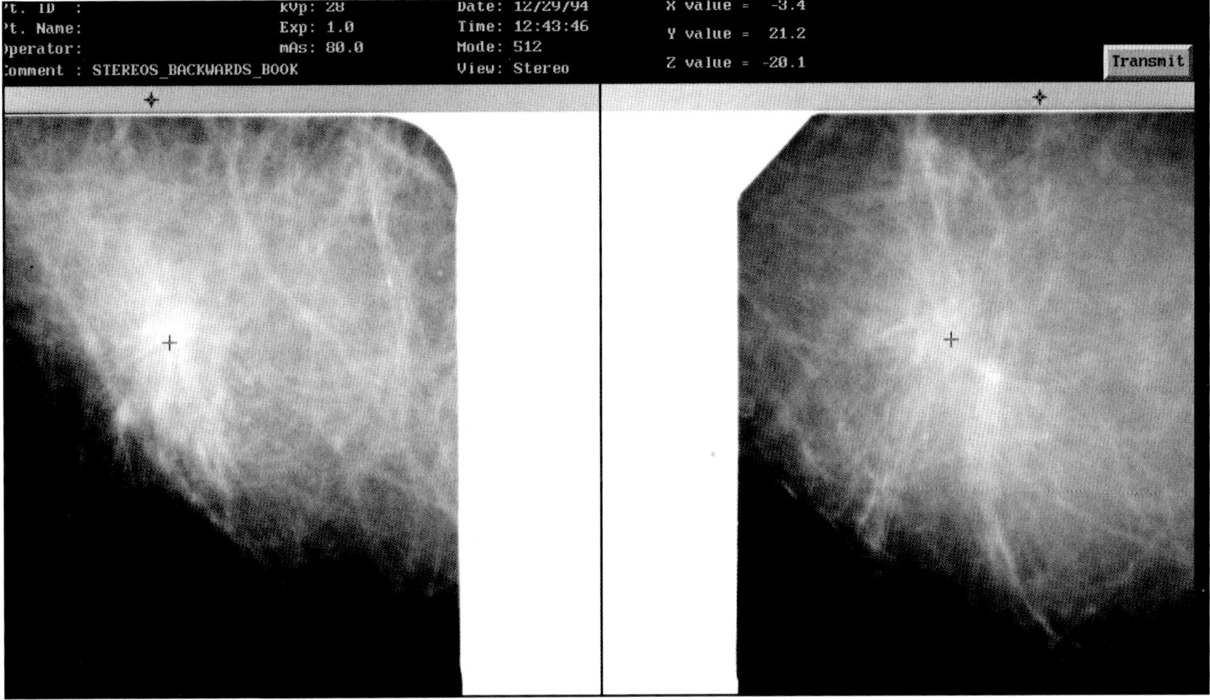

(b)

Figure 2.14 a and b. Direction of Shift**.** Note the position of the abnormality on the scout image **(a) (arrow)**. The inward shift of the abnormality (for this system, the abnormality should have shifted outward) on the stereo images is a visual cue that alerts the technologist to inappropriate order of stereo acquisition **(b)**. The error is also evident in the negative depth coordinate (upper right-hand corner).

Figure 2.14 continued.

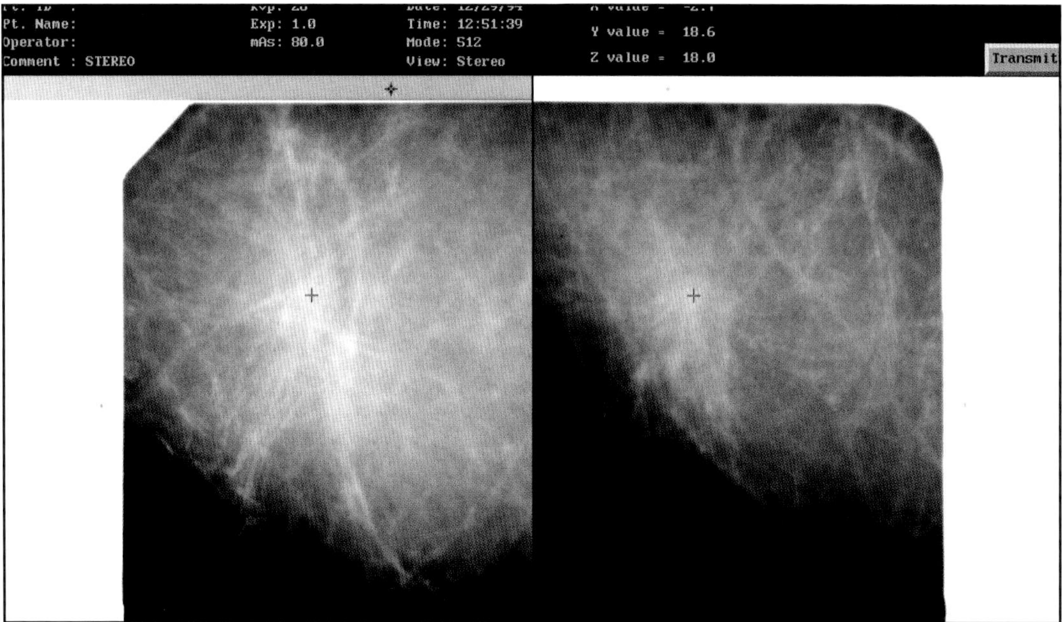

Figure 2.14c. Appropriate stereos demonstrate outward shift and an appropriate depth coordinate. Note the change in the X coordinate.

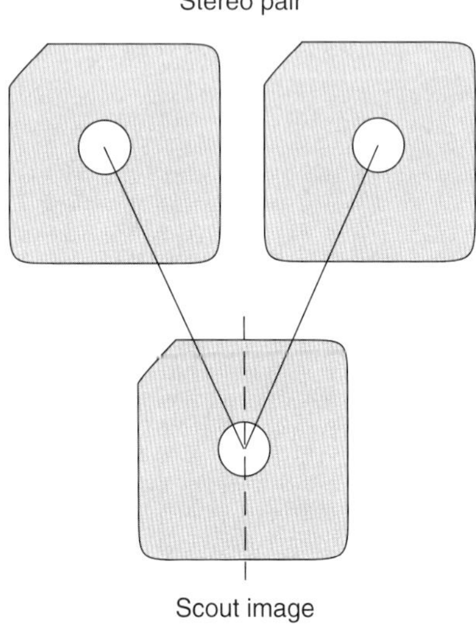

Figure 2.15. Equal Shift of the Abnormality**.** The abnormality will shift equally from the scouted position in each of the planar images. This is evident if the abnormality is well-centered in the biopsy field.

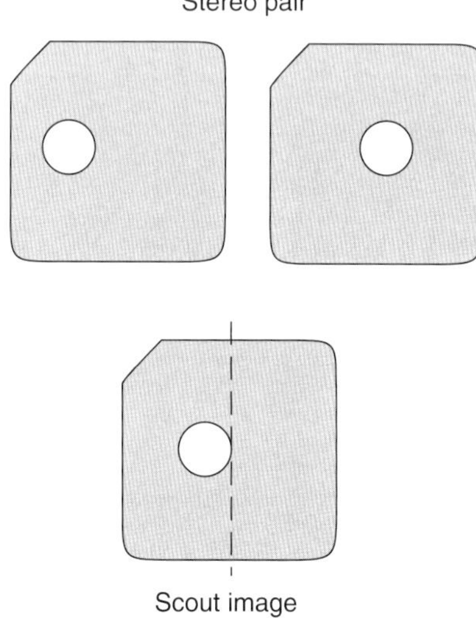

Figure 2.16. Less Evident Equal Shift. If the abnormality is not well-centered on the scout, the identical shift is less evident.

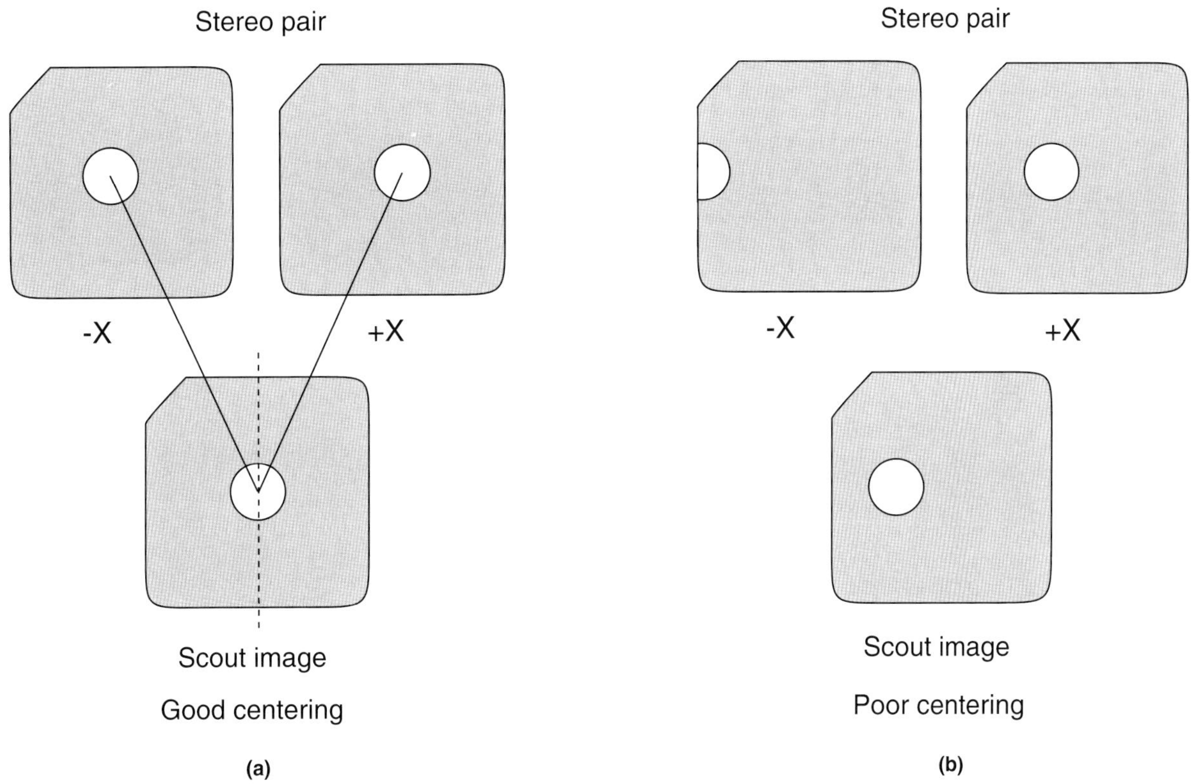

Figure 2.17 a and b. Horizontal Centering. Appropriate centering of the abnormality in the horizontal axis on the scout image will prevent nonvisualization of the abnormality **(a)**, whereas poor centering results in shift on the stereo images **(b)**.

Distance of Shift and Centering — The distance of abnormality shift on the +/- planar images from the scouted projection will vary from patient to patient, with compression thickness and abnormality depth relative to the breast support or compression plate. *However, in all cases, the abnormality will shift equally from the scouted position on both planar images* **(Figure 2.15)**. For example, from the scouted projection, if the abnormality shifts 10 mm on the (+) X image, then it will also shift 10 mm on the (-) X image. However, abnormality shape may change with different projections. This equal shift may not be as evident if the abnormality is not centered in the biopsy window **(Figure 2.16)**.

It is possible for the projected abnormality to shift outside the confines of the image receptor or x-ray field. Proper centering of the abnormality **(Figure 2.17)** in the horizontal plane (left-to-right axis) on the scout image will in most cases prevent nonvisualization (see *Shift and Nonvisualization*). *Centering in the vertical plane is not necessary*; however, it may facilitate access by the biopsy team.

Distance of Shift and Depth—The distance of abnormality shift depends on the depth of the abnormality relative to either the breast support or the biopsy/compression plate *and the stereotactic geometry of each manufacturer's system.* The two scenarios for abnormality shift are as follows:

1. In one system, an abnormality in closer proximity to the

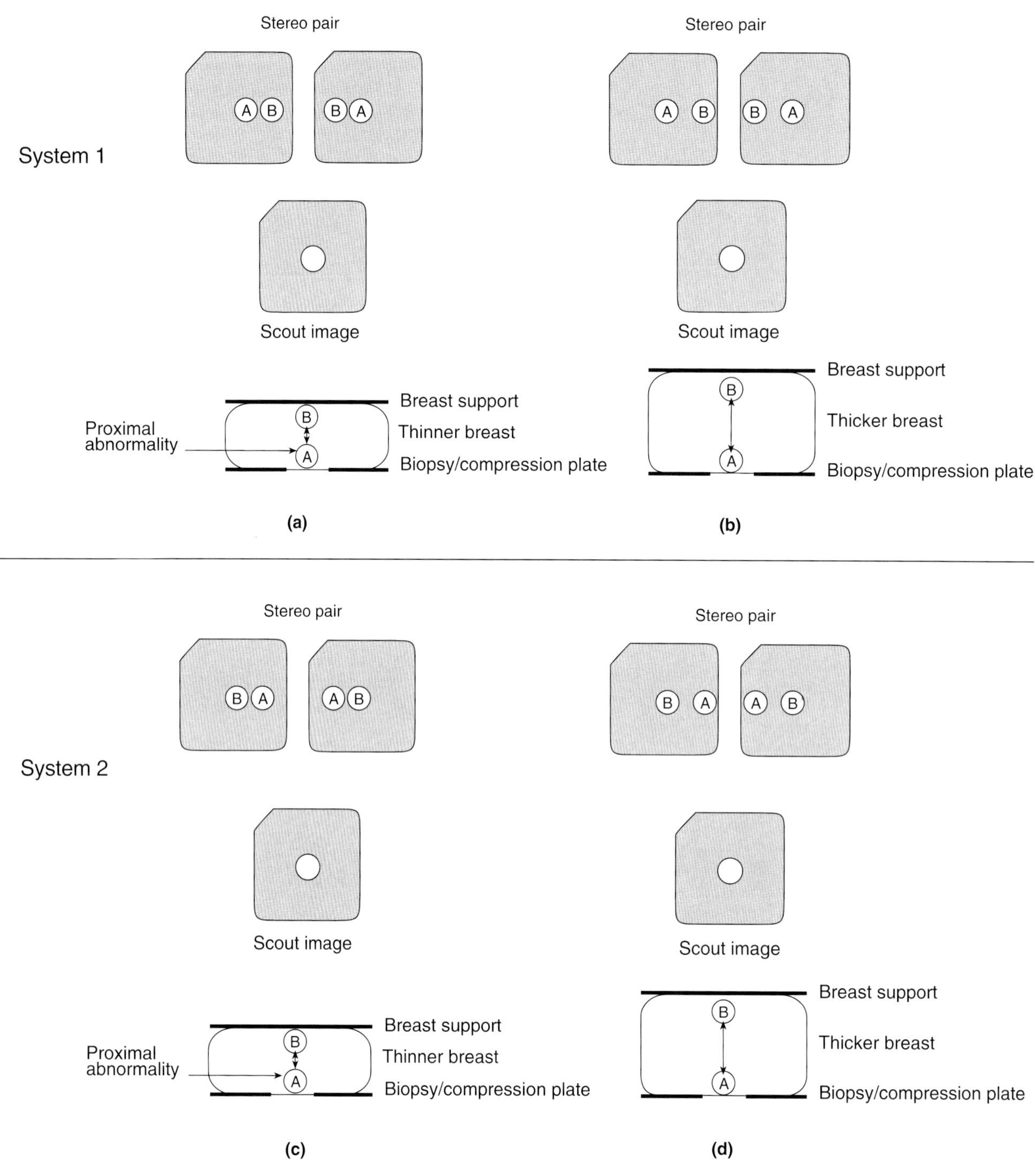

Figure 2.18 a-d. Distance of Shift in Two Systems. In System 1, an abnormality located closer to the biopsy/compression plate will shift *lesser* distance than an abnormality located closer to the breast support **(a)**. Increasing breast thickness increases the distance of shift **(b)**. In System 2, an abnormality located closer to the biopsy/compression plate will move a *greater* distance than an abnormality located closer to the breast support **(c)**. Increasing breast thickness increases the distance of shift **(d)**. This is the result of the stereotactic geometry of each system (see chapter 4).

biopsy/compression plate will move *less* distance in the imaging field than an abnormality closer to the breast support **(Figure 2.18a)**. The closer the abnormality is to the compression plate, the less it will move. As compression thickness increases, abnormality shift will increase **(Figure 2.18b)**.

2. In another system, an abnormality positioned in closer proximity to the compression plate will move a *greater* distance in the imaging field than an abnormality closer to the breast support **(Figure 2.18c)**. The closer the abnormality is to the biopsy/compression plate, the greater it will move. As compression thickness increases, abnormality shift increases **(Figure 2.18d)**.

An awareness of distance of shift relative to depth can be a useful guide for the biopsy team. For example, depending on the unit, extensive abnormality shift on the stereo images may indicate improper positioning **(Figure 2.19)**, contributing to *negative stroke margin* (discussed later in this chapter). For the clinician, understanding the *distance* and *direction* of shift is useful when identifying ill-defined abnormalities for targeting. When examining the stereo images for the abnormality, the clinician should search only that portion of the image where the abnormality is known to have shifted **(Figure 2.20)**.

Shift and Nonvisualization—Due to the design of the breast support and field limitations with some units, it is possible that an abnormality cannot be biopsied because it is partially visualized, or it is outside the field of view on one or both stereo images, despite accurate centering.

Appropriate centering of the abnormality in the imaging field becomes even more critical with this equipment, however, the geometry of the unit will be the limiting factor. If both stereo images do not demonstrate the abnormality, or the same portion of the abnormality, then appropriate targeting cannot be performed and biopsy should be canceled.

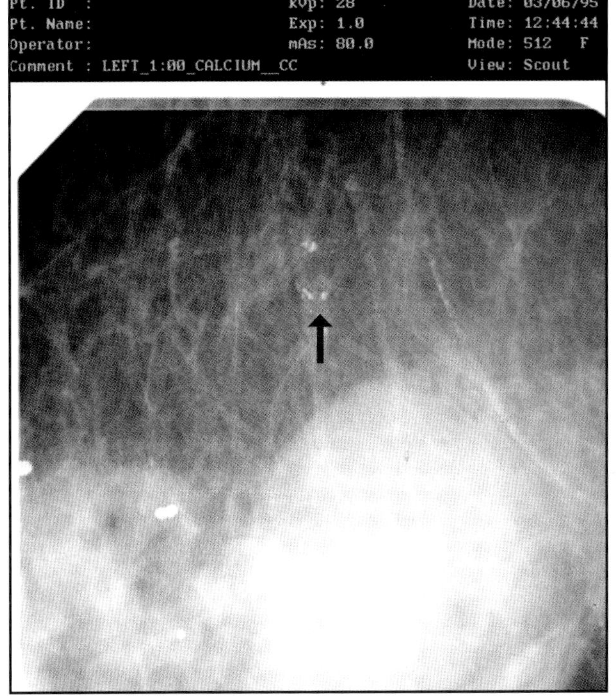

(a)

Figure 2.19 a-e. Shift and Depth. The scouted abnormality **(arrow) (a)** in the CC projection shifts a great distance on the stereo images **(arrow) (b)**, indicating (for this SBB system) that the abnormality is positioned *distal* to the biopsy/compression plate. Coordinate calculation (upper right hand corner) **(c)** indicates a depth of 51 mm with a total breast compression of 56 mm, inadequate for the stroke of the biopsy instrument. The breast is repositioned in a CC-FB projection **(d)**. The new stereos **(e)** demonstrate minimal shift, which means (in this SBB system) that the abnormality is more *proximal* to the biopsy/compression plate. Coordinate calculation indicates depth to be 29.7 for the compression of 56 mm, allowing ample room for stroke, with a 5 mm prefire postion.

Figure 2.19 continued.

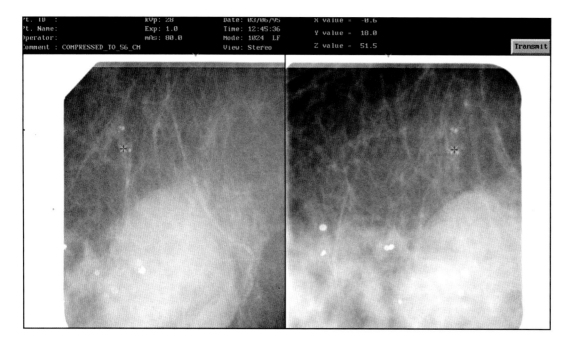

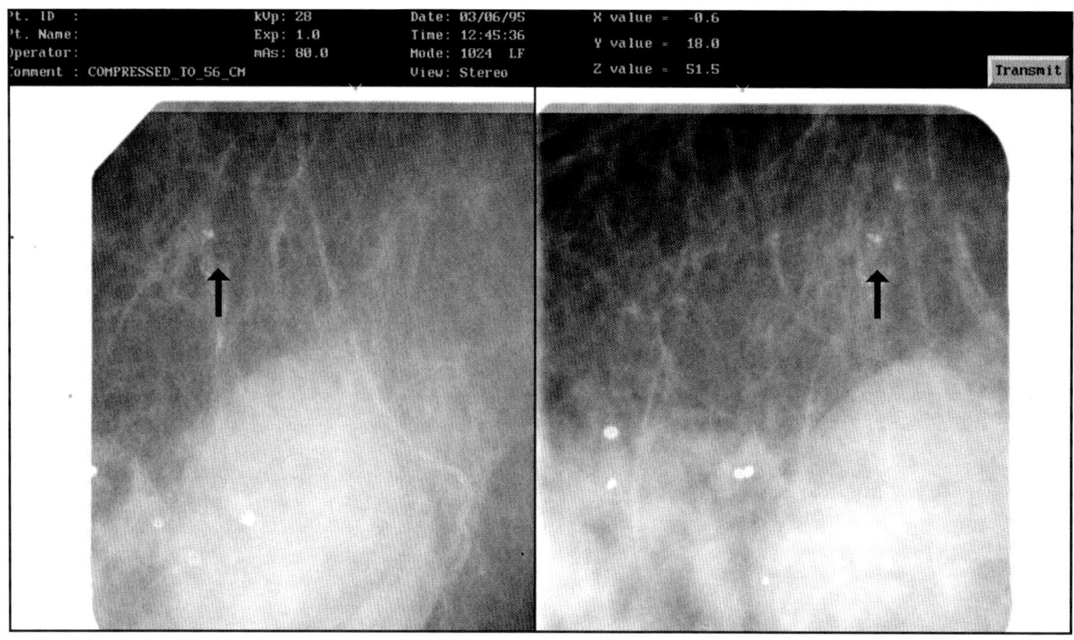

(b)

(c)

Figure 2.19 continued.

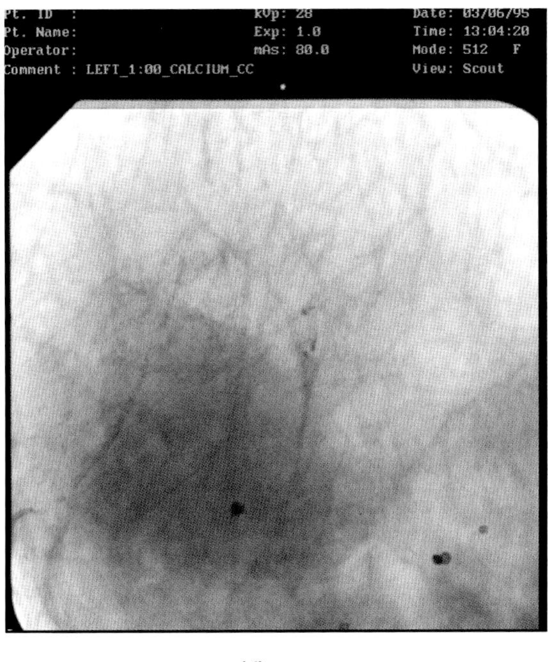

(d)

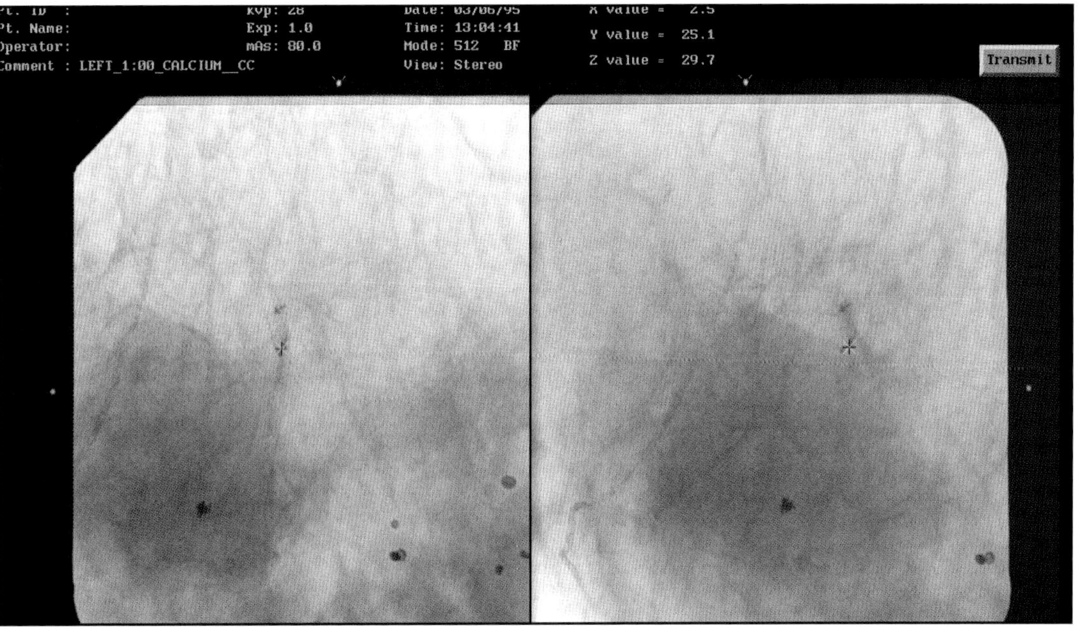

(e)

Nonvisualization is more likely to occur if the SBB equipment allows a proximal abnormality (positioned closer to the biopsy/compression plate) to shift a greater distance compared with a distal abnormality **(Figure 2.21)**. Core biopsy requires positioning of the abnormality as close to the biopsy/compression plate as possible (for easier access, accuracy, and stroke margin), thereby increasing the possibility of nonvisualization. Furthermore, the occurence of nonvisualization increases in those units with a fixed breast support. However, *systems with a movable breast support will maintain the abnormality in the field of view.*

Nonvisualization also occurs at greater breast thickness, usually 6 cm or more, depending on the geometry of the unit. Determining the compression thickness at which nonvisualization occurs will allow the clinician and technologist to choose a viable projection that provides compression thickness within the imaging confines of the SBB unit.

The mathematical algorithm for three-dimensional localization is designed for a particular set of stereo angles, therefore, never change the angle of stereo acquisition for coordinate calculation, unless recommended by the manufacturer. See chapter 4 for a discussion on angle of stereo acquisition.

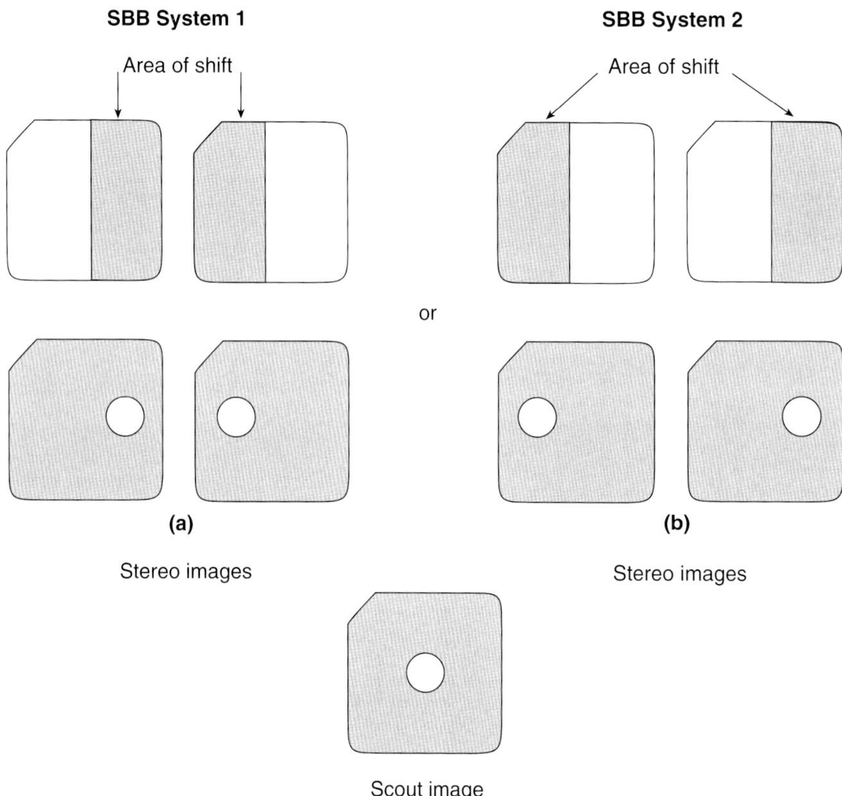

Figure 2.20 a and b. Area of Shift. When trying to identify ill-defined abnormalities, the clinician should search the imaging field only in the area to which the abnormality characteristically shifts (this depends on the unit.) In SBB System 1, the abnormalities will appear to shift toward one another, therefore, the shaded areas will be the area of search **(a)**. In SBB System 2, the abnormalities will appear to shift away from one another, thus, the shaded areas will be the area of search **(b)**.

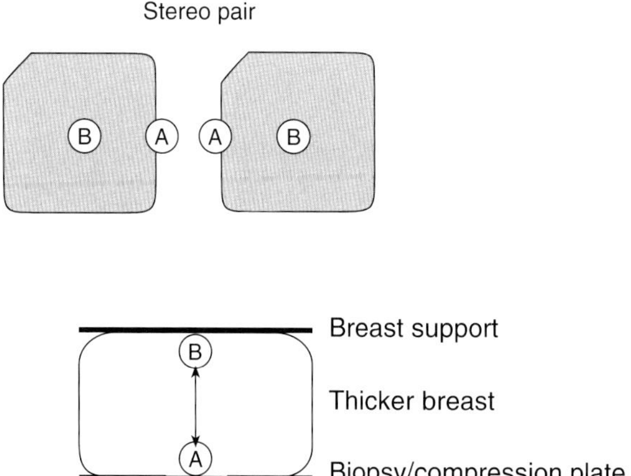

Figure 2.21. Shift and Nonvisualization. If the abnormality closer to the biopsy/compression plate shifts the greater distance (and no movable breast support is available to maintain visualization), then as compression thickness increases the abnormality will shift out of view on the stereo images, prohibiting biopsy.

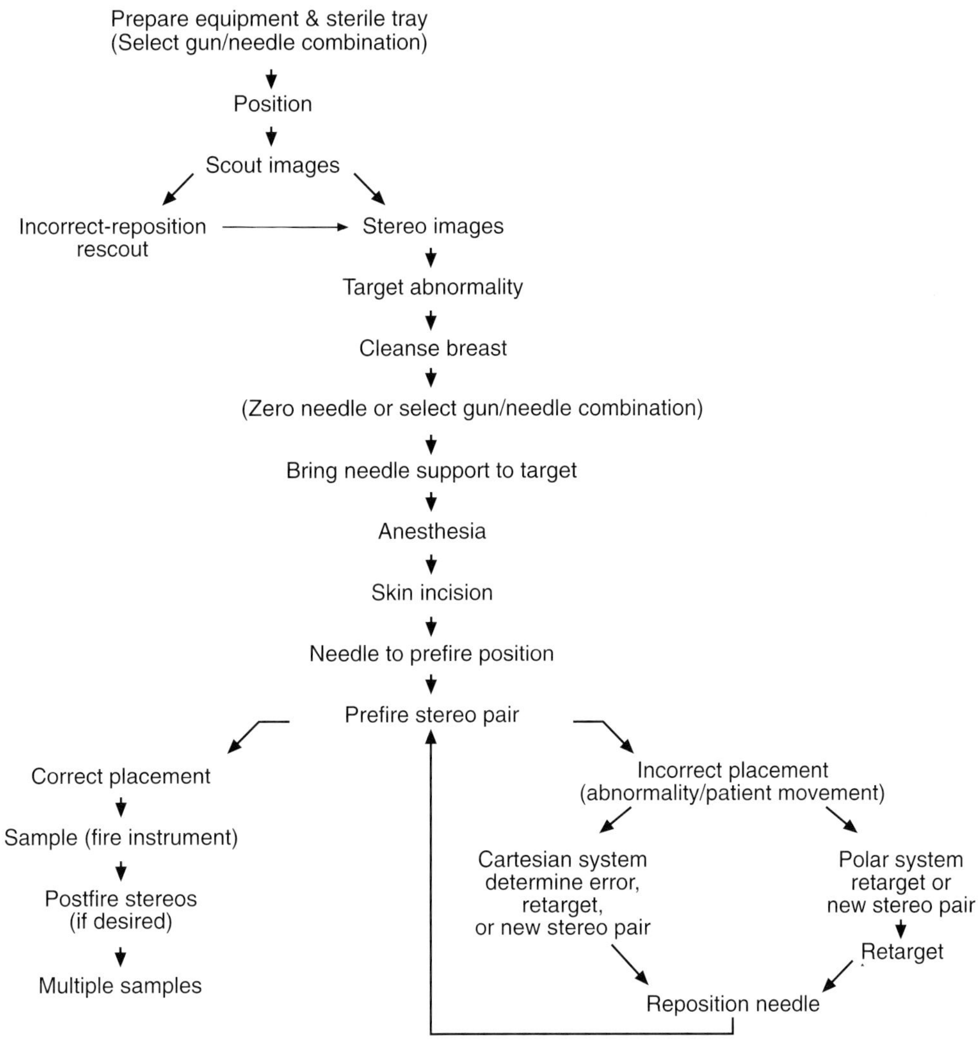

Figure 2.22. Flow Chart for Typical Stereotactic Core Biopsy Procedure.

The Core Biopsy Procedure

This section and the illustrations that follow describe a typical biopsy procedure, step-by-step, as outlined in **Figure 2.22**.

Prior to Patient Arrival

1. Check calibration. Perform a quality control test daily to check calibration of the targeting system, prior to scheduled biopsies or before each procedure, depending on the manufacturer's recommendations (**Figure 2.23**).

2. Review the mammogram. The clinician and technologist should decide the most effective approach for accessing the abnormality. This initial projection may be modified during actual patient positioning.

3. Prepare equipment for the patient and the procedure.

4. Program the unit for needle length and the stroke of the biopsy instrument. This step may be done at this point, or later in the procedure, depending on the manufacturer's recommendations.

When the Patient Arrives

1. Prepare sterile tray **(Figure 2.24)**. A list of necessary items can be found in appendix B.

2. Complete necessary paperwork and requisitions.

3. Obtain consent.

4. Have patient change clothes and use the lavatory.

5. Remove eye glasses and earrings.

Position and Scout

1. Position the patient **(Figure 2.25a)**. Selecting the appropriate approach to the abnormality can be straight-forward or complicated, depending on a number of factors (see chapter 6 on positioning). The patient body position, c-arm rotation, and visualization of the abnormality in both scout and stereo images are all issues that require attention. It is also critical to provide for *positive stroke margin* (described in the next section).

2. Obtain the scout image **(Figure 2.25b)**. The first step in the imaging process is to ensure adequate centering and visualization of the abnormality in the biopsy window. Acquire the scout image with the c-arm normal (perpendicular) to the image receptor. It may be necessary to reposition the breast or adjust technical factors, and repeat the scout image to obtain the final working image.

Acquire the Stereo Pair

Acquire the two images that form the stereo pair, according to the manufacturer's recommendations **(Figure 2.26)**. If the abnormality is not identifiable on either one of these images, the technologist can vary the technique accordingly, or reposition, rescout, and repeat the stereo images.

Determine Coordinates

Each manufacturer specifies the steps for targeting of the abnormality for coordinate calculation **(Figure 2.27)** (described in the next section).

Transfer Coordinates

The task of transferring the coordinates can be manual or electronic **(Figure 2.28)**. With manual transfer (usually with an upright SBB system), the actual biopsy platform or stage that holds the biopsy instrument is moved to correspond to the coordinates. Electronic transfer provides for the *display* of all three coordinates, with subsequent positioning of the biopsy platform or stage at a later point. Verification of the coordinates among the biopsy team is critical to ensure correct transfer.

Sampling

1. Precautions—Take universal precautions as defined by OSHA† standards. If necessary, drape equipment and patient for blood spatter (especially important with upright systems).

2. Antiseptic—Lightly cleanse the area within the biopsy window, using alcohol or a povidone-iodine solution **(Figure 2.29)**. Remove excess solution with a sterile sponge.

3. Needle guide—Place sterile needle guide on the needle guidance system, according to the manufacturer's instructions **(Figure 2.30)**.

4. Secure the biopsy instrument—Secure the loaded biopsy instrument in the holder on the needle guidance platform or stage **(Figure 2.31)**.

5. Program the unit for needle length and the stroke of the biopsy instrument **(Figure 2.32)**. This may be done at this point, or earlier in the procedure, depending on the manufacturer's recommendations.

6. Needle guidance—The biopsy team uses automated or manual controls to match the needle guidance device with the target coordinates for the X and Y axes, to target the abnormality **(Figure 2.33)**.

7. Anesthesia—The needle is brought forward, accurately indicating the site for anesthesia **(Figure 2.34)**. Local anesthesia can be administered to the skin and subcutaneous tissues. An excessive amount of anesthesia can interfere with the visualization of the abnormality on subsequent images. Anesthetic volume may also displace the abnormality. To minimize the volume injected per anesthetic dose, 2% lidocaine hydrochloride can replace the 1% formulation.

8. Mark the skin for an incision **(Figure 2.35)**.

9. Skin incision—Bring the needle forward again to accurately indicate the site for incision. For core biopsy, a 3-4 mm skin incision will facilitate the entry of the biopsy needle, reducing skin drag on the outer cannula when the biopsy instrument is fired **(Figure 2.36)**. This same skin incision can be used to access multiple targets, however, the limit in any direction is about 4 mm. Most clinicians make a skin incision, while others use a slightly smaller (16-gauge) needle to make a skin opening for the 14-gauge needle. Some clinicians do not use an initial skin wound to facilitate the biopsy needle. With this latter method, 3-5 separate openings are made for multipass or multitarget core sampling.

† Occupational Safety and Health Administration

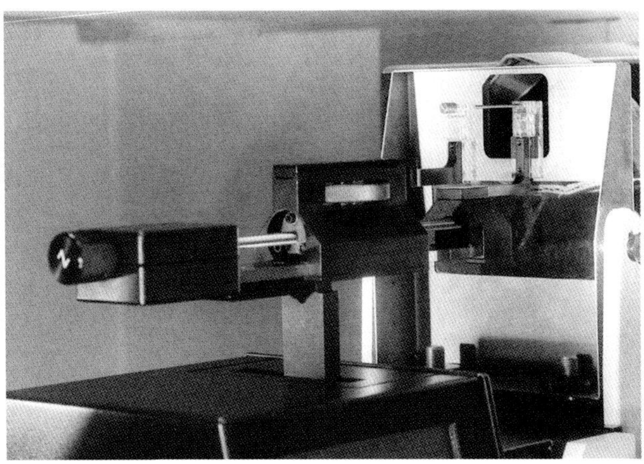

Figure 2.23. Check calibration.

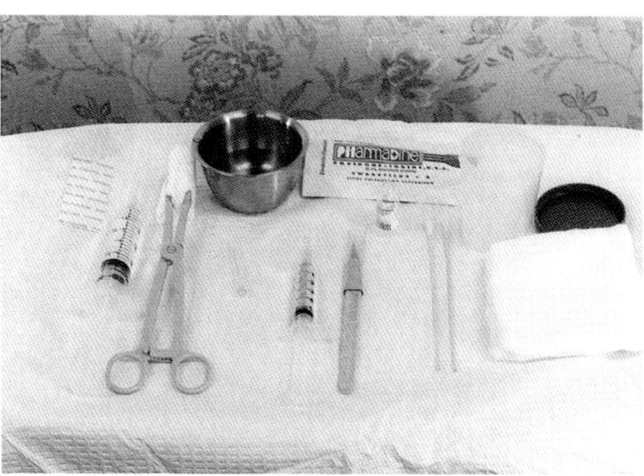

Figure 2.24. Prepare sterile tray.

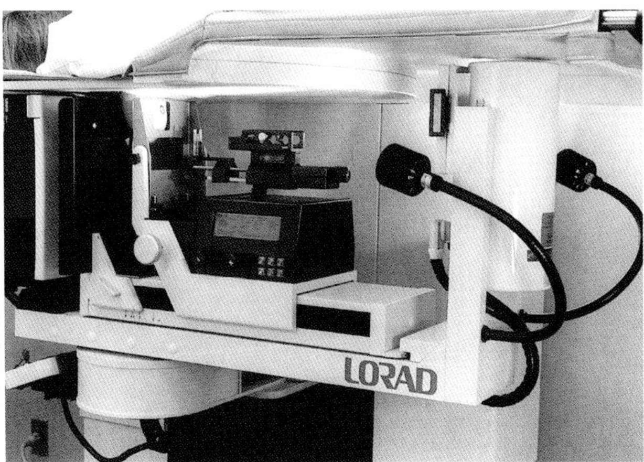

Figure 2.25a. Position the patient.

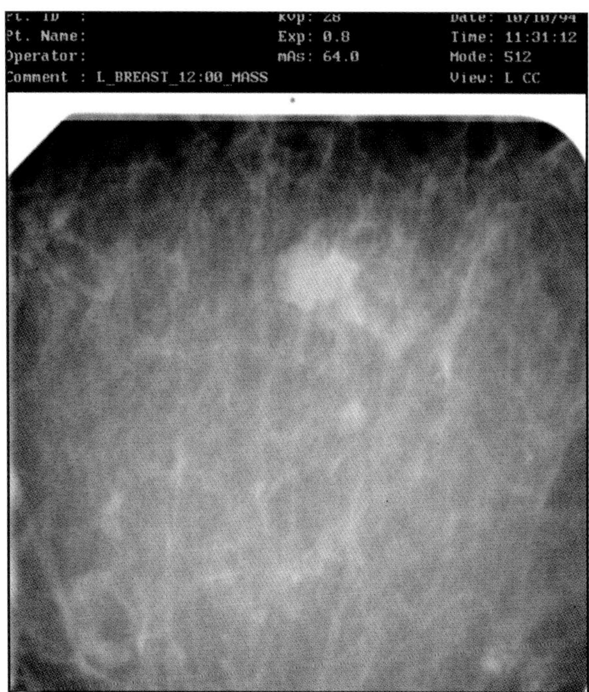

Figure 2.25b. Obtain the scout image. This scout image demonstrates a smoothly outlined abnormality, well-centered in the biopsy field.

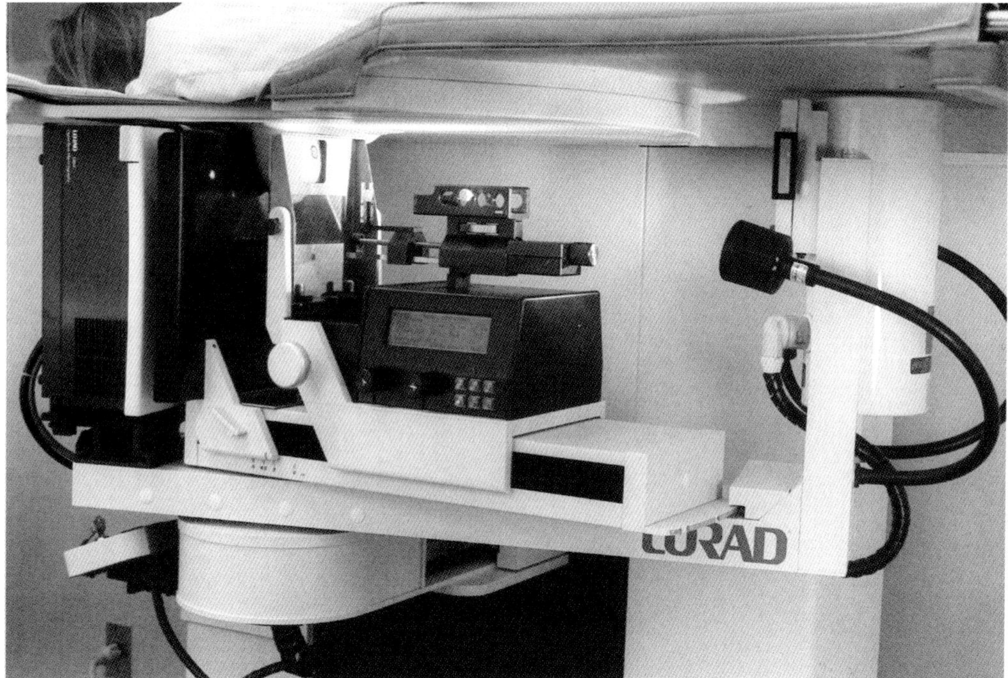

Figure 2.26a. Acquiring Stereo Images. Acquire two stereo images with the tube at different source positions. Note the shift of the c-arm.

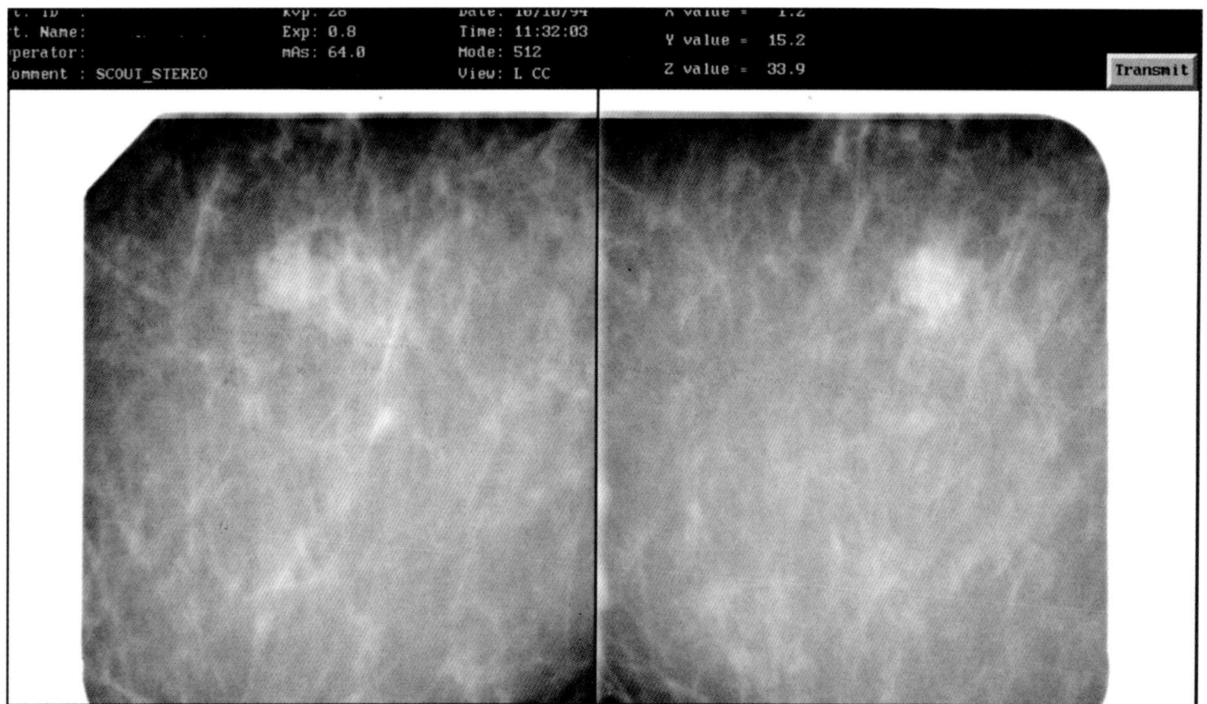

Figure 2.26b. Stereo Images. The abnormality can be easily seen on the stereo images, demonstrating proper directional shift.

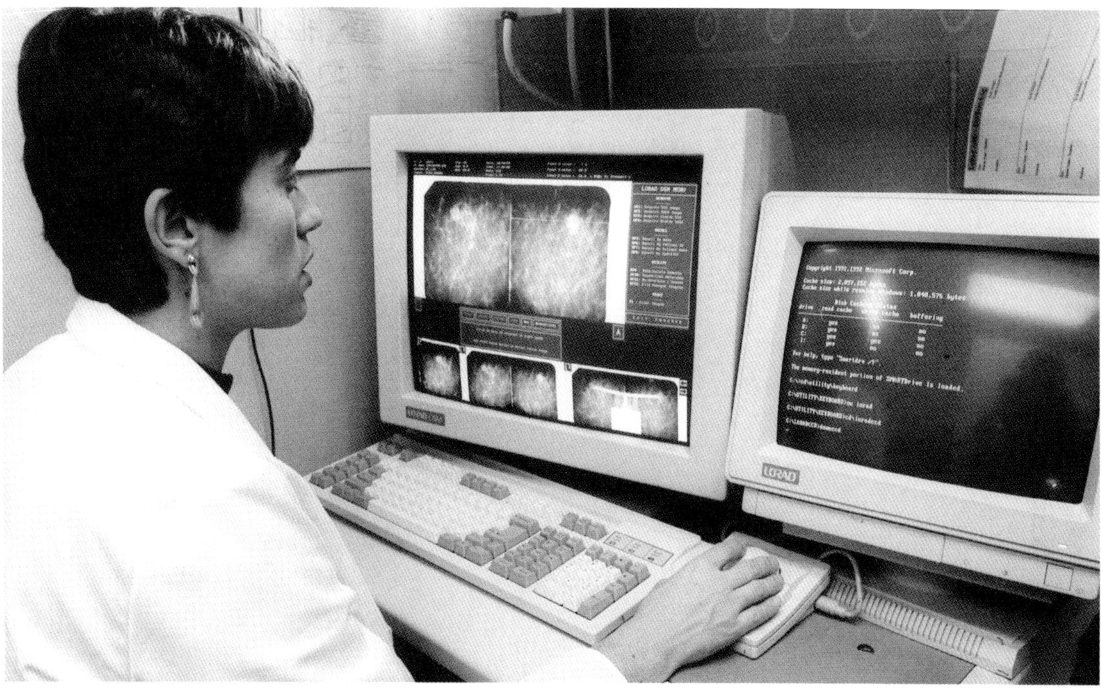

Figure 2.27a. Targeting the Abnormality. The clinician targets the abnormality for coordinate calculation.

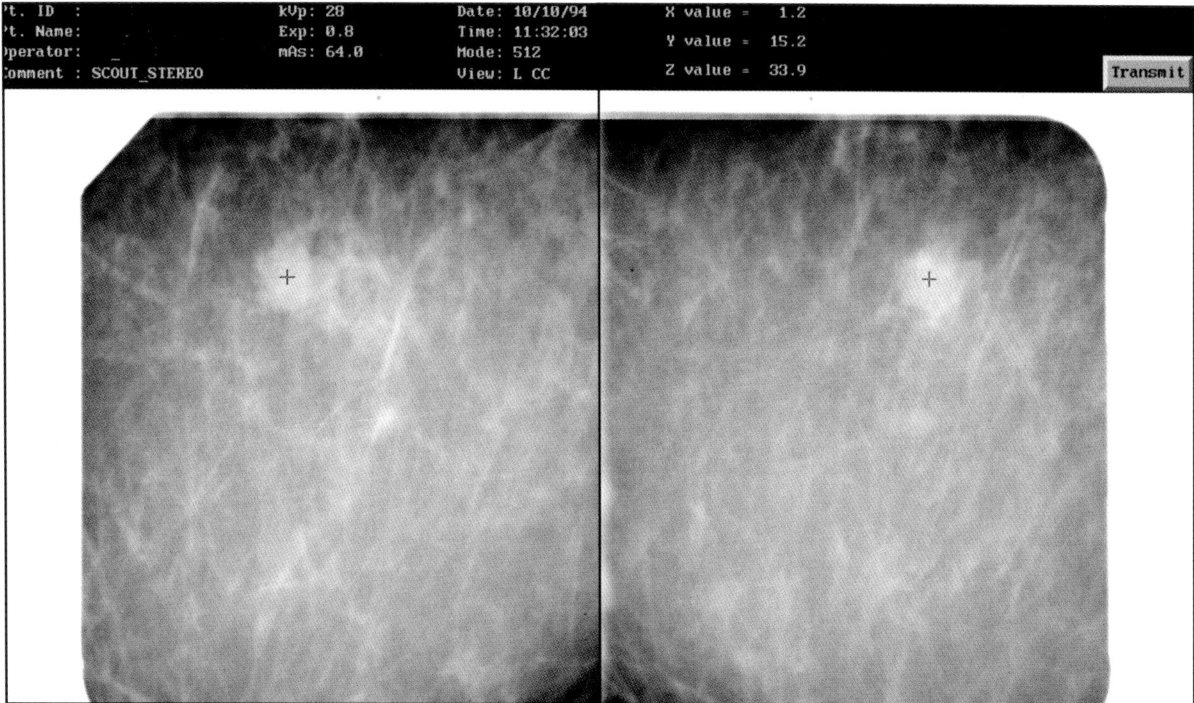

Figure 2.27b. Coordinate Determination. Based on targeting **(cursors)**, the computer determines coordinates for the abnormality (upper right-hand corner).

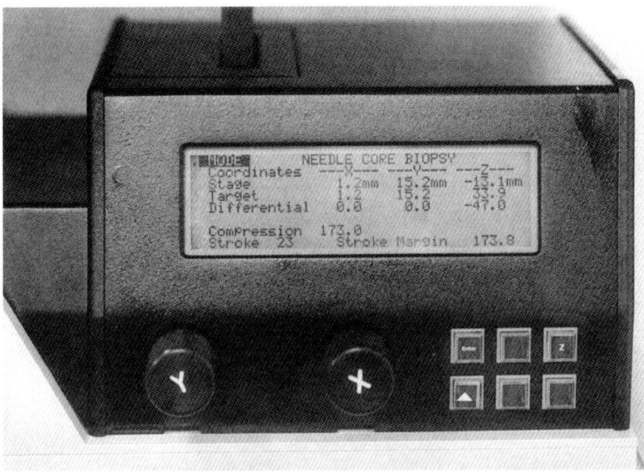

Figure 2.28. Transfer coordinates to the needle guidance system.

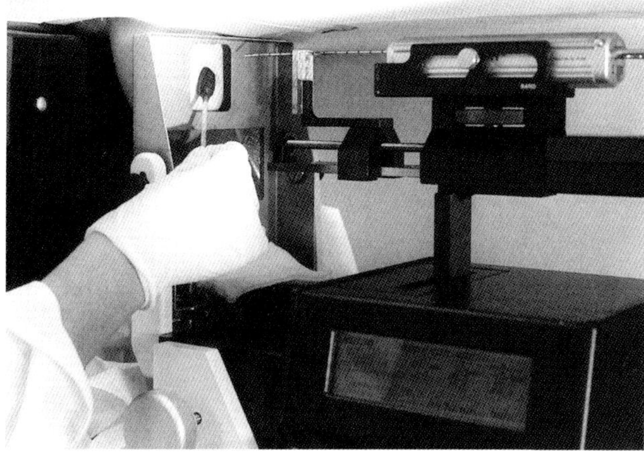

Figure 2.29. Apply antiseptic conservatively.

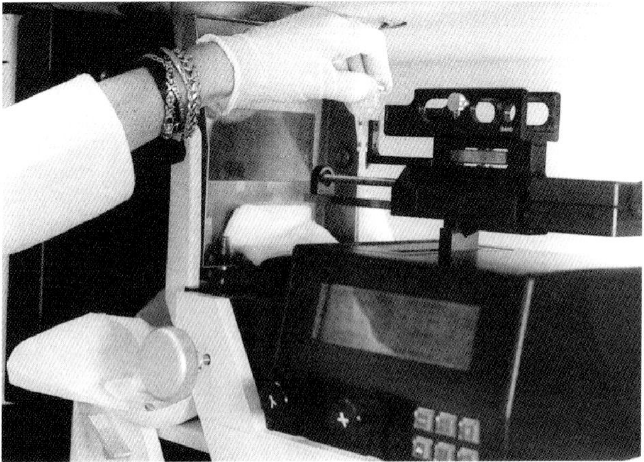

Figure 2.30. Place the needle guide. The forward needle guide maintains accuracy of needle placement.

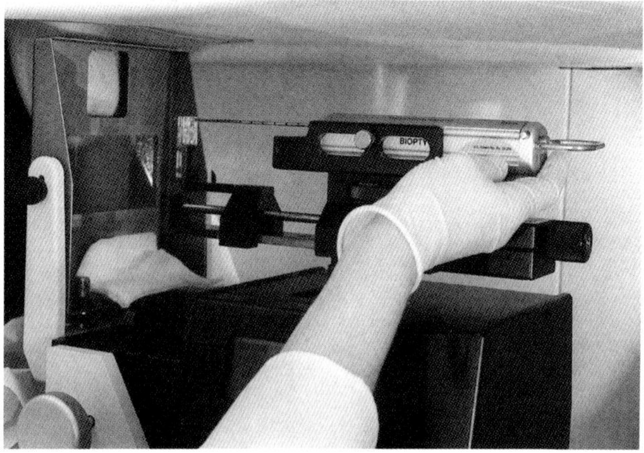

Figure 2.31. Place the biopsy instrument. Secure the loaded biopsy instrument into the holder.

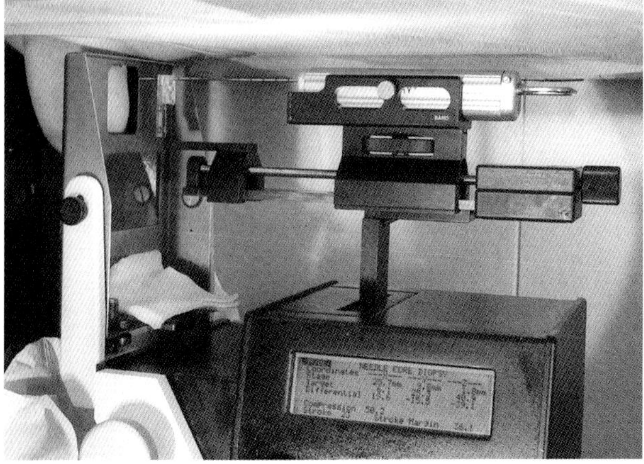

Figure 2.32. Calibrate needle length. Calibration for needle length ensures accuracy in reaching the depth coordinate.

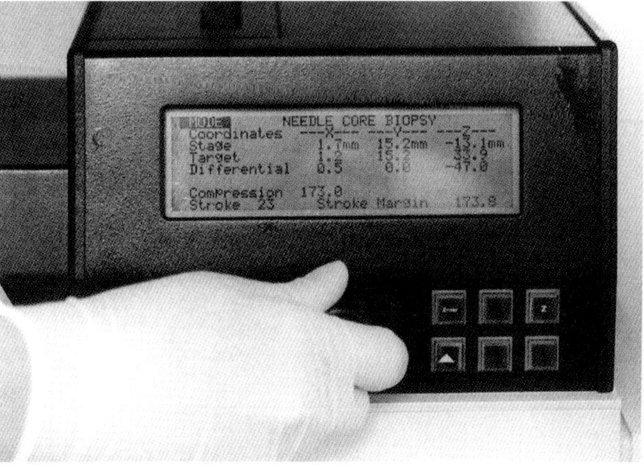

Figure 2.33. The clinician matches the platform needle guidance stage or platform with the abnormality coordinates.

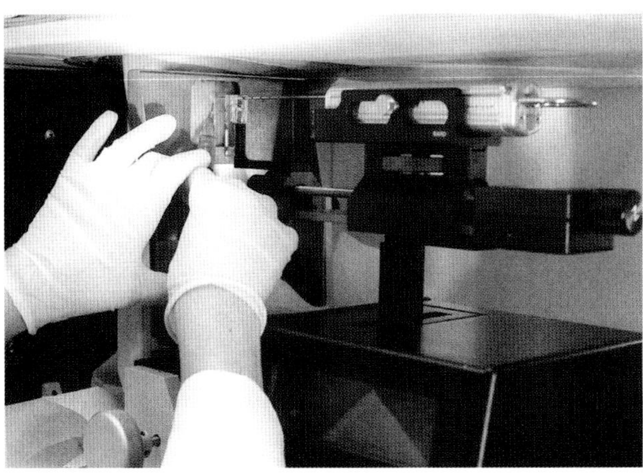

Figure 2.34. Move the needle forward to indicate the site for anesthesia of superficial and subcutaneous tissue.

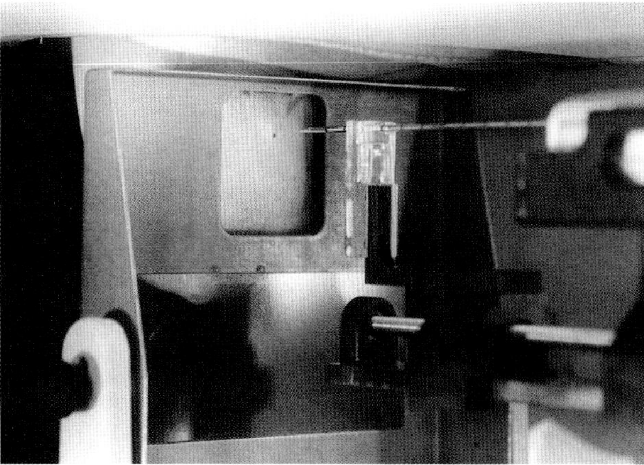

Figure 2.35. Mark the skin. Once a skin welt has been raised, bring the needle forward just far enough to make a mark on the skin.

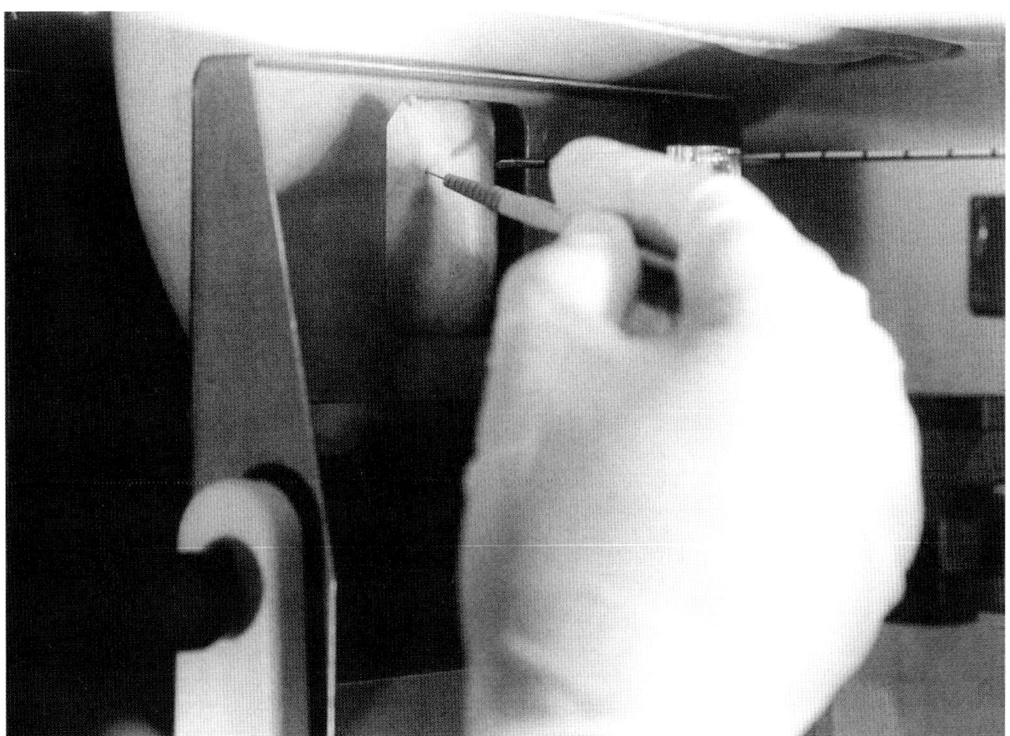

Figure 2.36. Make a skin incision. A small skin incision allows smooth passage of the biopsy needle through the skin.

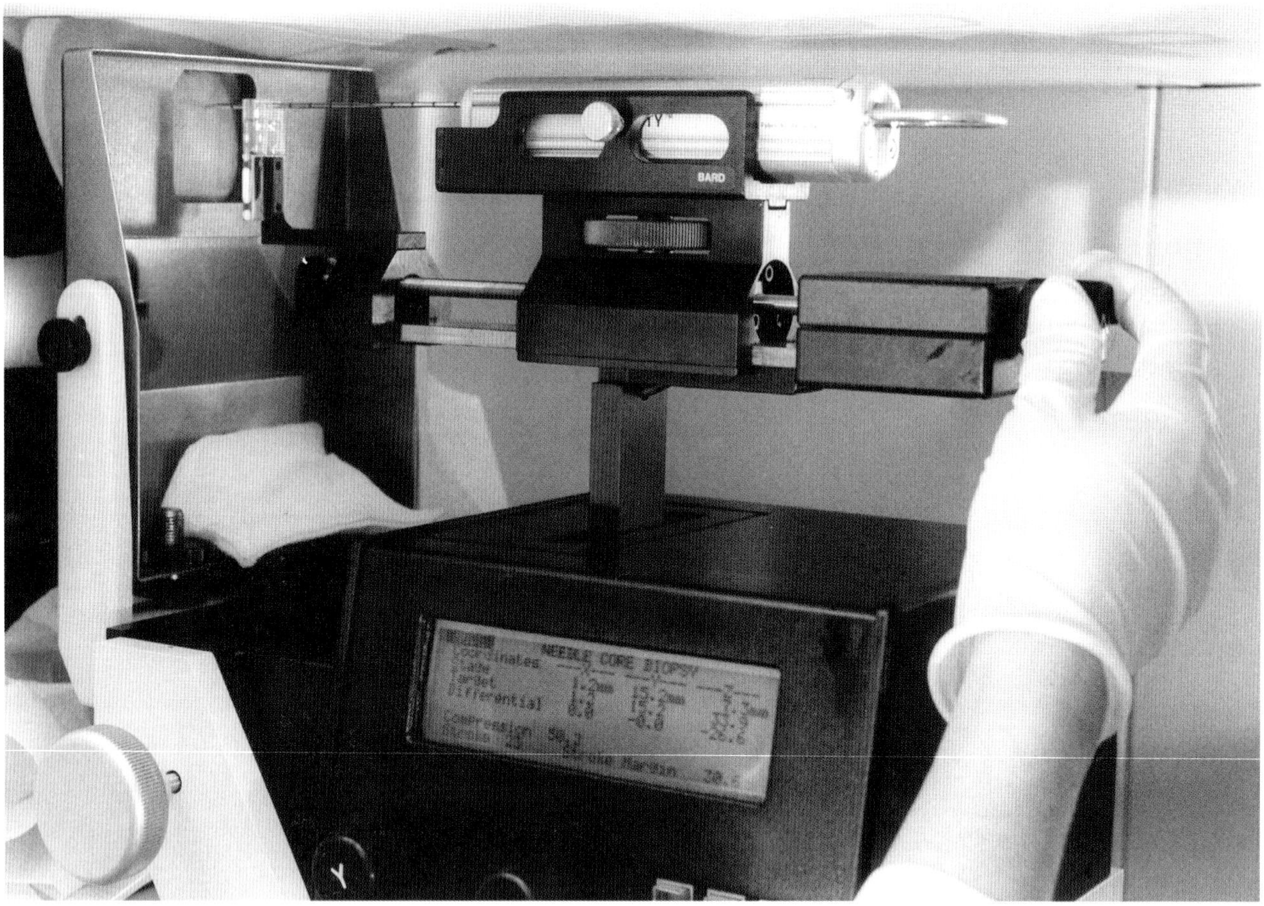

Figure 2.37. Placement of the Biopsy Needle. The clinician advances the biopsy needle into the breast to the appropriate depth.

Placement of the Biopsy Needle

The clinician guides the needle into the breast, advancing it to the desired depth. See later discussion on determining prefire depth **(Figure 2.37)**.

Confirmation (Prefire Stereo) Images

Acquire this stereo pair prior to firing the biopsy instrument to ensure correct needle placement and to check for abnormality movement (see later discussion) **(Figure 2.38)**. Retracting the anterior needle guide for prefire images will prevent superimposition over the area of interest.

First Sample

1. Check for proper seating of the biopsy instrument.

2. Make sure anterior needle guide is forward to provide accurate needle placement.

3. Ensure positive stroke margin, discussed later in this chapter.

4. Fire the biopsy instrument for the first sample.

Postfire Stereo Images

Acquire postfire images, if desired, immediately after firing the biopsy instrument to verify the needle has traversed the abnormality **(Figure 2.39)**. Abnormality movement and needle deflection are two possible problems that become evident on postfire images. This information may alter

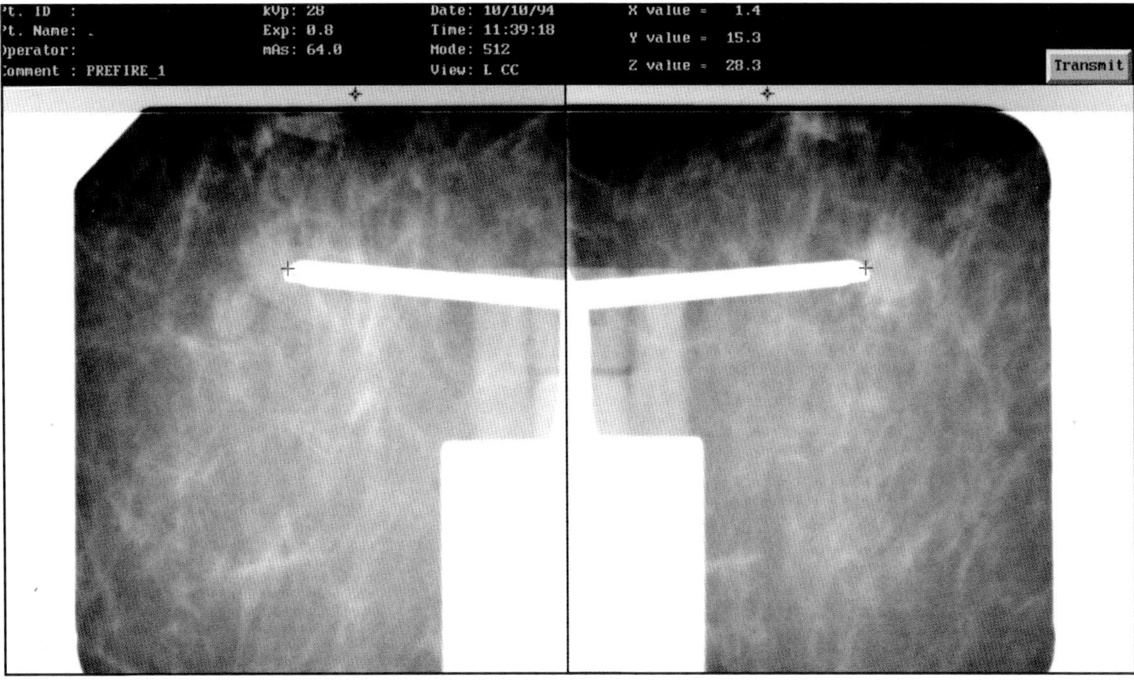

Figure 2.38. Acquire Confirmation Stereo Images. Confirmation stereo images verify placement of the biopsy needle. Targeting of the biopsy needle **(cursors)** indicates accurate placement to within 1 mm of the original targets (Figure 2.27b), with an allowance for a -5 mm prefire position on the Z coordinate.

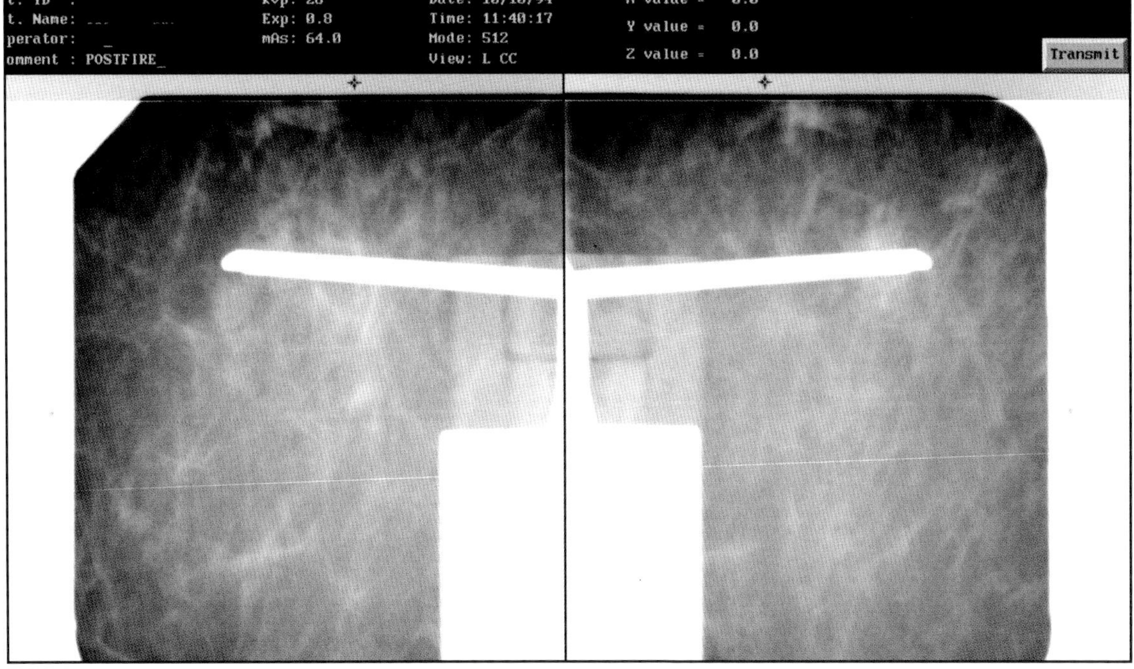

Figure 2.39. Acquire Postfire Stereo Images. Postfire images (optional) confirm the forward movement of the biopsy needle.

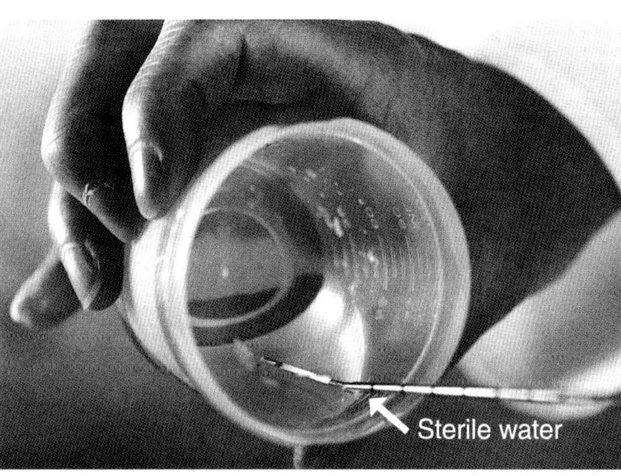

(a)

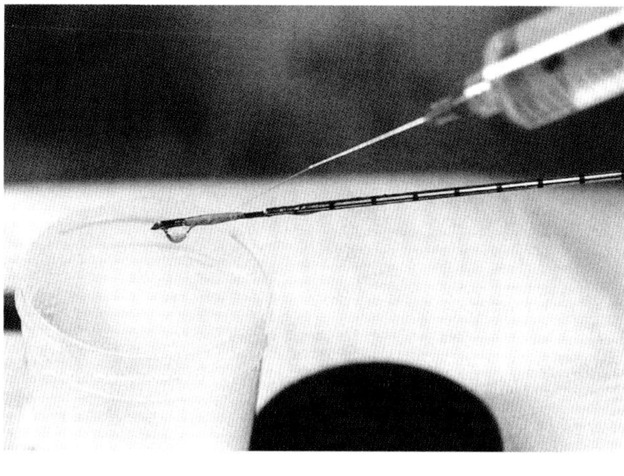

(b)

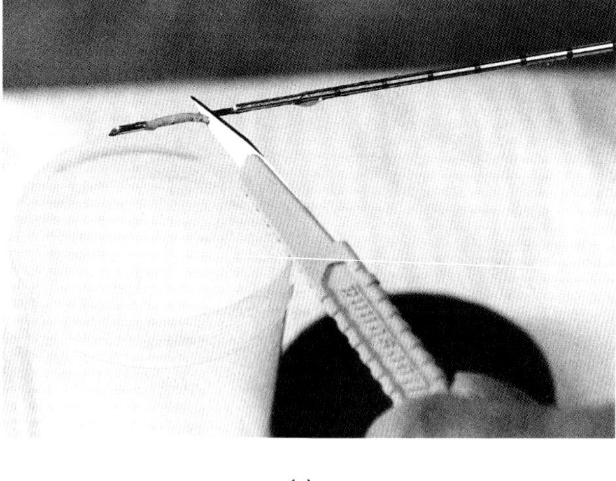

(c)

Figure 2.40 a-c. Remove the biopsy specimen. Three methods are demonstrated here. Shake off into sterile water and add formalin after sampling is complete **(a)**. Push off with a stream of water into formalin **(b)**. Edge off with blunt side of scalpel into formalin **(c)**.

subsequent needle positions for multiple sampling (see *Stereotactic Errors* in chapter 3).

Removal of the Specimen

Figure 2.40 demonstrates three methods for removing the core specimen from the needle. Delicate handling of the sample will keep it intact. Placing the specimen into sterile water requires the addition of formalin for preservation at the conclusion of the procedure. Direct placement into formalin requires care to avoid contamination of the needle.

Multiple Samples

The clinician can collect multiple (or offset) core specimens by varying the position of the biopsy needle. Three to five samples are taken of the suspicious area using the *same* needle, unless damaged or contaminated during the biopsy process. It is useful to wipe excess blood from the biopsy needle using a *damp* sponge, to allow smooth needle movement and to prevent back up of blood into the biopsy instrument. Further confirmation stereo images for each sample may be desirable, but are not always necessary to check needle placement. This is especially helpful after correcting original coordinates and when sampling microcalcifications. Early in the learning curve, confirmation and postfire stereo images for each core specimen will assure the clinician of proper needle placement.

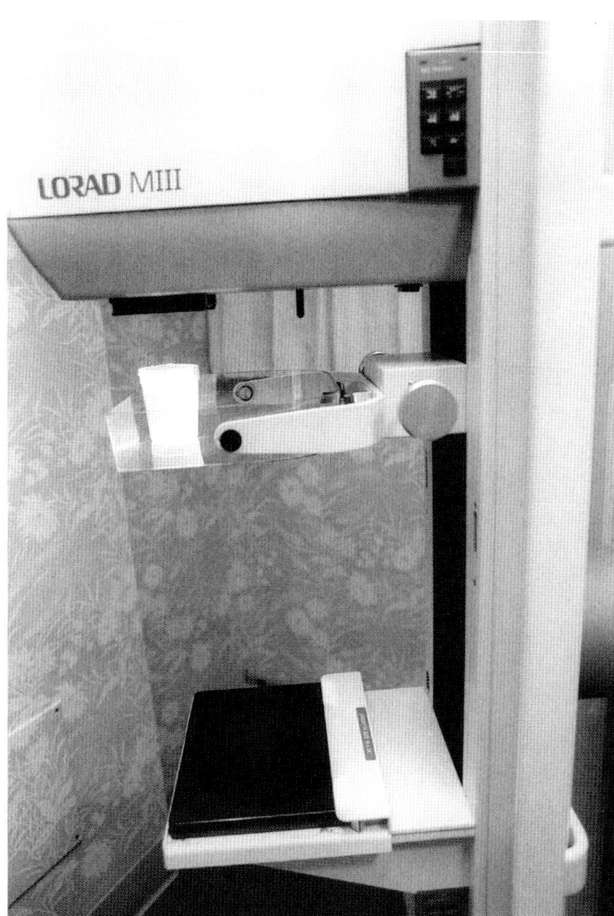

Figure 2.41a. Specimen Radiography. Prior to releasing the patient from the biopsy position, radiography of the specimen verifies removal of calcifications. Here, the specimen in sterile water is imaged with magnification.

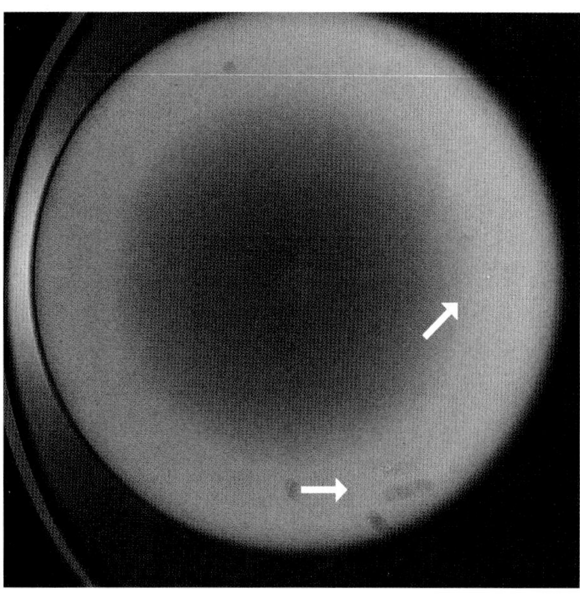

Figure 2.41b. This specimen demonstrates calcifications **(arrows)** after core biopsy.

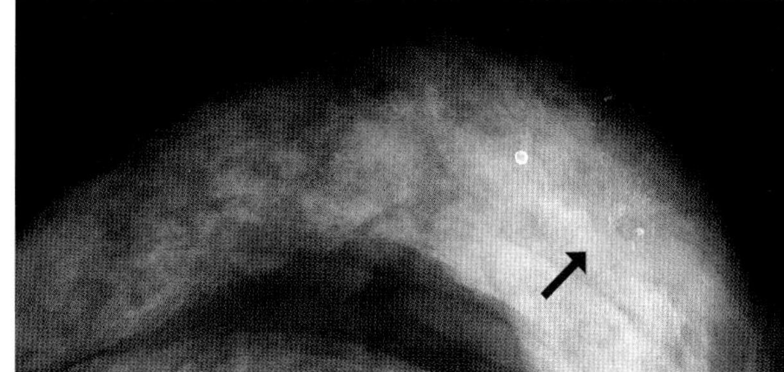

Figure 2.41c. The patient's screening mammogram indicates the original calcifications **(arrow)**.

Specimen Radiography

If the abnormality in question involves calcifications, specimen radiography can ensure adequate sampling **(Figure 2.41)**. Reviewing this image before releasing the patient from compression allows further sampling, if necessary.

Many methods are in use for specimen radiography. In general, a mammography unit with magnification capabilities can provide the necessary image. The greatest magnification factor is attainable by placing the specimen container on the compression plate and elevating this plate higher than the magnification device allows. Lower kVp (22 kVp) increases the contrast of the image. It is best to acquire two images, utilizing different cassettes, to distinguish dust or other artifacts from calcifications in the sample. Always use caution in handling and transferring core specimens.

Poststudy Image

Acquiring a poststudy image with the x-ray tube perpendicular to the breast support may document access to the abnormality. A recognizable reduction in the number of calcifications in comparison to the scout image can document sampling **(Figure 2.42a)**. In addition, lucencies resulting from the removal of tissue can confirm access to the abnormality **(Figure 2.42b)**.

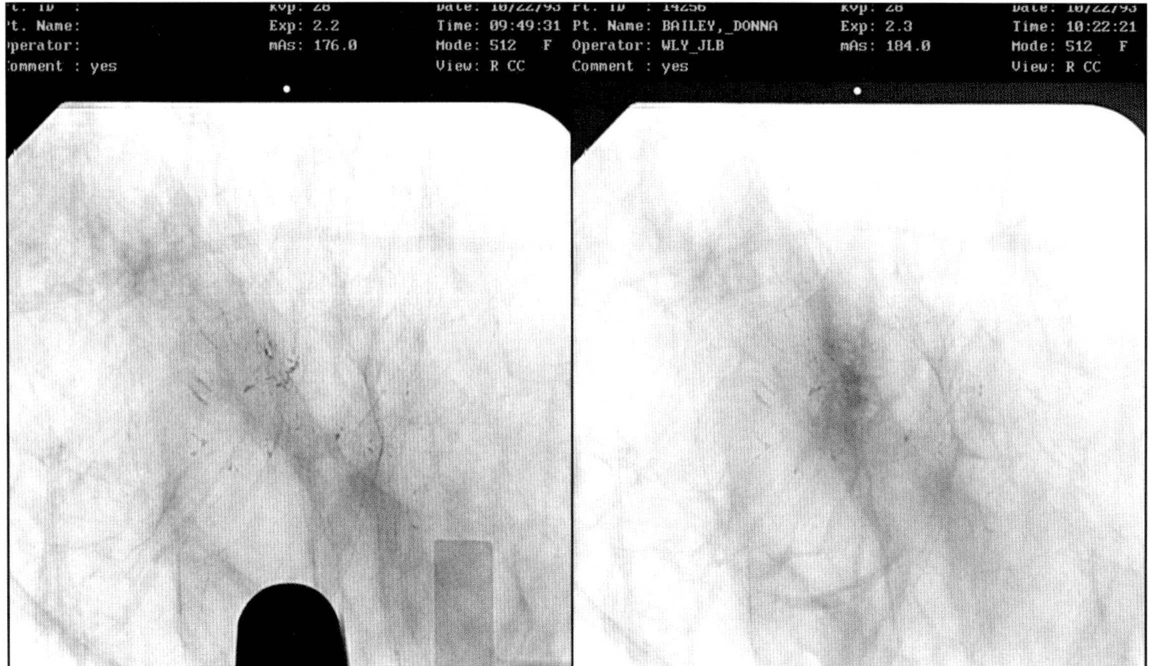

Figure 2.42a. Poststudy Image. The image on the left demonstrates the area of concern prior to core biopsy; the image on the right is the poststudy image, providing proof of removal of calcifications.

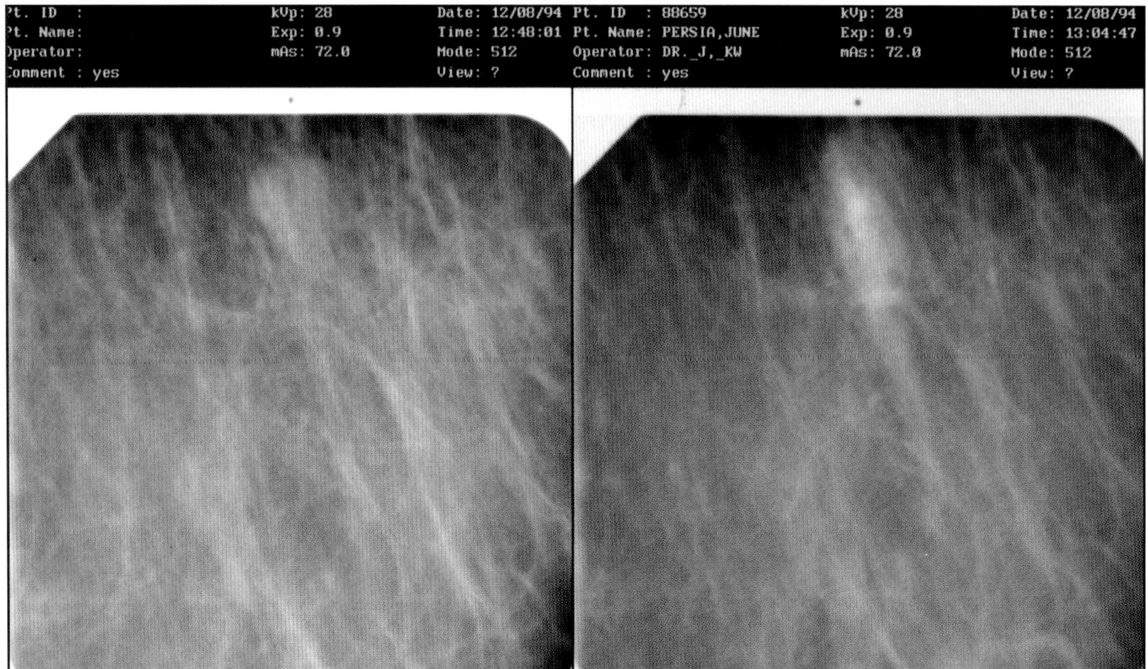

Figure 2.42b. The image on the left demonstrates a mass prior to core biopsy; the poststudy image on the right demonstrates lucencies, indicating tissue removal and confirming access to the abnormality.

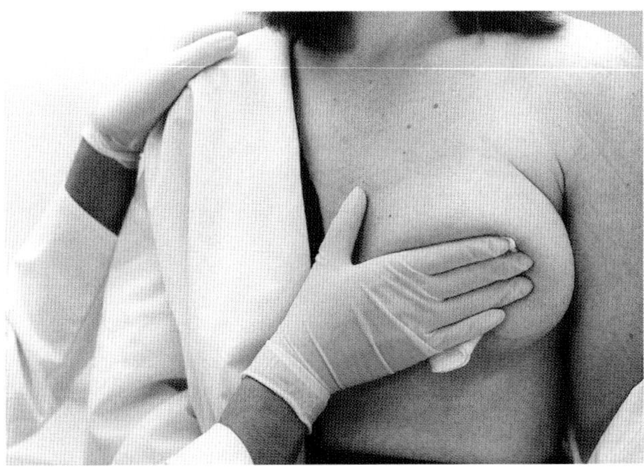

Figure 2.43. Apply pressure until bleeding ceases.

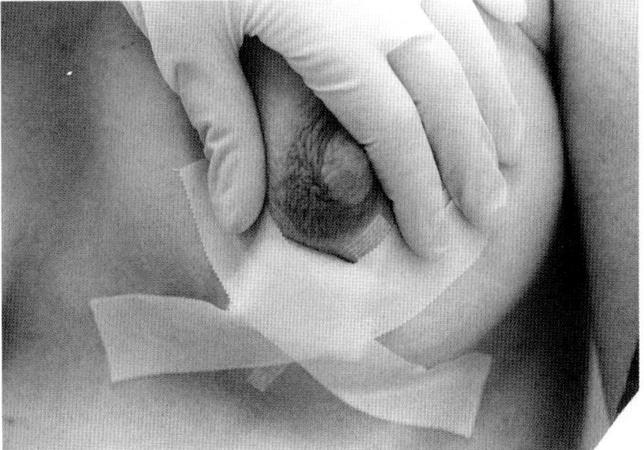

Figure 2.45. Place a pressure dressing over the wound to inhibit bleeding.

After the Procedure

1. *Postprocedure Patient Care*—After completion of the procedure, apply pressure between the skin nick and the abnormality location until bleeding ceases **(Figure 2.43)**. Place a steristrip over the wound to draw the skin edges together for healing **(Figure 2.44)**. Application of an antibiotic ointment may be desirable. Placing a pressure dressing over the wound for the remainder of the day may inhibit bleeding **(Figure 2.45)**. The patient should have verbal and written instructions for postbiopsy care, which should include a contact person in the event complications occur. Possible complications, although rare, are hematoma and infection.

2. *Postbiopsy Follow-up*—Next day contact with the patient, by phone or in person, helps to ensure the biopsy site is stable.

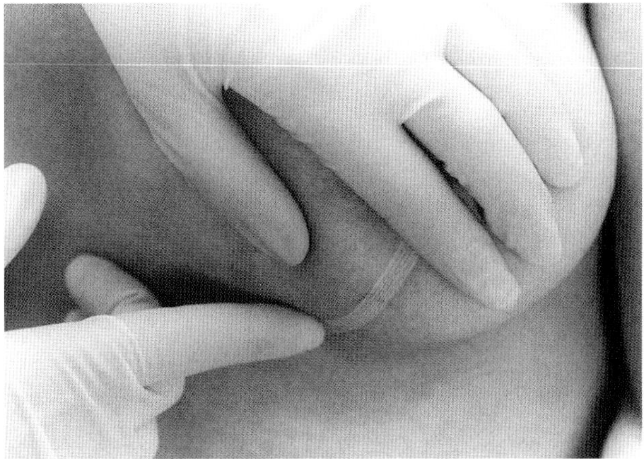

Figure 2.44. Use a steristrip to draw skin edges together.

Principles of Stereotactic Core Biopsy

The Biopsy Instrument

Reusable and disposable single-patient biopsy instruments are available. Each biopsy instrument (gun) consists of a spring-loaded system with a cocking device and firing button **(Figure 2.46)**. An automatic or manual safety feature should be standard on all instruments to prevent premature or accidental firing. The anterior and posterior carrier blocks of the biopsy gun hold the hubs of each part of the biopsy needle **(Figure 2.47)**. The design of the mechanism allows high-velocity firing of the carrier blocks that hold the two-piece needle. The distance that the gun moves the needle, from the starting (or cocked) position to the home (or fired) position, is the **stroke** (or throw) of the instrument **(Figure 2.48)**. Stroke varies from 11-23 mm, depending on the manufacturer and the model. With shorter throw instruments, less of the sample notch is available for sampling **(Figure 2.49)**. Strokes of 22-23 mm are most popular. While most biopsy instruments have a single-stroke length, others provide multiple-stroke movements that are useful for breasts of thinner compression widths.

The efficiency of the biopsy instrument is critical to obtaining a good core specimen. The following characteristics contribute to the effectiveness of the gun.

1. *Spring force and velocity*—The *velocity* of movement, governed by the instrument's *spring force,* will determine the efficiency in obtaining a useful core of tissue. This is

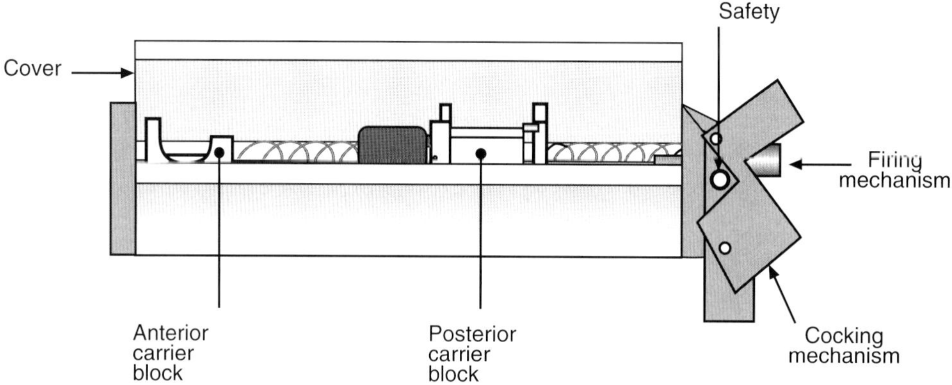

Figure 2.46. The Biopsy Instrument.

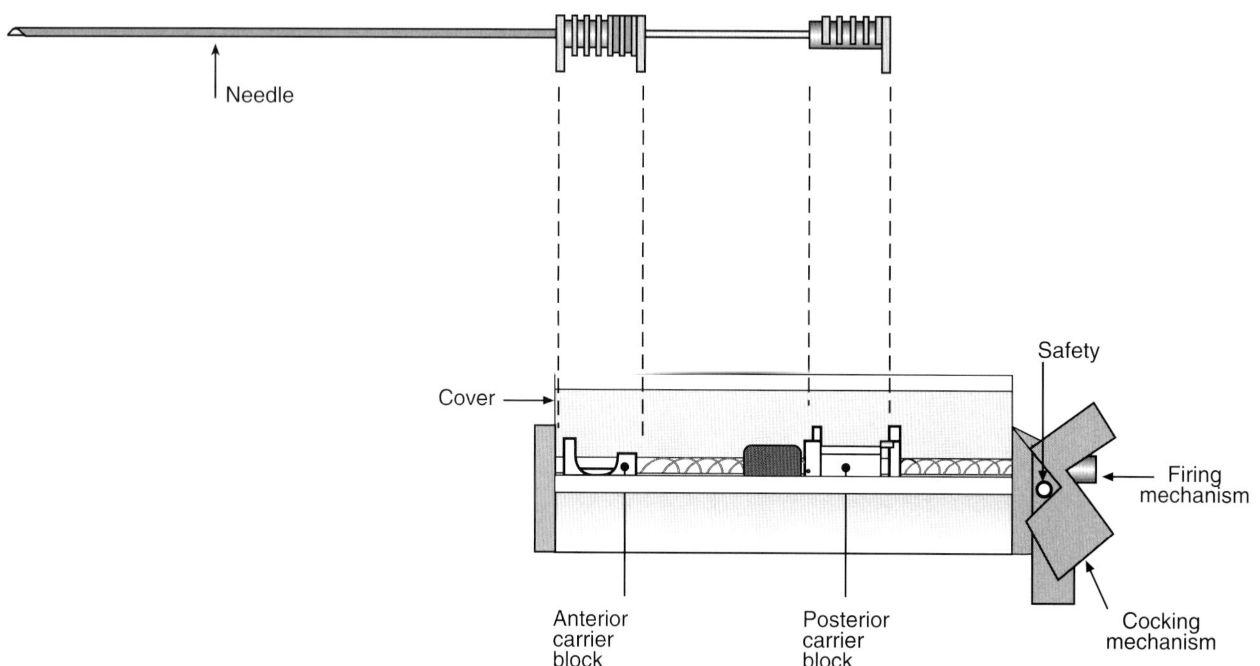

Figure 2.47. Biopsy Instrument/Needle Combination.

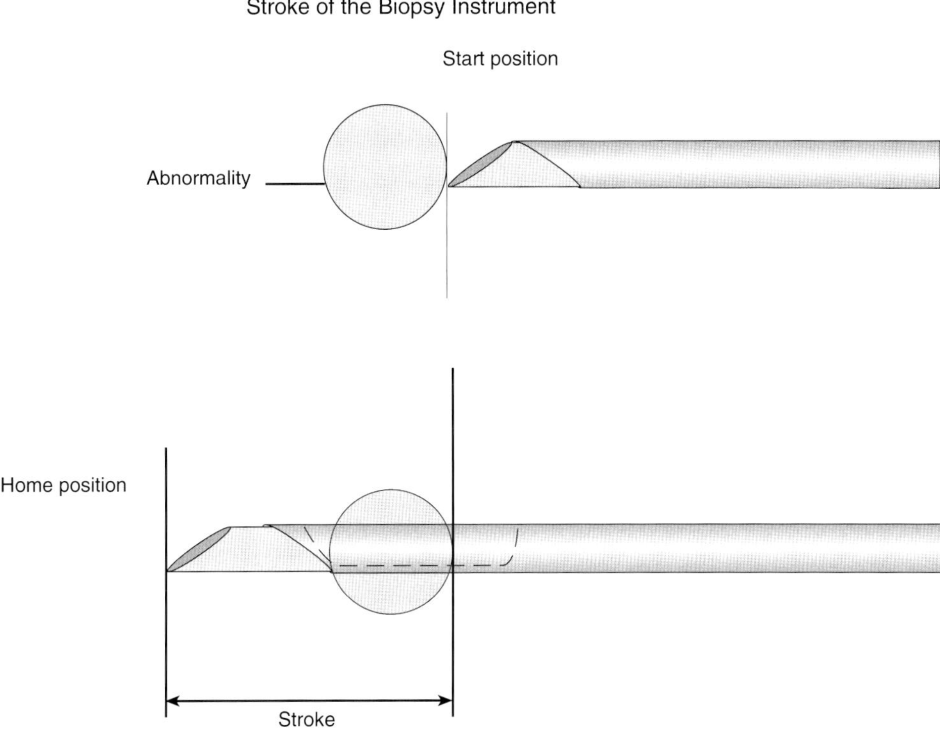

Figure 2.48. Stroke of the Biopsy Instrument. The stroke of the biopsy instrument is the distance the needle moves from the starting (cocked) position to the home (fired) position.

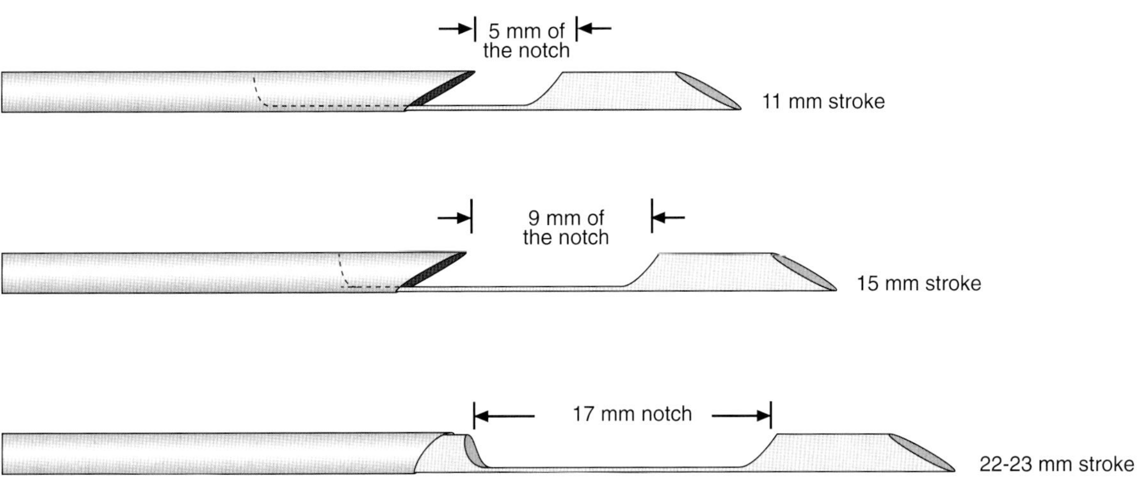

Figure 2.49. Stroke and Available Sample Notch. The stroke of the biopsy instrument determines the length of available sample notch.

particularly important when sampling extremely firm abnormalities. Deflection of the needle is more likely to occur with less velocity, which results from weaker springs. This may also contribute to missing the abnormality.

2. *Maintenance of spring force*—The gun's mechanism may become weak with multiple use. Interval quality control testing by the gun manufacturer will assure consistency in spring force. Before choosing a single-patient disposable gun, investigate the effectiveness of the spring system to ensure that subsequent firings maintain the same spring force as the first firing.

3. *Weight*—A heavy biopsy instrument may be awkward to handle.

4. *Cocking mechanism*—Some biopsy instruments are easier to prepare for firing than others. A double-cocking mechanism allows the first motion to expose the sample notch for specimen removal, and the second motion to prepare for firing. With this feature, removal of the needle will not be necessary after each core sample.

5. *Safety features*—An automatic safety to prevent accidental firing of the biopsy instrument is critical and should be available on all instruments.

Firing Mechanism—The firing of the biopsy instrument occurs in two stages. The posterior carrier block holding the notched stylet portion of the needle fires first. This causes the anterior carrier block to drive the cutting cannula forward over the stylet. The core of tissue is taken during this excursion **(Figure 2.50)**. The movement of the posterior carrier block triggers the movement of the anterior carrier block. If for some reason the posterior block does not make its full movement, the anterior block holding the cutting cannula will not fire. The open sample notch is left in the breast, causing complications to the procedure. This may occur from mechanical failure, or negative stroke margin. Hard or fibrous tissue may also "heap up" in front of the bevel, which may stop the movement of the needle in cases of very minimal stroke margin.

Needles for Core Biopsy

The biopsy needle in use for core biopsy has two parts – an inner stylet, cut with a sample notch for specimen acquisition, and an outer cutting cannula **(Figure 2.51)**. The needles typically have a beveled tip, however, a pencil-point needle† was recently introduced.

The biopsy needle must be compatible with the biopsy instrument. Although the needle hubs may fit well in the carrier blocks of the biopsy instrument, the *alignment* of the stylet and cannula may be incorrect **(Figure 2.52)**. Misalignment may result in difficulties during needle excursion, such as fragmented core samples, drag on the biopsy needle, tearing of tissue inside the breast, and hematoma.

Needle Gauge—Needles in use for core biopsy typically range from 14 to 18-gauge. The most popular size for core biopsy is 14-gauge. (The larger the gauge number, the smaller the needle size.) The gauge of the needle will affect the size of the biopsy specimen and has a direct correlation with the effectiveness of the histologic interpretation[1,2].

Needle Length—Needle lengths range from 10-16 cm. The following criteria should be taken into consideration when choosing needle length:

1. *Available length*—Due to the guidance system of SBB units, shorter needle length may limit the depth that can be accessed. For example, a 16-cm needle will access greater depths than a 10-cm needle.

2. *Superimposition of the biopsy instrument in the biopsy window*—With shorter needle length, a greater portion of the biopsy instrument will impinge on the radiographic field. This may obscure or interfere with imaging the abnormality during pre- and postfire studies.

3. *Limited space*—The physical characteristics of upright units may limit needle length.

Stroke Margin

Breast thickness must be of sufficient width to accept the motion of the needle from the prefire position to the home position, without exiting the breast and striking the breast support. ***The distance from the home position of the needle to the breast support, usually with an allowance of 4 mm for safety, is referred to as the stroke margin*** **(Figure 2.53).**

The calculation of stroke margin is critical. *Positive stroke margin* indicates ample thickness for needle excursion. *Negative stroke margin* indicates the needle will exit the breast and strike the breast support. If the biopsy needle impales the breast and strikes the breast support, it will injure the underside of the breast and possibly end the procedure. The following can also occur: the needle tip may be damaged from impact (if removal of the needle is not possible from the entrance site, decompression of the breast will be necessary to remove the needle from the underside of the breast), or the outer cannula may not fire the notch sample. Unsuccessful sampling, tearing of breast tissue, hematoma, and discomfort to the patient are all possible complications.

† Harper needle, EMS Medical Systems, Indianapolis, Indiana

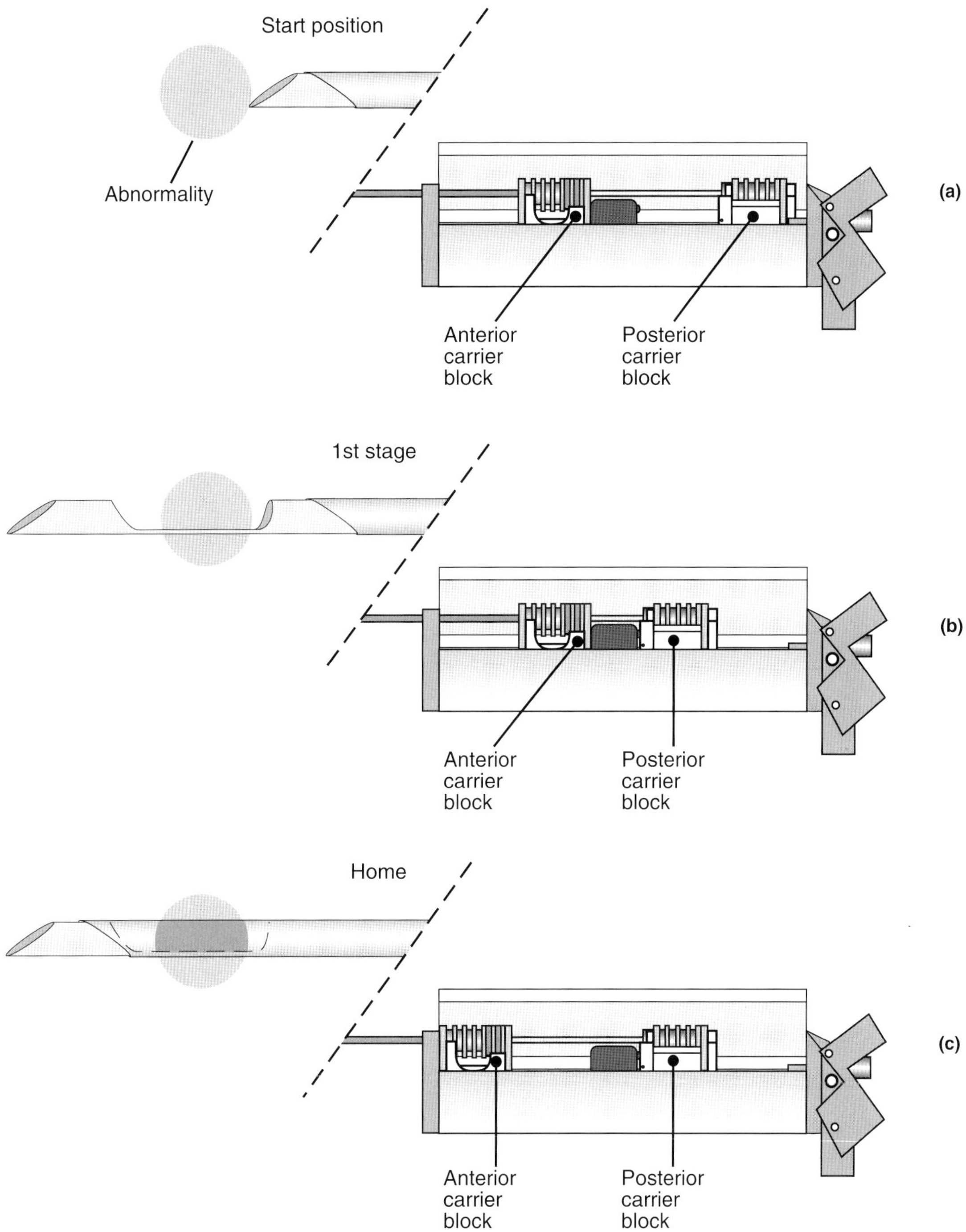

Figure 2.50 a-c. Two-Stage Firing Mechanism. Firing the biopsy instrument occurs in two stages. The posterior carrier block holding the stylet **(a)** fires first, advancing the sample notch into the abnormality **(b)**. This triggers the firing of the anterior carrier block that holds the cutting cannula, allowing the removal of tissue **(c)**.

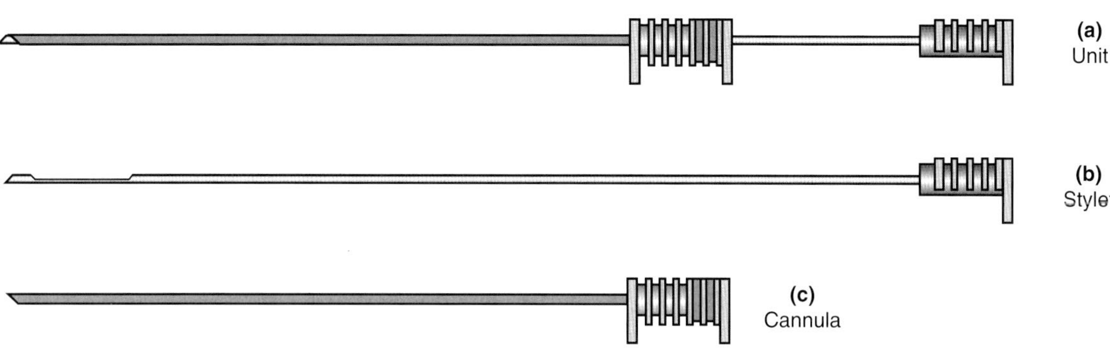

Figure 2.51 a-c. Core Biopsy Needle. The core biopsy needle **(a)** has two parts, the inner stylet with sample notch **(b)** and the outer cutting cannula **(c)**.

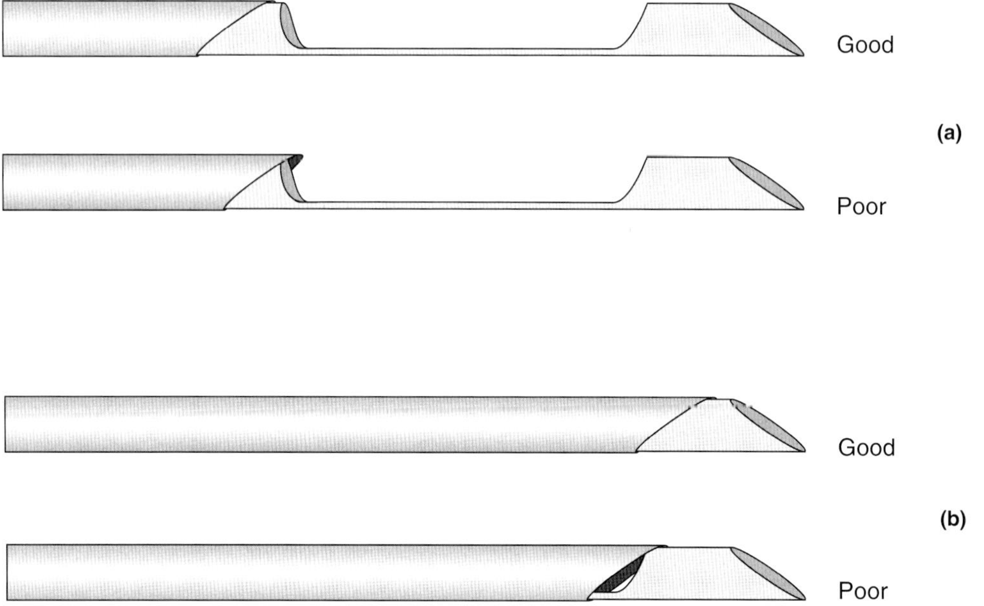

Figure 2.52 a and b. Biopsy Instrument and Needle Compatibility. Although the hubs of the biopsy needle may fit into the biopsy instrument, the sample notch may not open to its fullest extent **(a)**, or some part of the sample notch may be inadequately covered by the cannula **(b)**, which may cause tearing of tissue.

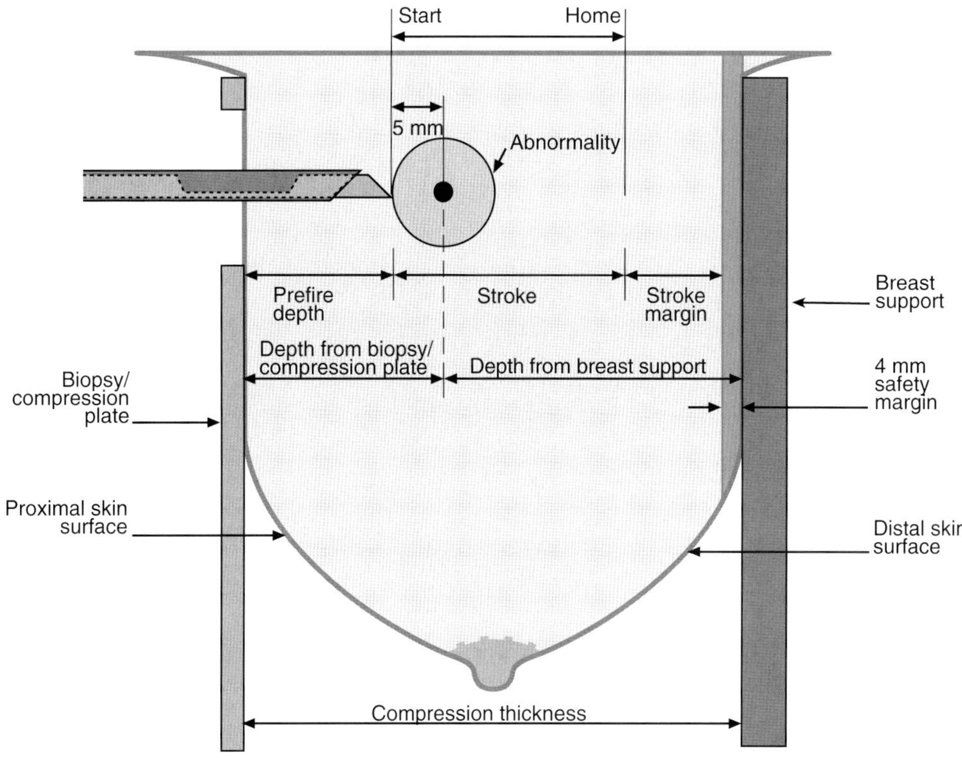

Figure 2.53. Stroke Margin.

The clinician may manually calculate the stroke margin, or the computer of the SBB unit will perform this task. Regardless, the team, including the technologist, must be aware of the calculation of the stroke margin. However, visual indicators are equally important. For example, if the computer or manual calculations determine positive stroke margin but visual cues indicate otherwise, recheck the calculations; errant information keyed into the computer, or a misread figure, could be at fault. The following general formulas help determine stroke margin, however, always follow the manufacturer's recommendations.

When depth is determined from the *proximal* aspect of the compressed breast,

Stroke margin = (compression thickness - 4 mm) - (prefire depth + stroke).

When depth is determined from the *distal* aspect of the compressed breast,

Stroke margin = (prefire depth - stroke) - 4 mm.

Altering the prefire position of the needle tip, using a shorter stroke biopsy instrument, or repositioning the breast, may be necessary to counter a negative stroke margin (see chapter 6 on positioning).

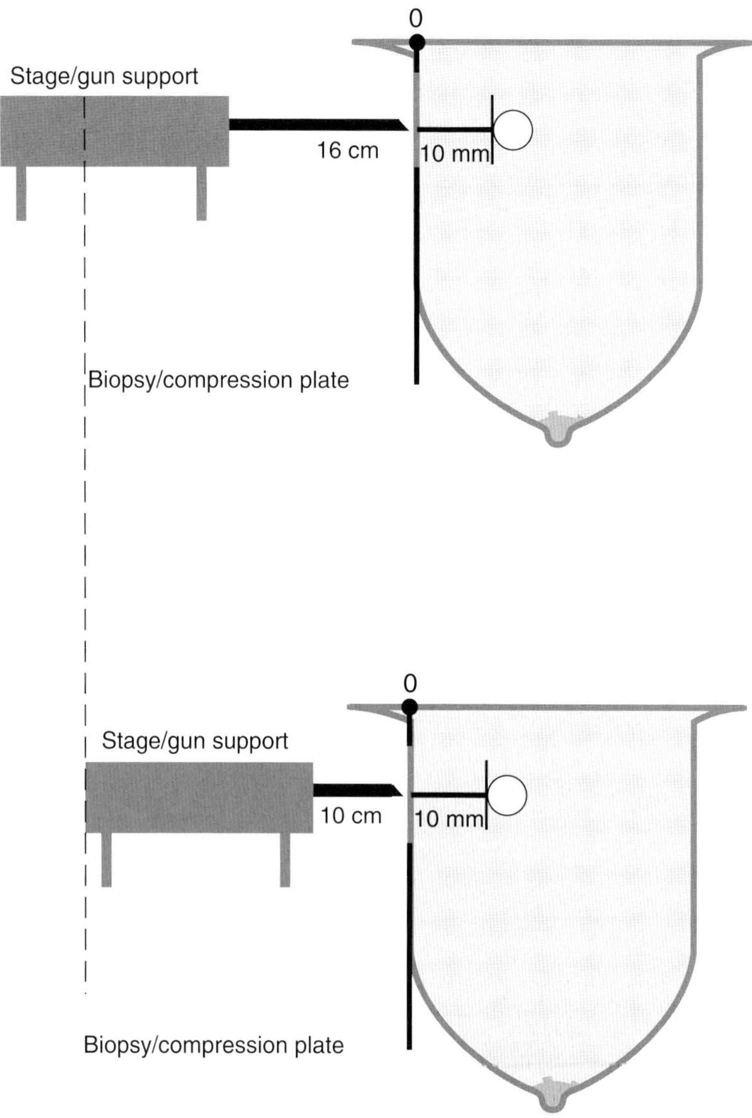

Figure 2.54. Needle Calibration. Needle length must be calibrated to achieve correct depth. This illustration demonstrates how the needle guidance stage must be at different starting points for different length needles to ensure reaching the depth coordinate.

Programming Needle Length and Stroke

To arrive at an accurate depth coordinate and to ensure accurate calculation of stroke margin, programming needle length (sometimes expressed by the length of the needle/gun combination) and biopsy instrument stroke is necessary **(Figure 2.54)**. Programming the *stroke* simply requires entering a number into the computer or into a calculation. The programming of *needle length* is somewhat more complicated.

There are two methods to factor the needle length into the system. However, the *needle calibration*, or *zero process*, is

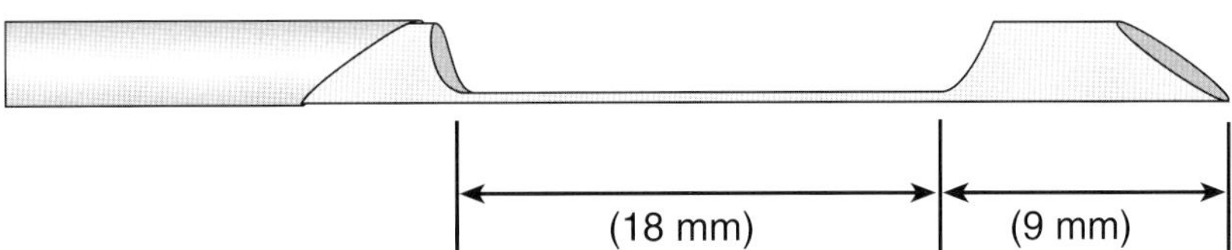

Figure 2.55. Needle Instrument. Calculating the prefire position involves knowing the measurement of the sample notch and the length of the needle from sample notch to the tip of the needle.

specific to each unit, therefore, follow the manufacturer's instructions. A one time default setting for various needles or gun/needle combinations is one method. The unit will provide a selection menu for choosing the appropriate combination. Another method programs needle length on a case-by-case basis using *actual needle length* utilized for each patient. The latter method is more reliable, as a +/- 2 mm manufacturing deviation in the needle is possible. This method also ensures that any other variables interfering with depth accuracy are taken into consideration.

Needle length may be expressed within the depth coordinate. Another technique "zeros" the gun support for the needle length, using this 0 as a starting point to reach the depth coordinate.

Determining Prefire Position

Ideally, firing of the biopsy instrument will place the center of the sample notch in the center of the abnormality, thereby obtaining the maximum amount of tissue possible in the core sample. This may require placing the needle proximal to the depth coordinate, prior to firing.

Calculating prefire position, or "back-off," depends on the following criteria.

1. Stroke of biopsy instrument.

2. Distance from tip of needle to sample notch **(Figure 2.55)**.

3. Length of sample notch measured at inferior aspect (Figure 2.55). Measurement should be made by the clinician, rather than relying on package measurements, as manufacturers differ in how they measure the sample notch.

It is important to remember that for shorter stroke instruments, only a portion of the sample notch is available (Figure 2.49).

The formula to determine prefire back-off is as follows:

$$\textit{Prefire Back-off} = S - \left(\frac{L}{2} + NT\right)$$

where S=stroke, L=length of available sample notch, and NT=length of needle tip.

Parker[3] and Hendrick[4] recommend placing the needle 5 mm proximal to the depth coordinate. For example, if the Z or D coordinate is 24 mm, the prefire position would be 19 mm. While this standard is adequate for most of the longer stroke (22-23 mm) biopsy instruments, it is inaccurate for shorter throw instruments. **Figure 2.56** demonstrates a comparison. Parker and Hendrick also report that the abnormality will move forward with needle impact. If the clinician feels that the abnormality will move forward a significant amount, he or she should reduce the calculated number accordingly.

Calibration of the Stereotactic System

The manufacturer calibrates the stereotactic system at installation of the unit. However, daily verification is necessary. The testing procedure will analyze the accuracy of the biopsy system, including the targeting device, digitizing system, and coordinate calculation. Daily testing (or more frequent if necessary), prior to the first procedure, will ensure the unit's accuracy. Deviation from normal limits requires at least one repeat test. If retesting affirms the error, recalibration is required. Neglect of this very important test can complicate as well as jeopardize procedures.

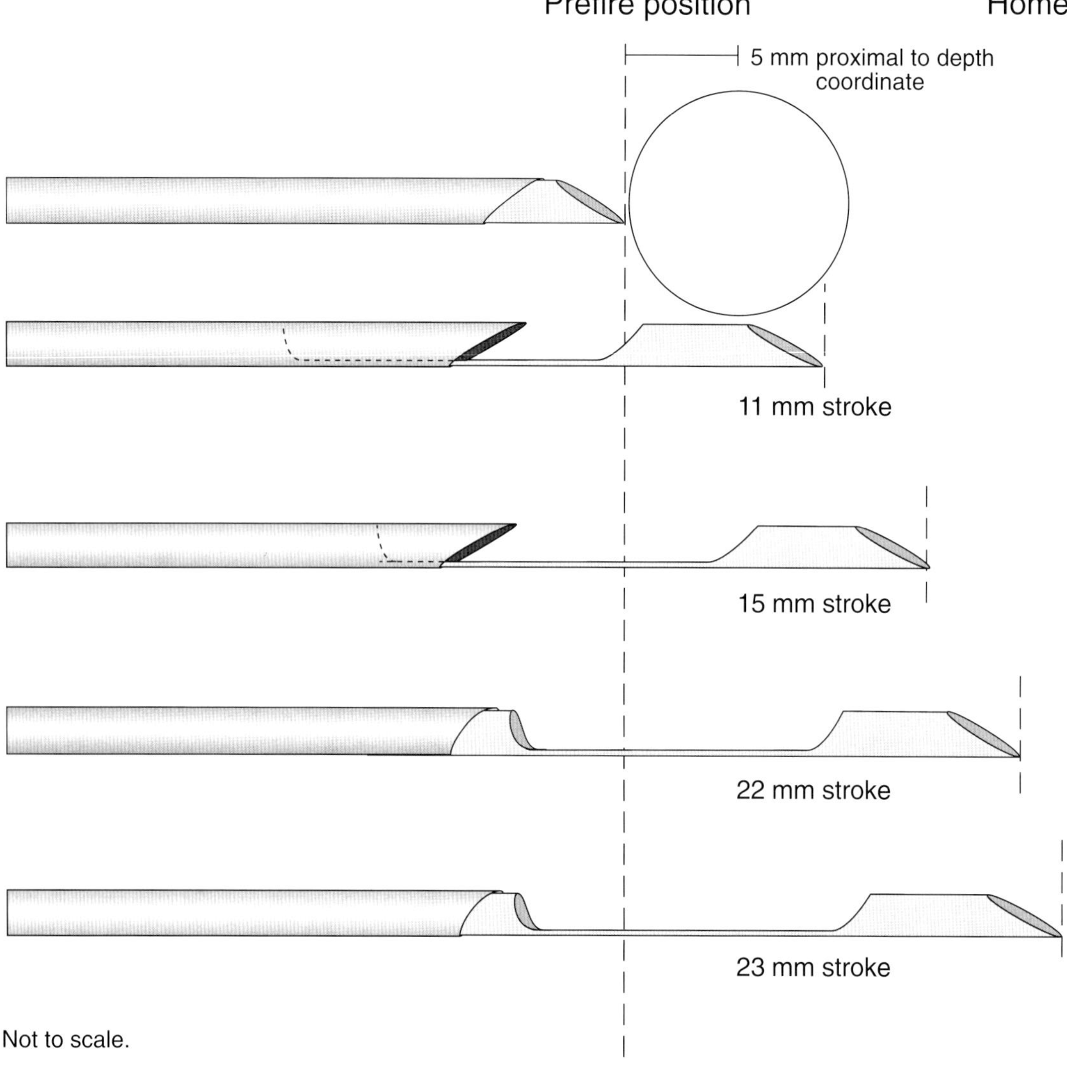

Figure 2.56. A Comparison of Biopsy Instrument Prefire Positions. Prefire position, or "back-off," will vary with the stroke of the biopsy instrument and needle measurements. The accepted 5 mm prefire position proximal to the depth coordinate will be satisfactory for 22 or 23-mm throw instruments, but not for shorter throw instruments. This figure illustrates how the abnormality could be missed with shorter throw instruments.

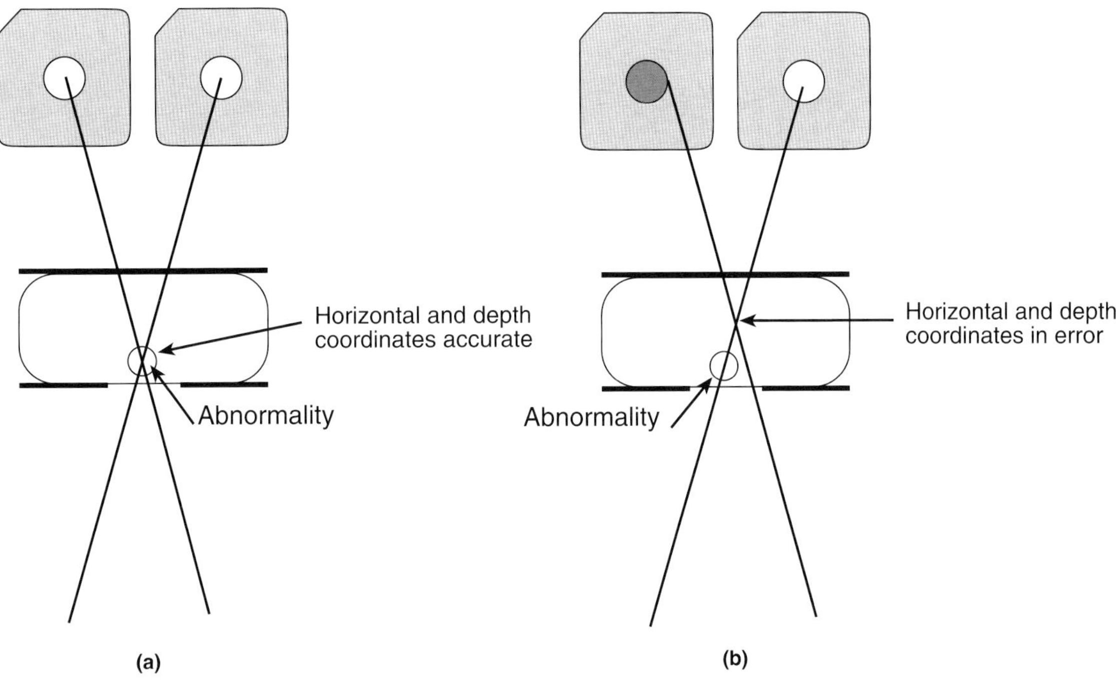

Figure 2.57 a and b. Targeting the Abnormality. The abnormality is well-visualized on both stereo images **(a)**, providing for accurate targeting and yielding accurate results.The abnormality is not seen well on the left-hand stereo image **(b)**. Guessing the position of this abnormality for targeting will yield incorrect horizontal and depth coordinates.

Targeting

Accurate targeting of the abnormality is critical for precise stereotactic localization. *The essence of stereotactic localization involves targeting the same point in space (or as near to it as can be estimated) on both planar images* **(Figure 2.57)**. This necessitates correct display, shift, and identification of the abnormality on both planar images. The clinician must also identify a unique point within the abnormality on both planar images. The identification process is not always as easy as it may seem **(Figure 2.58)**. For example, identifying a unique point within a well-rounded mass presents little challenge. However, choosing a unique point for odd-shaped masses, diffuse areas of distortion, or calcifications may be very difficult. Principles of shift and display will aid in appropriate targeting **(Figure 2.59)**. *Under no circumstances should a study continue if the clinician cannot identify the abnormality, or a unique point, on both stereo images.* Selecting alternative projections may solve this dilemma. Radiologic consultation may be necessary to help identify the abnormality when a nonradiology clinician is performing the exam. In addition, if the patient has not had a suitable work-up prior to biopsy, it is useful to consult with a clinician regarding the viability

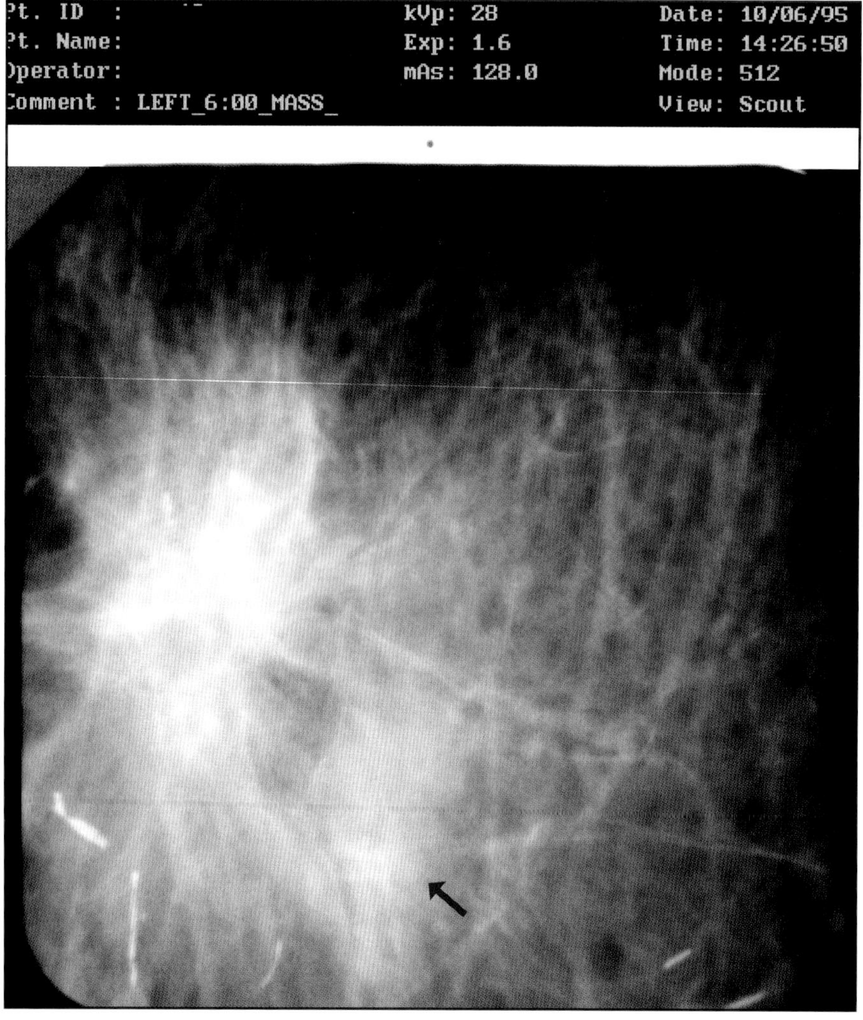

(a)

Figure 2.58 a-c. Targeting and Abnormality Identification. This patient, following lumpectomy and irradiation, demonstrated a new mass. The scout image **(a)** demonstrates this abnormality **(arrow)** well. On the stereo images **(b)**, the abnormality is well-visualized on the left-hand image but not on the right. Repositioning in a new projection provides stereos **(c)** that demonstrate the abnormality on both the left and right image, allowing for accurate targeting. Histology positive for recurrence.

Figure 2.58 continued.

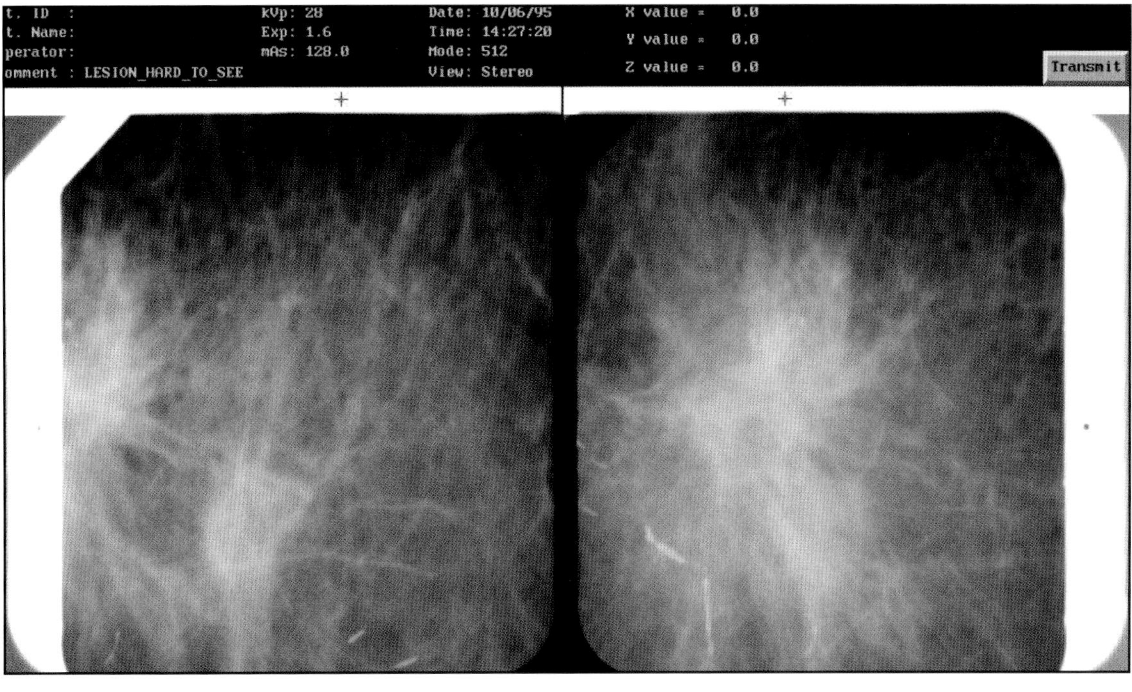

(b)

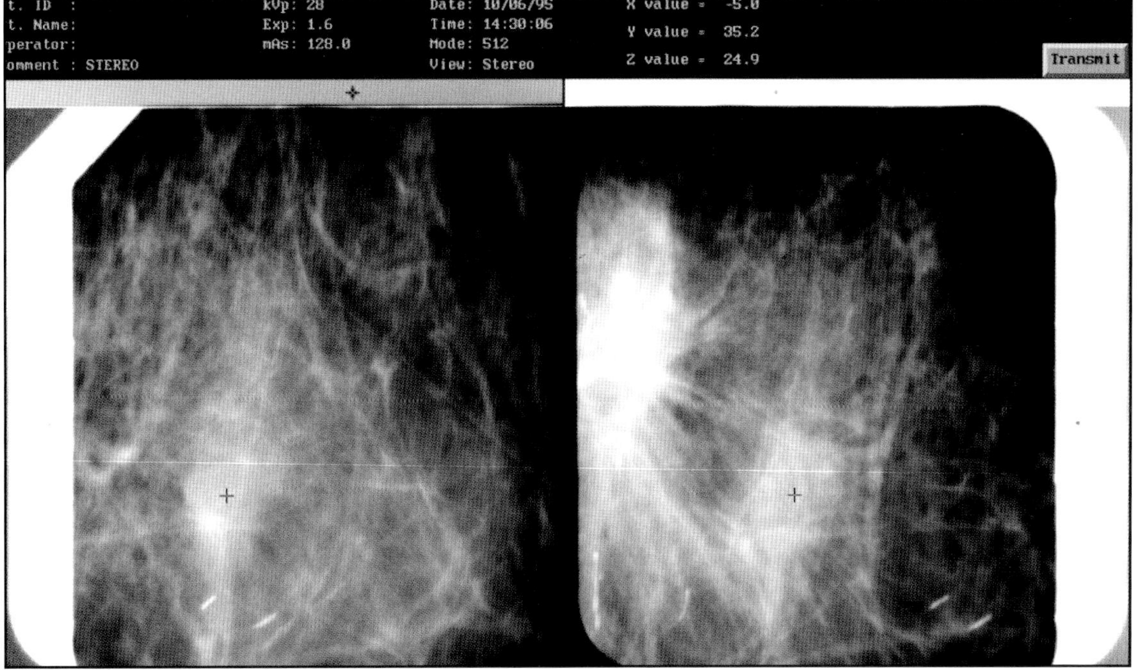

(c)

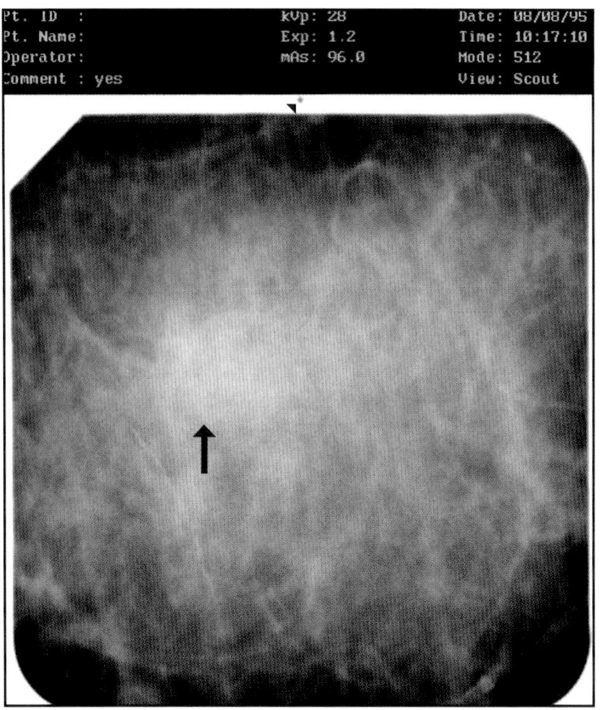

(a)

Figure 2.59 a-d. Applying Principles of Shift for Accurate Targeting. Failed aspiration of a cyst in the right breast under ultrasound in a patient post-left breast mastectomy resulted in hematoma. The aspiration was then attempted under stereotactic guidance. The scout image **(a)** demonstrates the cyst **(arrow)** to the left of the reference cursor **(arrowhead)**. On the stereos **(b)**, the right-hand image demonstrates the cyst well; *note the wide shift of the abnormality*. The wide area of density on the left stereo image makes it difficult to correctly identify the abnormality. The edge effect **(arrowheads)** seems to indicate this area to be the cyst **(arrow)**. However, the distance of shift should be the same in each stereo image, alerting the clinician that this density is not the cyst. The cyst is actually to the left of this density **(cursor)**. Figures **(c)** and **(d)** demonstrate the mammogram preaspiration **(arrow)** and post-successful aspiration.

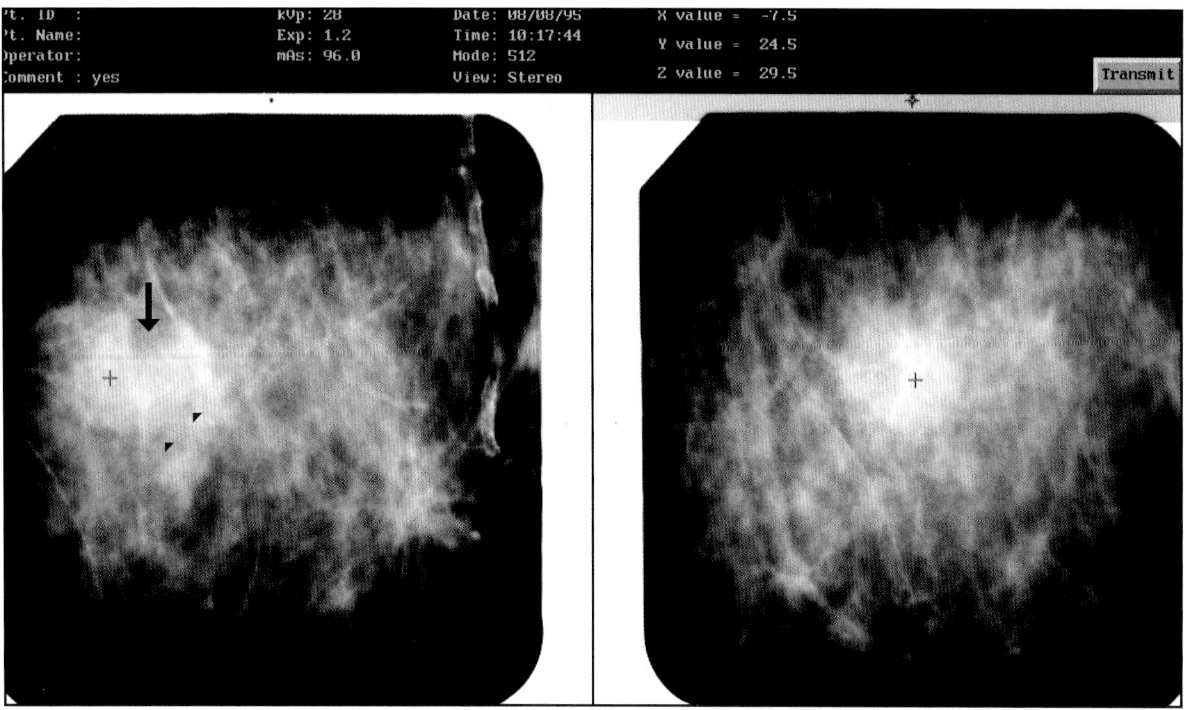

(b)

Figure 2.59 continued.

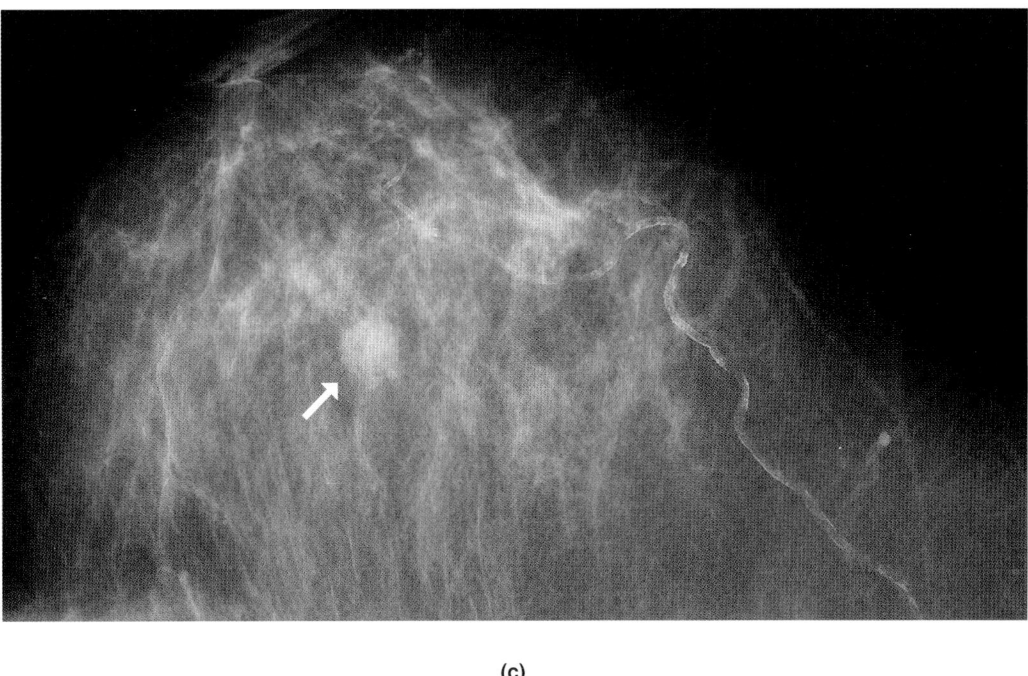

(c)

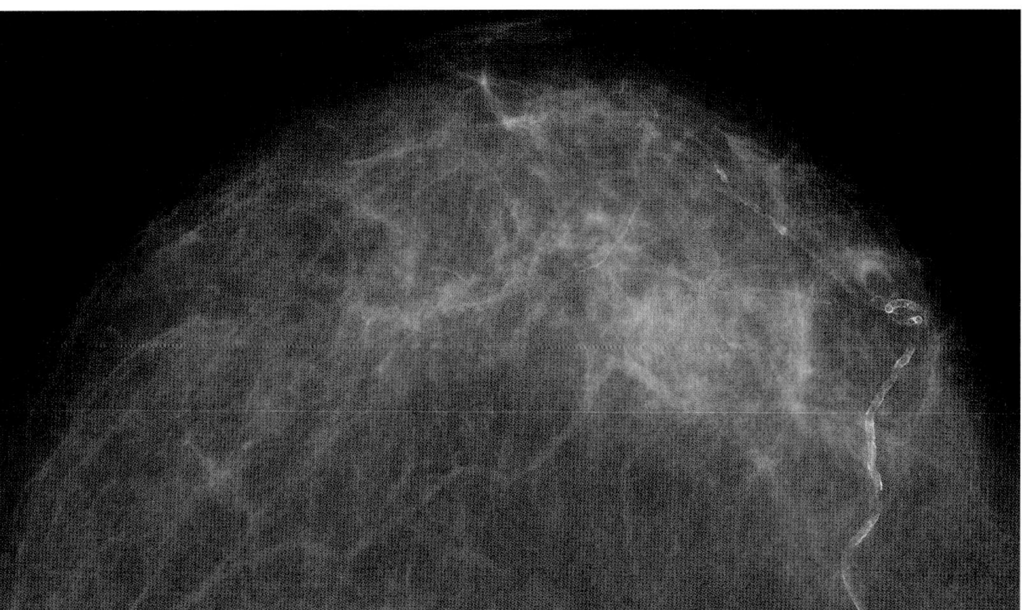

(d)

of the procedure. This will save a great deal of time and patient stress in searching for a pseudo mass that disappears on one or both stereo images.

Targeting Procedure—The manufacturer will recommend a targeting sequence to achieve accuracy. In most cases, there is a prompt for sequencing within the digitizing unit. With digital devices, the computer program maintains sequencing. When targeting the abnormality, adhere to the following specific rules:

1. *Identify the reference point(s) and indicate with a cursor.* This may be accomplished using the computer. Never attempt to complete targeting if the reference points cannot be found. This will result in faulty calculations **(Figure 2.60)**.

2. *Maintain the same vertical axis.* Between stereo projections, the abnormality will not shift in the vertical direction unless the patient moves between images. Therefore, when identifying or targeting, always remain on the same vertical axis (Y axis) from one planar image to the other **(Figure 2.61)**. When using a screen-film system, a straightedge is helpful. With digital units, a horizontal line appears on the monitor to maintain the same vertical plane.

3. *Indicate the targets on both planar images, utilizing the cursor.* If using a screen-film system, use a pen to mark the targeting point on both planar images. This will be helpful when comparing with confirmation prefire stereos, and if retargeting becomes necessary.

Targeting Accuracy—There are a number of methods to ensure safe, effective biopsy and to improve and check targeting accuracy.

Prior to targeting, review scout and stereo images:

1. Check the scout image for superimposed vessels that may be punctured during sampling **(Figure 2.62)**.

2. Check scout for proper centering.

3. Check both stereo images for the abnormality **(Figure 2.63)**. Recheck centering on the scout image and technical factors, if the abnormality is not visualized.

4. Check stereo images for direction of abnormality shift.

After targeting:

5. Verify that coordinates have been transmitted or transferred accurately.

6. Check the scout image for abnormality position in the biopsy window and correlate with the calculated X and Y coordinates; they should match.

7. Compare depth coordinate with mammographic information. If the depth coordinate of the abnormality is outside the expected depth, it is possible that identification of the abnormality, or targeting, was incorrect.

8. With most SBB systems, the depth coordinate should be a positive number, in which case, a negative depth coordinate would indicate an error.

If detection of an error is not possible at this point, confirmation (prefire) stereo images may allow the clinician to recognize and correct for targeting errors.

Confirmation (Prefire) Stereos

Acquire the confirmation stereo pair with the needle at the exact depth coordinate, or at the prefire position. These images will verify the accurate placement of the needle. **Figures 2.64-2.66** demonstrate possible errors. Unfortunately, there are a number of causes that can result in these same visual errors. Faulty targeting, patient or abnormality motion, and calculation errors all have the same visual appearance.

X or Y errors are readily discernible but are not measurable (due to the magnification factor) on the prefire images, and foreshortening of the needle gives a false impression of the actual position of needle depth. Rather than relying on the appearance of the stereo image, and estimating an error, use the computer or microprocessor to check for inaccuracies by targeting the needle tips. If the coordinates of the needle position do not match the original calculated coordinates (allowing for prefire placement), then an error of needle placement is most likely due to a mechanical or computer error **(Figure 2.67)**.

In some cases, the error will be in millimeters; this errant needle position is useful as an offset target. Other errors require repositioning of the needle. A correction factor can be calculated by determining the *difference* between the coordinates of the needle and the abnormality coordinates. If the needle position is accurate but an error is visible, then abnormality movement is most likely at fault **(Figure 2.68-2.70)**.

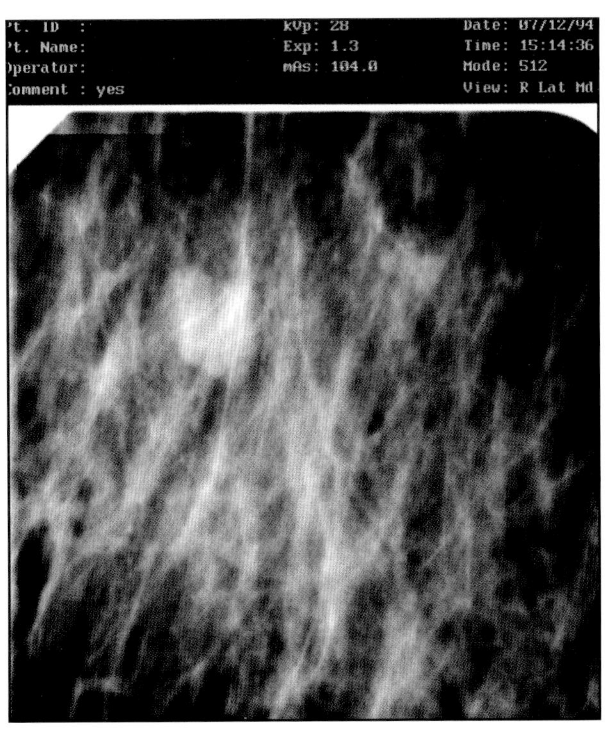

(a)

Figure 2.60 a and b. Identification of Reference Points. Reference points incorrectly marked on stereo images yield inaccurate coordinates. Comparing the position of the abnormality on the scout image to the resulting coordinate will ensure accurate targeting. In this case, the abnormality is positioned in the scout image **(a)** in the negative half of the biopsy window, at about -9 mm. The horizontal coordinate (upper right-hand corner) determined from the stereo images **(b)** yields an inaccurate -2.8 mm position. The depth coordinate also yields a negative number, another indication for this system that targeting was inaccurate. The depth coordinate will not always be negative in false reference marking, so it is best to check all coordinates.

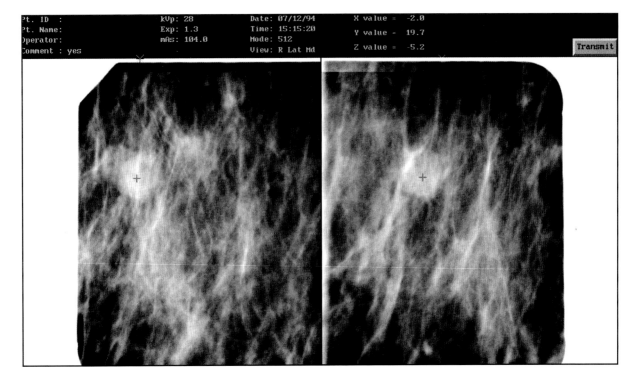

(b)

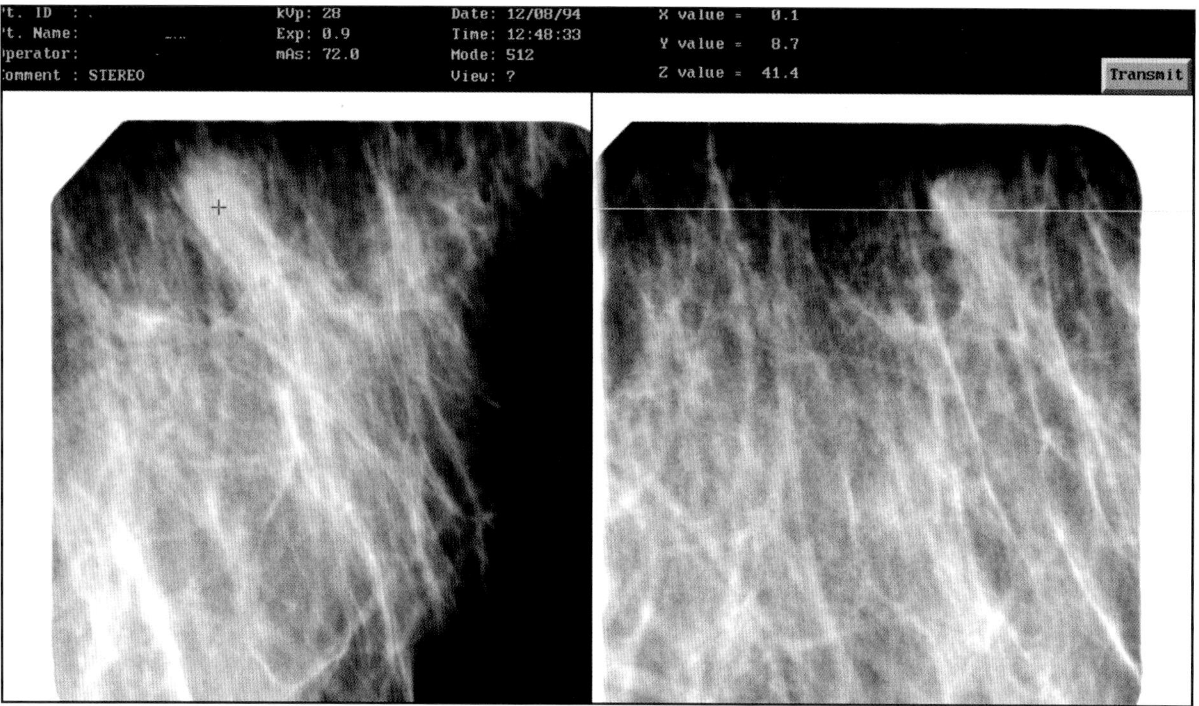

Figure 2.61. Maintaining a Vertical Axis. Unless the patient or abnormality has moved a great distance between stereo images, the abnormality will remain on the same vertical axis. With a digital unit, a hortizontal line appears on the monitor to maintain the same vertical axis.

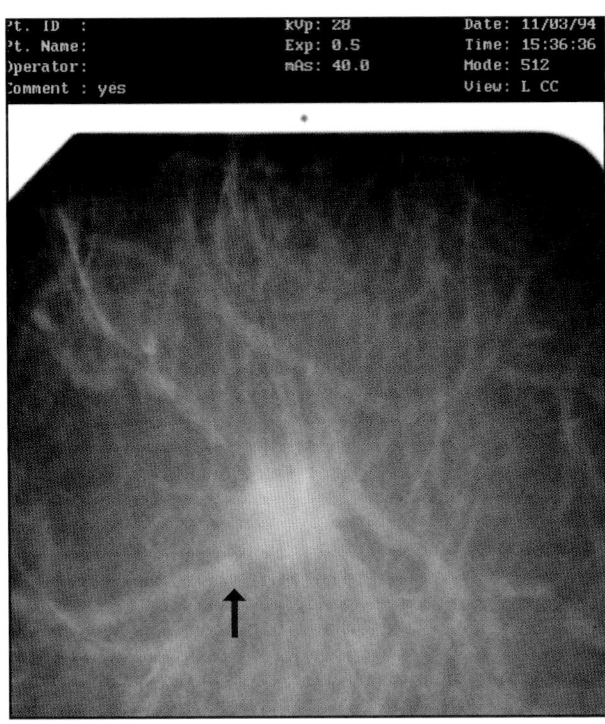

(a)

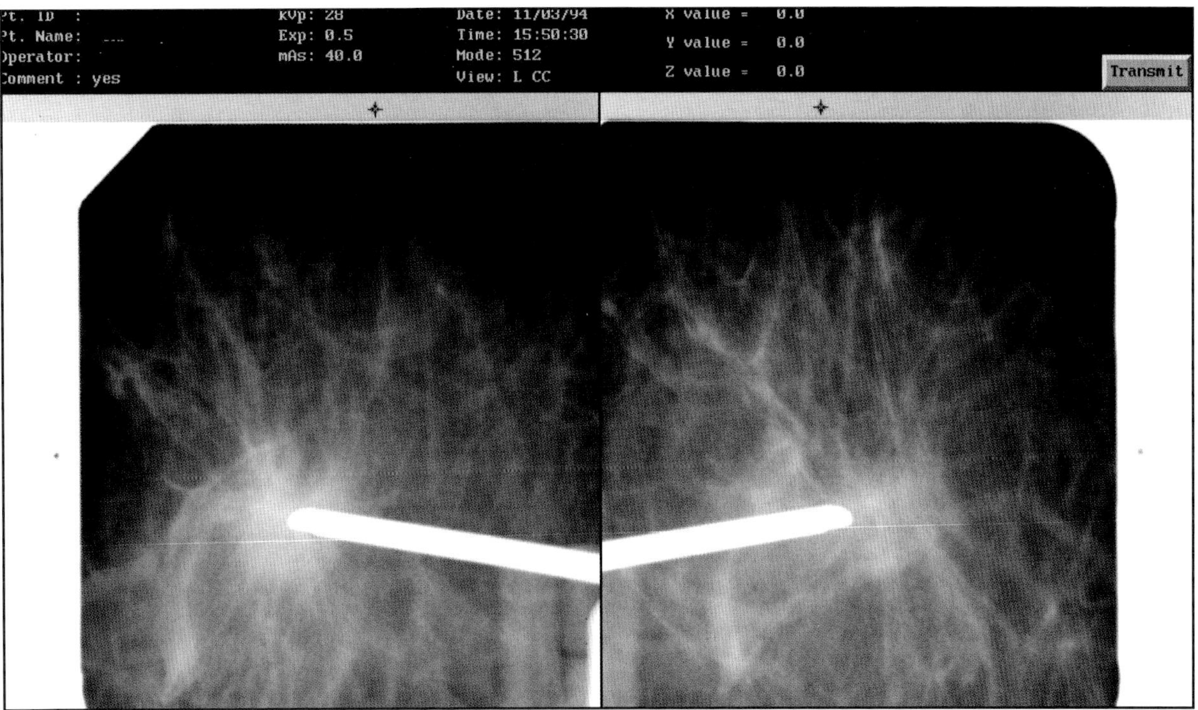

(b)

Figure 2.62 a and b. Avoiding Vessels. The scout image should be checked for overlapping blood vessels. A blood vessel **(arrow)** over the abnormality of interest on the scout image **(a)** is punctured at needle insertion causing hematoma **(b)**. This not only increases patient bleeding but also can obscure the area of interest.

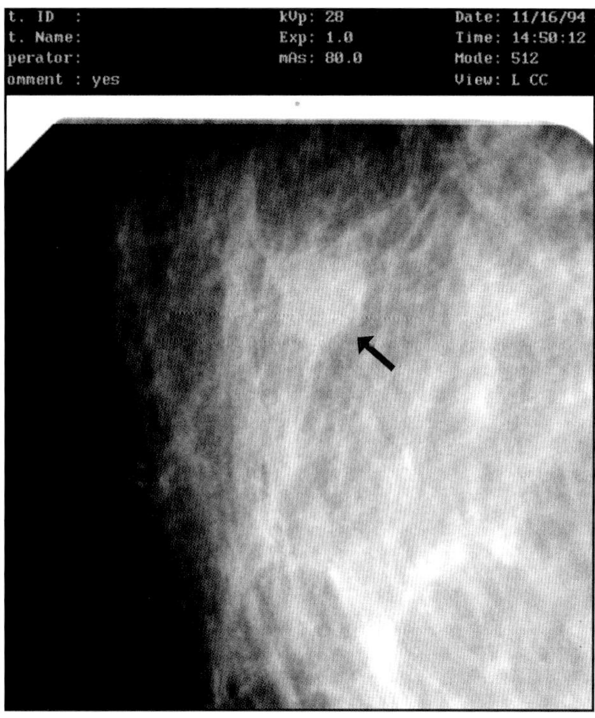

(a)

Figure 2.63 a-d. Checking Both Stereo Images for Abnormality Visualization. A low-density abnormality well-visualized on the scout image **(a) (arrow)** can only be seen on one side of the stereo pair **(b) (arrow)**. Repositioning and rescouting **(c) (arrow)** allows visualization on both stereo images **(d) (cursors)**.

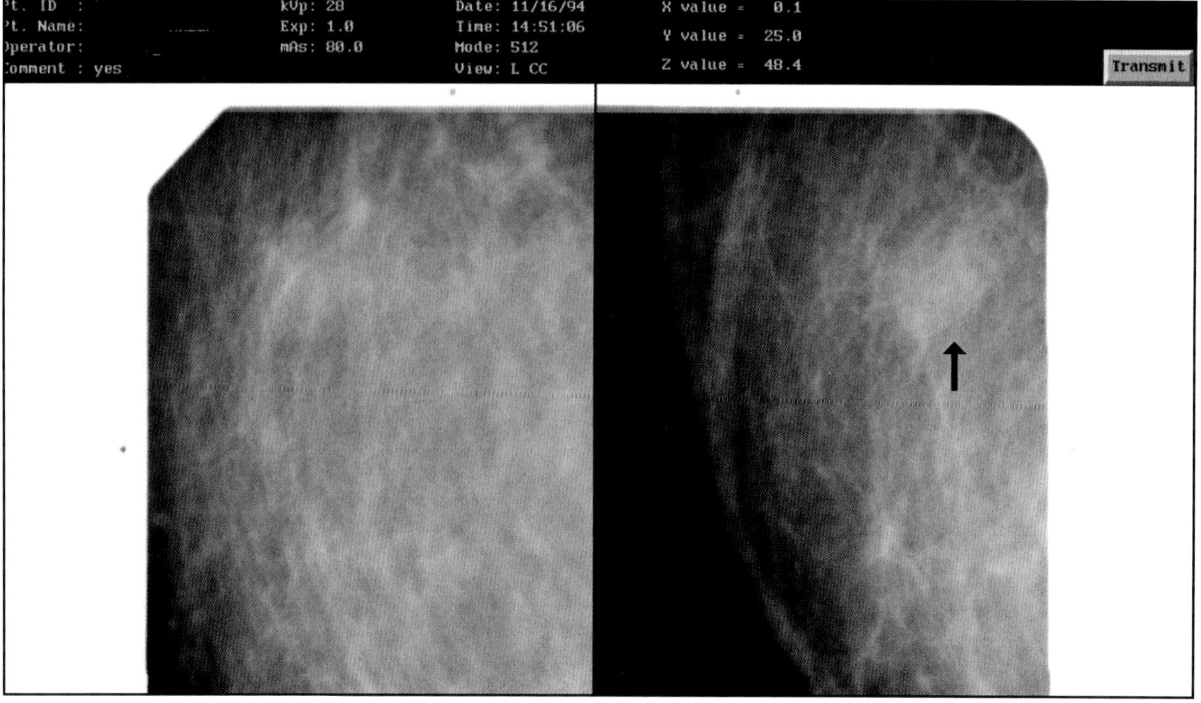

(b)

Figure 2.63 continued.

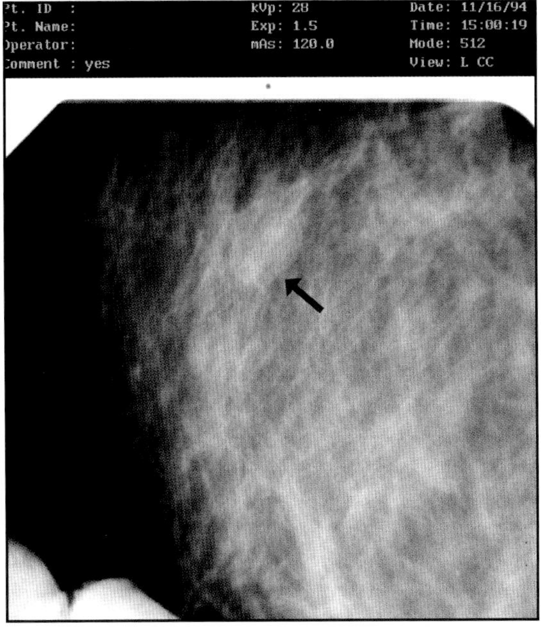

(c)

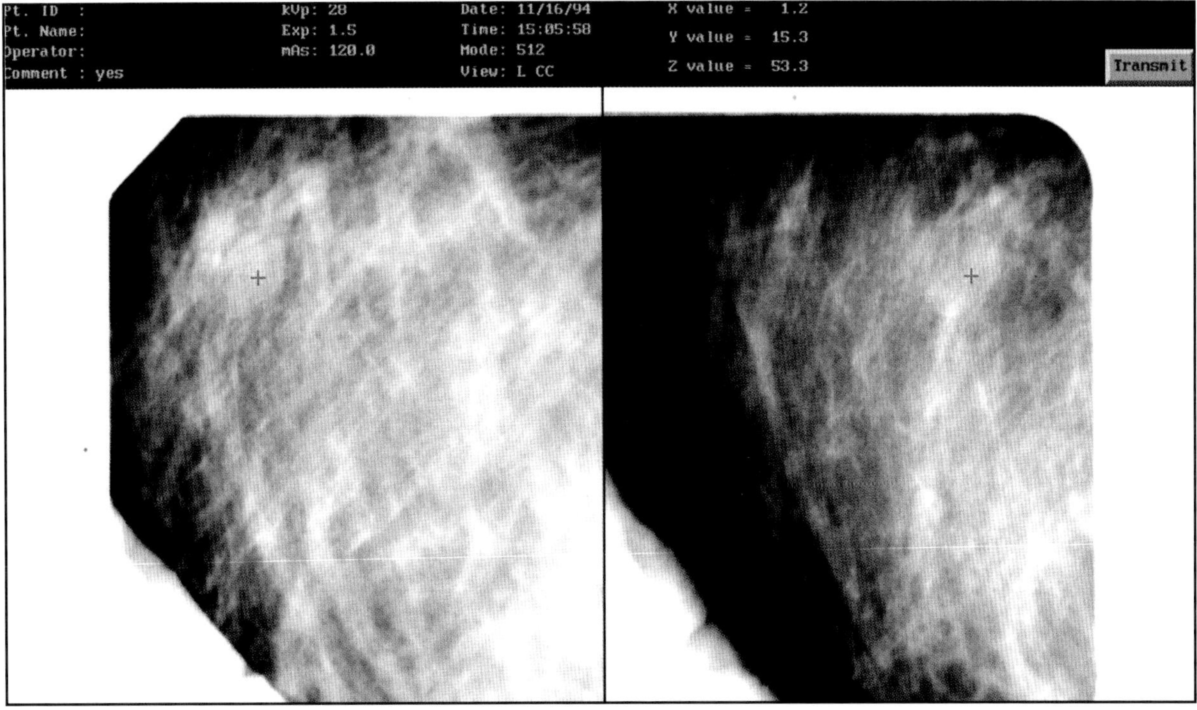

(d)

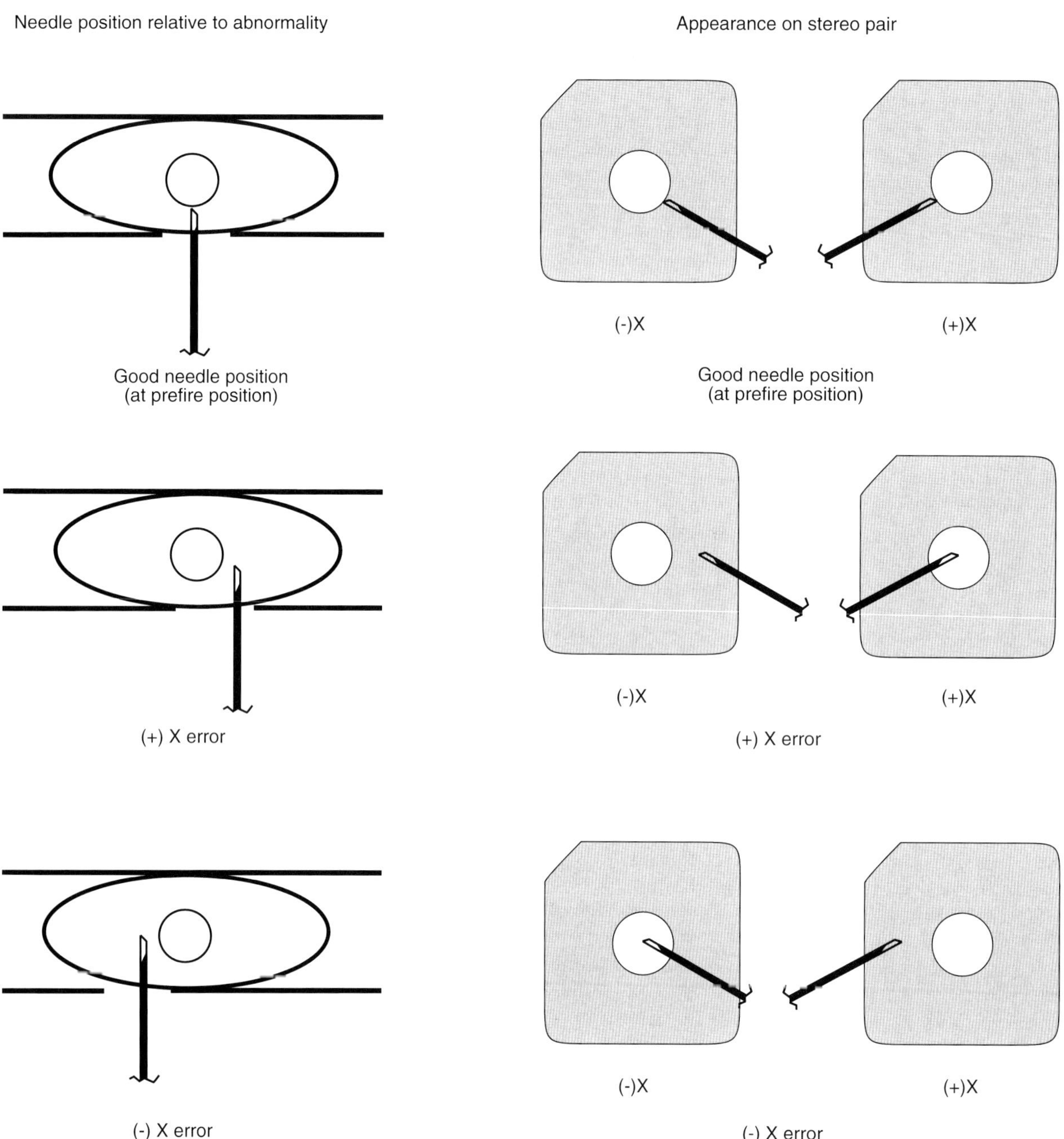

Figure 2.64. Examples of Horizontal Errors.

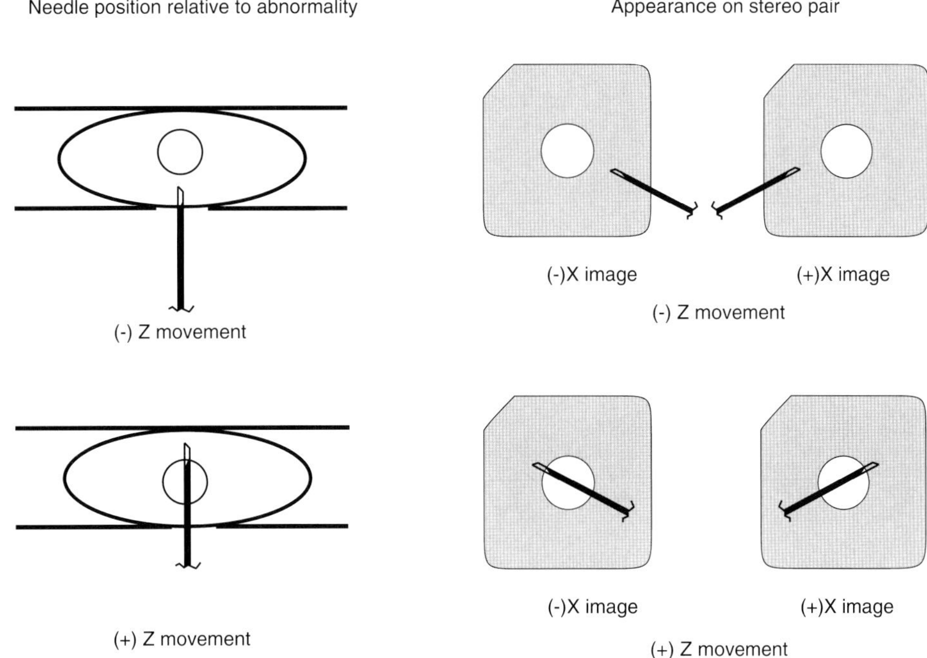

Figure 2.65. Examples of Depth Errors.

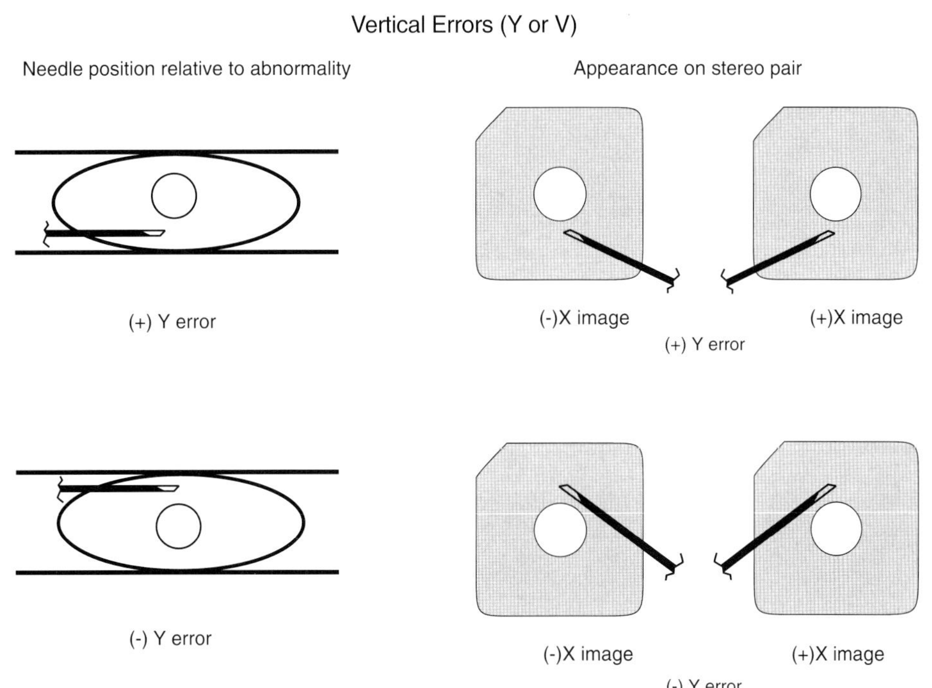

Figure 2.66. Examples of Vertical Errors.

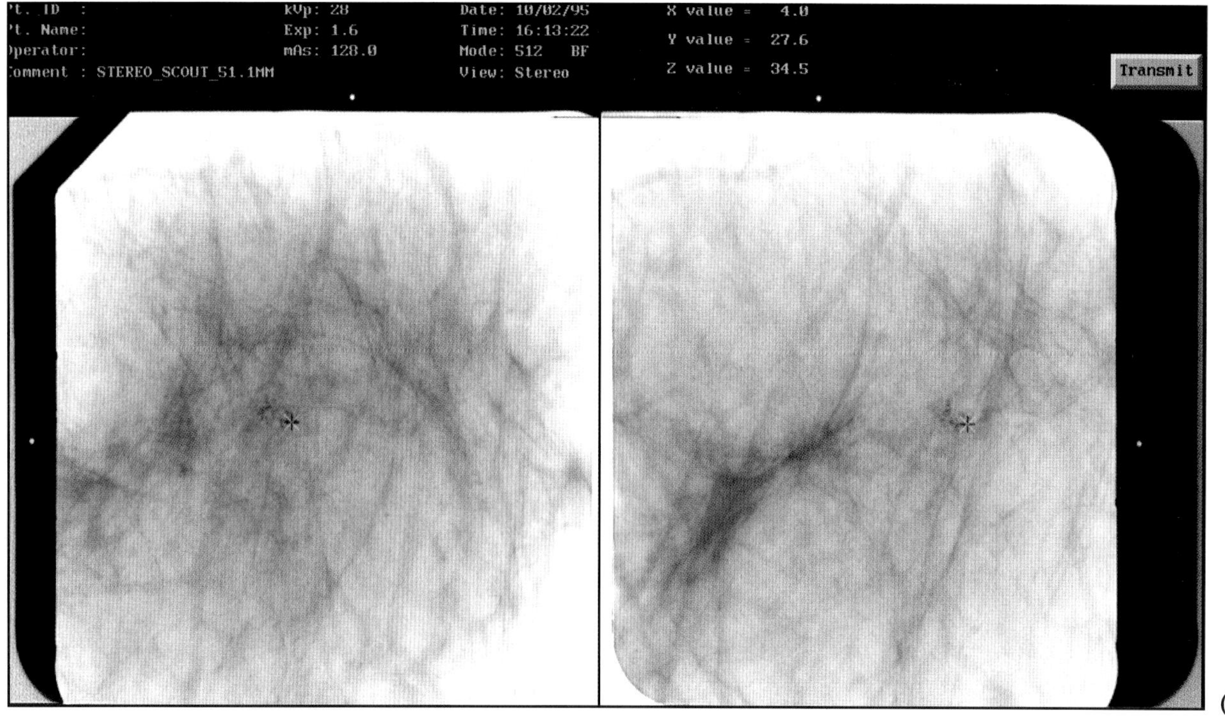

(a)

Figure 2.67 a and b. Inaccurate Needle Placement. The stereo images **(a)** yield coordinates as shown (upper right-hand corner). Confirmation stereos **(b)** demonstrate a horizontal error. Targeting over the needle tips **(cursor)** indicates the needle guidance system is inaccurate (upper right-hand corner). The biopsy/compression plate was not placed correctly. A correction factor was determined and sampling completed.

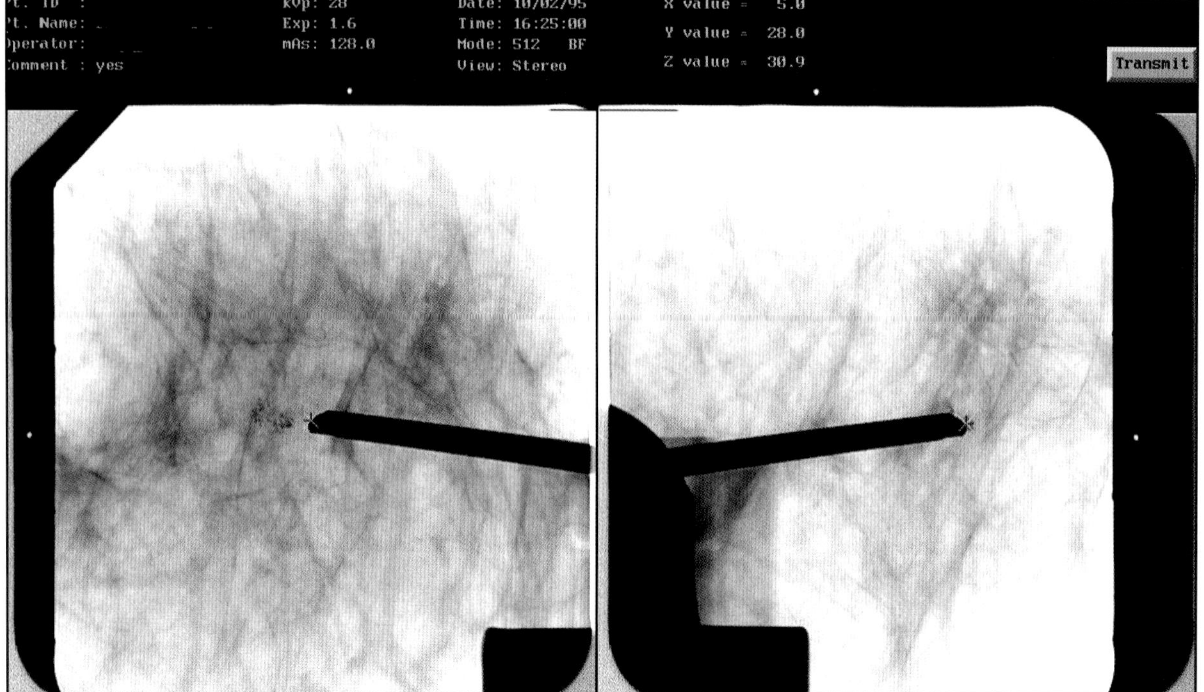

(b)

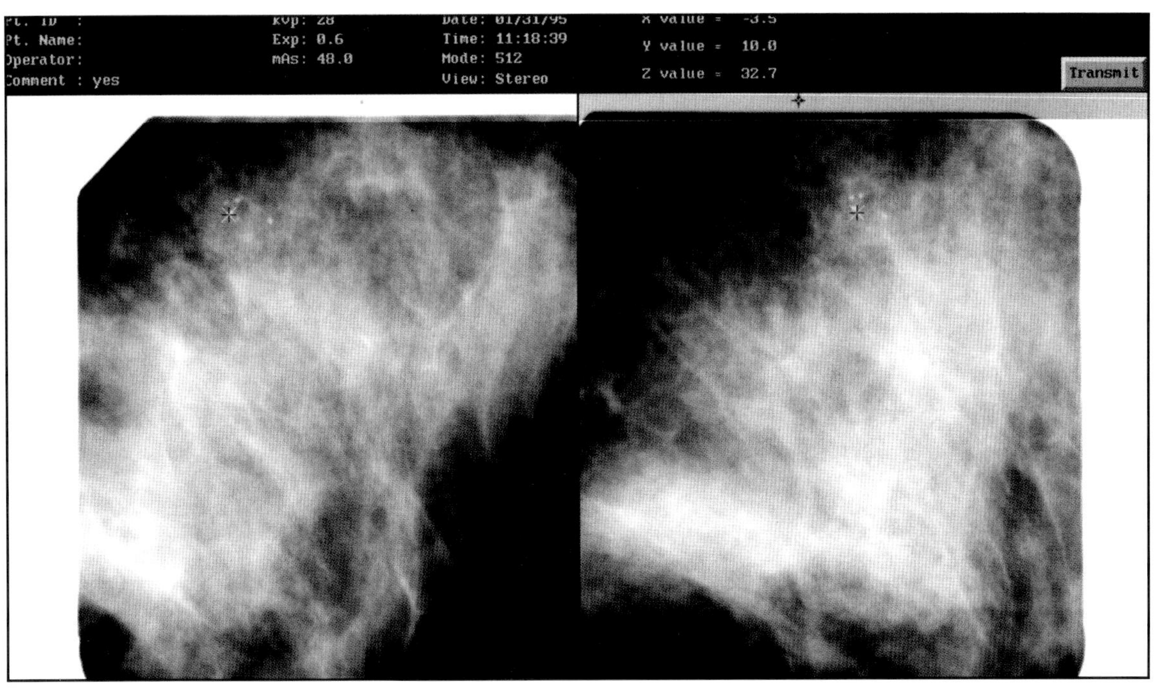

(a)

Figure 2.68 a and b. Abnormality Movement. The stereo images **(a)** yield coordinates as indicated (upper right-hand corner). Confirmation stereos **(b)** demonstrate a vertical error. After targeting the needle position (allowing for a -5 mm prefire position), needle placement is accurate as indicated by the first set of coordinates (upper right-hand corner), when compared with the original determined coordinates (a). The abnormality has moved. Because the abnormality is well-seen on these stereos, retargeting was performed, as indicated by the second set of coordinates.

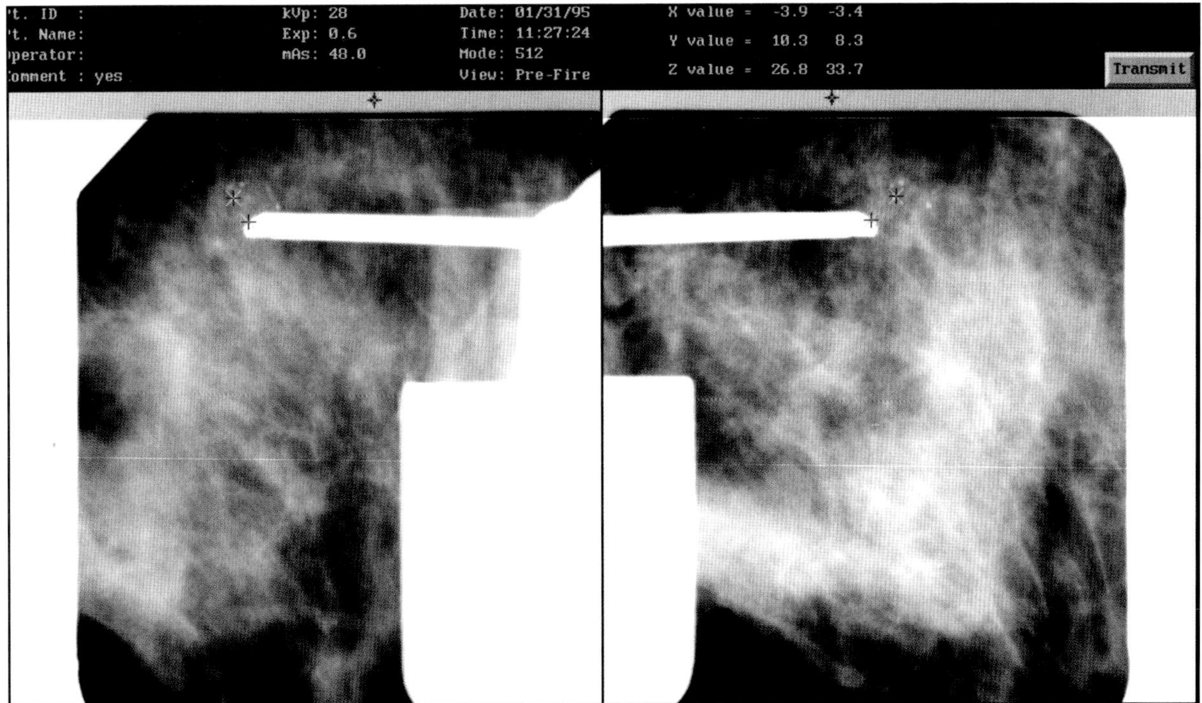

(b)

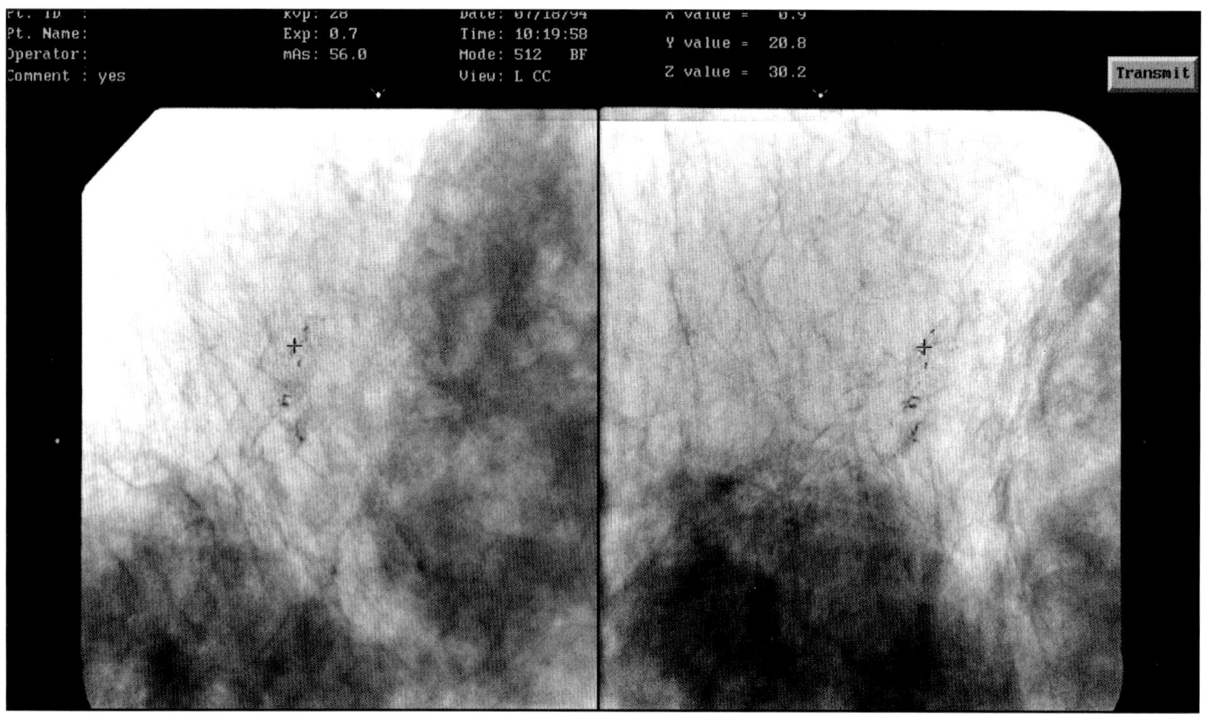

(a)

Figure 2.69 a and b. Abnormality Movement. Stereo images **(a)** demonstrate abnormality coordinates (upper right-hand corner). Confirmation stereos **(b)** indicate a horizontal error. Targeting of the needle indicates accurate placement (upper right-hand corner).The abnormality has moved. The stereos were repeated after removal of the needle and new coordinates were obtained.

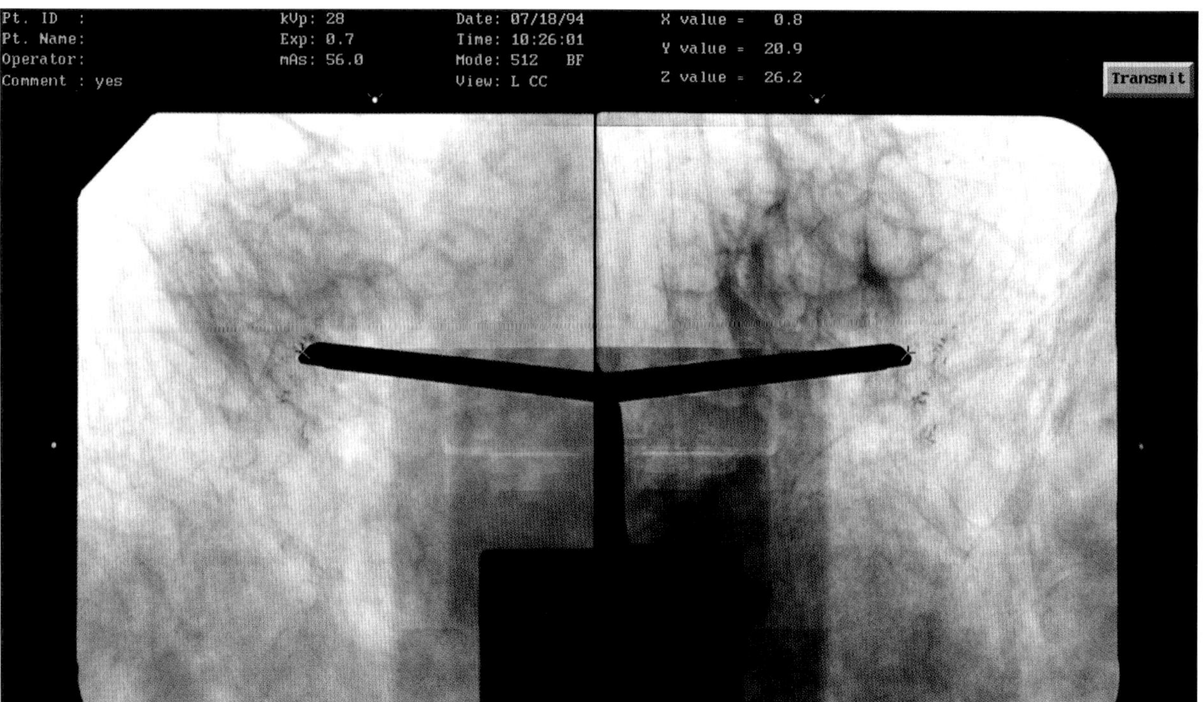

(b)

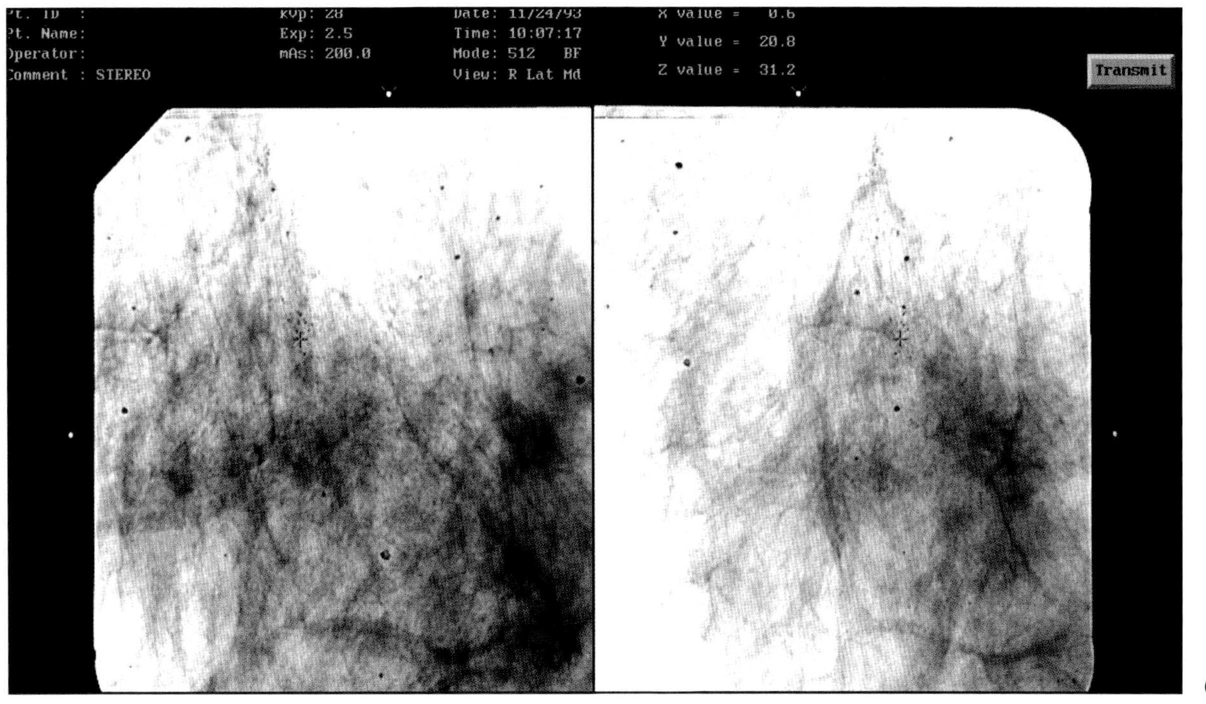

Figure 2.70 a and b. Abnormality Movement. Stereo images **(a)** demonstrate abnormality coordinates (upper right-hand corner). Confirmation images **(b)** demonstrate horizontal and vertical errors. Retargeting of the abnormality yields new coordinates (upper right-hand corner), substantiating that these errors are due to abnormality movement.

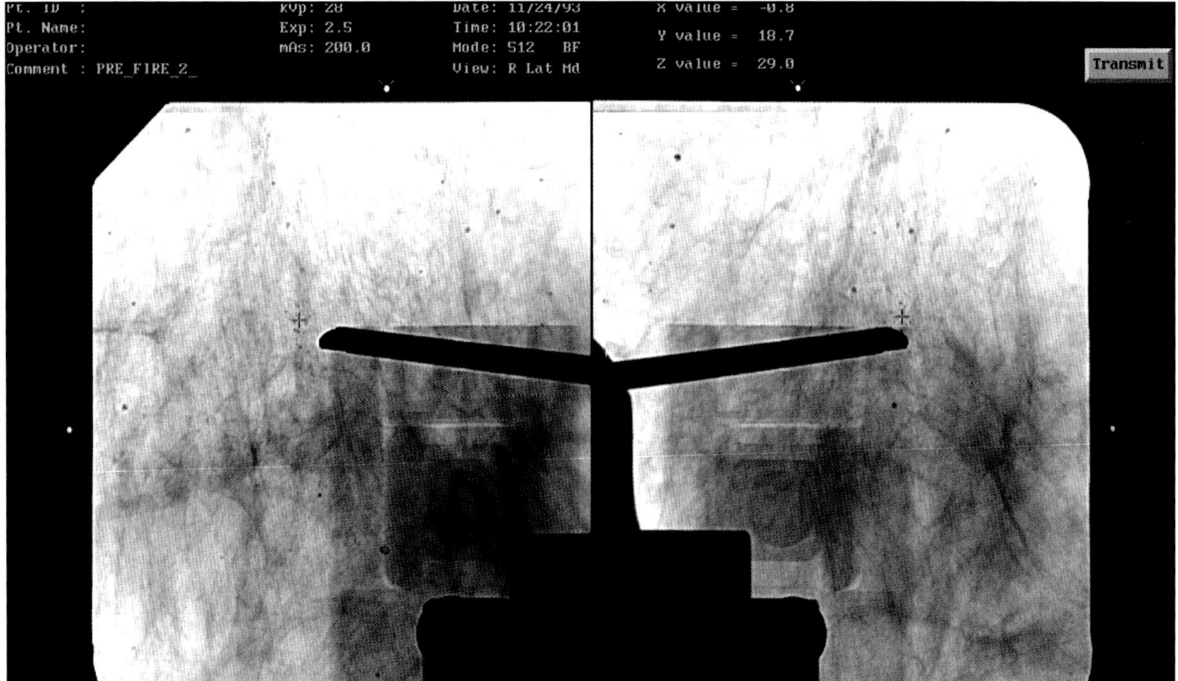

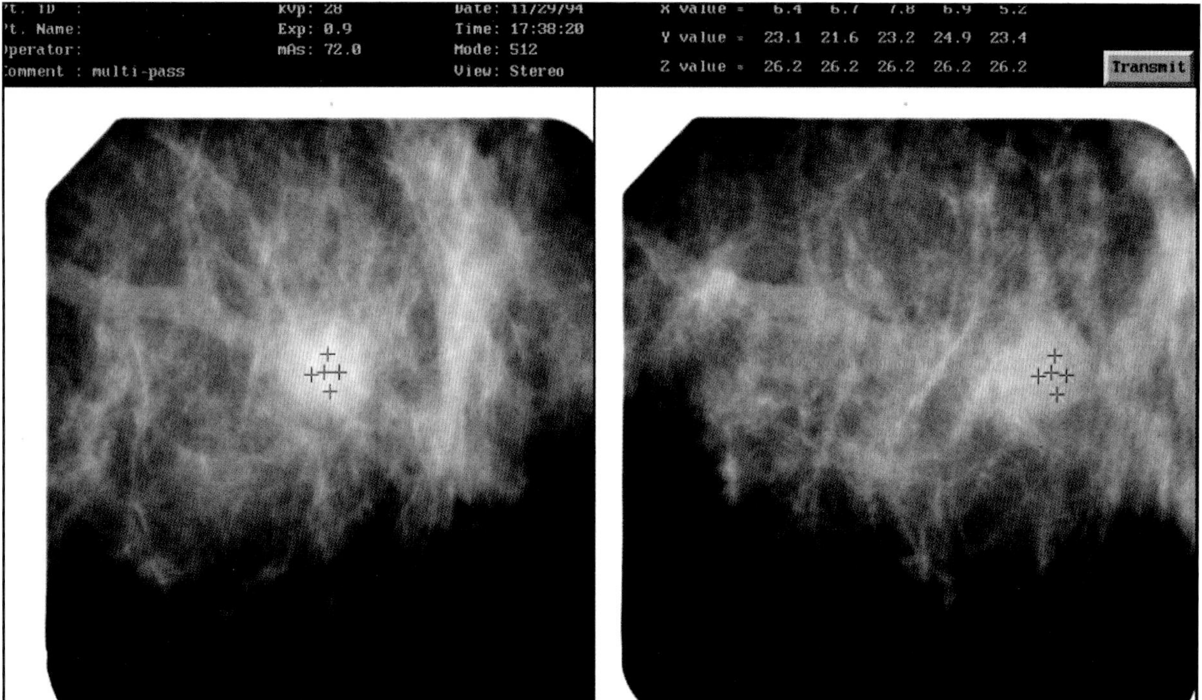

Figure 2.71. Multple Passes. The clinician indicates on one side of the stereo image multiple vertical and horizontal positions for multiple sampling, maintaining the same depth coordinate as indicated in the upper right-hand corner of this stereo image.

Less common, but possible, is errant targeting of the abnormality. Again, this needle position may be useful as an offset target. If the abnormality is visible on both the prefire stereo images, then retargeting is possible to determine the abnormality's new location. If the abnormality is not visible on one or both images (sometimes the needle obscures the abnormality), then it is necessary to repeat the stereo pair after removal of the needle. Retargeting will give the new location of the abnormality. A new set of confirmation stereos will confirm needle placement. Chapter 3 provides realistic methods to contend with targeting issues.

Multiple Sampling

There are various methods for subsequent sampling. The clinician can choose multiple passes simply by varying the horizontal and vertical position of the needle from the original target coordinates, based on the size of the abnormality. A digital SBB system will allow identification of the "offsets." Because the depth coordinate remains the same, these points are indicated on one side of the stereo image, yielding new X and Y coordinates (**Figure 2.71**). In a polar coordinate system, indicating new X and Y offsets will also yield new depth coordinates. However, this is to compensate for the needle arc when changing vertical or horizontal placement, and should not be perceived as giving multiple depths. Various depth coordinates can only be determined by targeting a unique point on both planar images. This is known as a *multitarget* option, and should be used only in those cases where the clinician can choose the same unique point on both stereo images (**Figure 2.72**). Multitargeting is especially useful for calcifications that may be at different depth planes.

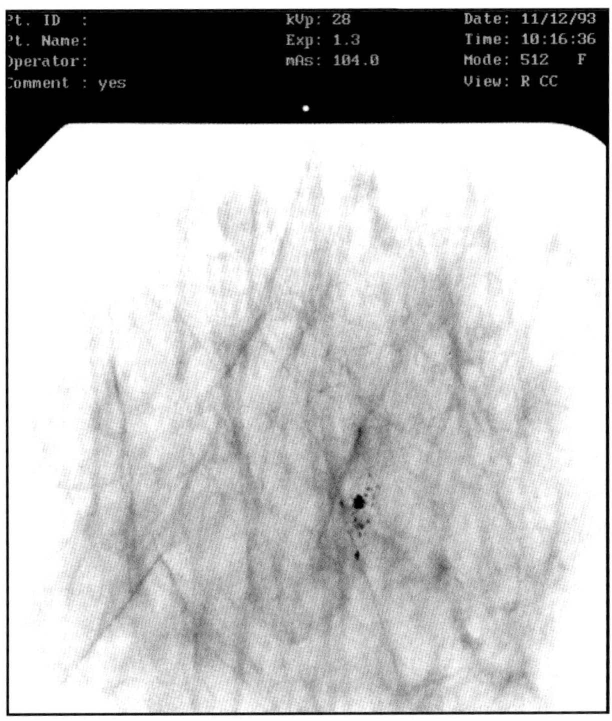

(a)

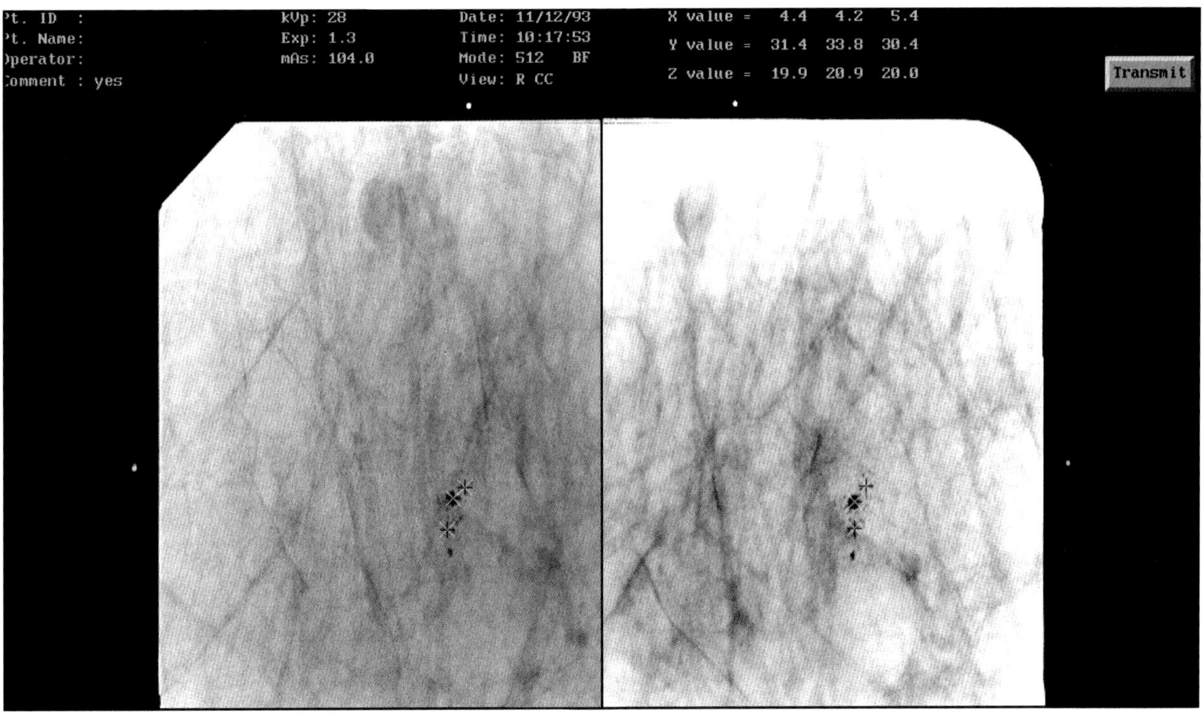

(b)

Figure 2.72 a and b. Multitargeting. Multitargeting is useful for calcifications that may be at different depths. The scout image **(a)** demonstrates calcifications. The clinician can vary horizontal, vertical, and depth coordinates of multiple samples. This can be accomplished by targeting on a unique calcification on both stereo images **(b),** yielding new coordinates.

References

1. Dowlatshahi, D., Yaremko, M.L., Kluskens, L.F., Jokich, P.M. 1991. Non-Palpable Breast Lesions: Findings of Stereotaxic Needle-Core Biopsy and Fine Needle Aspiration Cytology. *Radiology* 181:745-750.

2. Parker, S.H., Lovin, J.D., Jobe, W.E., Luethke, J.M., Hopper, K.D., Yakes, W.F., Burke, B.J. 1990. Stereotactic Breast Biopsy with a Biopsy Gun. *Radiology* 176 (September) (3):741-7.

3. Parker, S.H. and Jobe, W.E. 1993. *Percutaneous Breast Biopsy* New York: Raven Press.

4. Hendrick, R.E. and Parker, S.H. 1994. Stereotaxic Imaging, In Syllabus: A Categorical Course in Physics, Technical Aspects of Breast Imaging. Radiological Society of North America Publications.

Problems and Pitfalls in Core Biopsy

Paul R. Fisher, M.D.

3

Clinicians learn to perform procedures, such as stereotactic breast biopsies, by first understanding the underlying principles (such as those outlined in this text), then through actual clinical experience. Certainly, expertise cannot be claimed in any procedure until lessons from real world successes, and failures, are incorporated into procedural methodologies. This section presents some of the pitfalls the clinician may encounter while performing stereotactic biopsies. While it is expected that novices will be less confident and a little slower in the beginning, it is hoped that the experiential learning curve will be much shortened, so that users may more rapidly achieve a high level of proficiency. Early clinical successes may also help convince skeptical clinicians of the utility and reliability of the procedure, and may partially disarm possible detractors from stereotactic core biopsy.

General Errors

General errors are those that are common to many other radiologic procedures, such as mislabeled images, loss of power during a procedure, lost reports, etc. This chapter will deal only with those pitfalls specifically related to stereotactic breast biopsy.

Classes and Types of Errors

There are five *classes or categories* of errors that clinicians will encounter for this procedure: patient selection errors, stereotactic errors, sampling errors, insufficient errors, and analysis errors. Within each classification, errors are further divided into three types. This chapter explains how easily most errors can be avoided.

Some errors merely require awareness and attention to detail, referred to as a *Type I error*. A *Type II error* is a tradeoff pitfall, for which the clinician can arbitrarily reduce its likelihood, but at some cost in money, time, or diagonistic yield. A *Type III error* is essentially unavoidable.

Clinicians should monitor for each of these error types before and during the procedure. If a serious error is detected, the confidence in the results must be lowered. This does not mean, however, that the procedure must be halted, or its results ignored. As explained in the section on analysis errors, false positive pathology results are rare because the core biopsy sample offers the pathologist the same histologic information as obtained from an open biopsy. Thus, positive results can be relied upon even when obtained during a substandard biopsy. Of course, we should not trust negative biopsy results obtained by such problematic cases. Furthermore, we usually have the option of subsequent open surgical biopsy to rely upon in these cases.

Patient Selection Errors

Not all patients with nonpalpable breast abnormalities are good candidates for stereotactic biopsy. Thus, many problems can be avoided by properly selecting patients. This is especially true when first learning this procedure.

Weight

Some patients are too large to be accommodated on the stereo table. Therefore, patient weight and the weight limit of each unit is an important consideration. (Type I)

Compressed Thickness of the Breast

The breast must be thick enough when compressed to allow

the full throw of the gun. For a typical 23-mm throw gun, the breast should measure at least 42 mm. (Type I) Some abnormalities in smaller breasts can be biopsied using a shorter throw gun. However, the yield from such guns is often scanty, increasing the chances for a nondiagnostic result. (Type II)

Always be aware of the stroke margin, and know the particular alarm for the unit in use for negative stroke margins. The alarm indicates a needle position so deep that the needle will approach or pass through the far side of the breast after firing. For example, the stroke margin alarm at one site was changed from a continuous beep to a short series of beeps during an upgrade, without informing some of the mammographers. This led to confusion and could have resulted in perforation of the distal breast skin surface, or damage to the x-ray detector.

Superficial Abnormalities

Abnormalities just under the skin may pose technical problems. For example, the tip of the needle should be optimally placed 5 mm before the center of the abnormality, but the cutting edge of the outer cannula should be through the skin nick before firing. There are a number of techniques that can be tried in these cases (see the section entitled *Cutting Edge at/or Proximal to Dermis* later in this chapter). Some abnormalities are so superficial that they may be best referred to surgical biopsy. If an abnormality is truly centered in the skin, it is usually benign and palpable. (Type II)

Diffuse Abnormalities

Accurate three-dimensional localization is possible only when an abnormality can be identified on *both* stereo images. A vague asymmetric density **(Figure 3.1 a and b)**, or a large group of indistinguishable calcifications, cannot reliably generate useful coordinates, even if the abnormalities are fairly large. For example, in one case, a stereotactic biopsy was performed on a patient with very suspicious calcifications over an entire quadrant of her breast. Despite 9 passes, no diagnostic calcifications were found in the specimens, and pathologic review indicated severe ductal atypia. A subsequent open biopsy revealed comedocarcinoma, consistent with the radiographic diagnosis. In retrospect, the localization was hampered because no individual calcification or tight cluster could be identified on the stereo pair. (Type I)

Patient Cooperation

Patient motion can invalidate localization data, especially if the motion occurs in the time interval between the localization stereo pair and needle placement. This motion may be gross, as in breast retraction following a cough, or may be subtle and go unnoticed unless the technologist and clinician carefully watch the patient and her breast position (see the section entitled *Stereotactic Errors* later in this chapter).

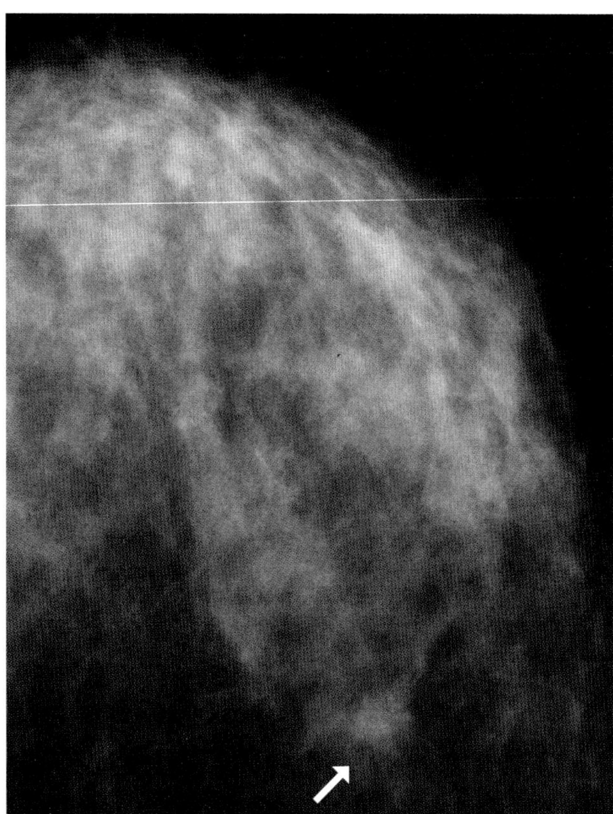

Figure 3.1a. Diffuse Abnormalities. A vague region of asymmetric density and mild distortion **(arrow)** was seen on the diagnostic work-up images .

When reviewing patients for this procedure, remember that their cooperation will be important to achieve reliable results. Women who cannot remain prone for the duration of the procedure (20-40 minutes) are not good candidates. This includes people with heart failure, arthritis, or extreme emotional liability or psychosis. To achieve true informed consent, patients must be capable of understanding the procedure. Thus, cognitively impaired patients are not typically good candidates. Even if consent is obtained from their guardians, we cannot expect a patient to help us perform this (or any) procedure if she does not understand why it is being performed. (Type I) Some patients may seem to be good candidates, but for any number of reasons are unable to cooperate at the time of biopsy. (Type III)

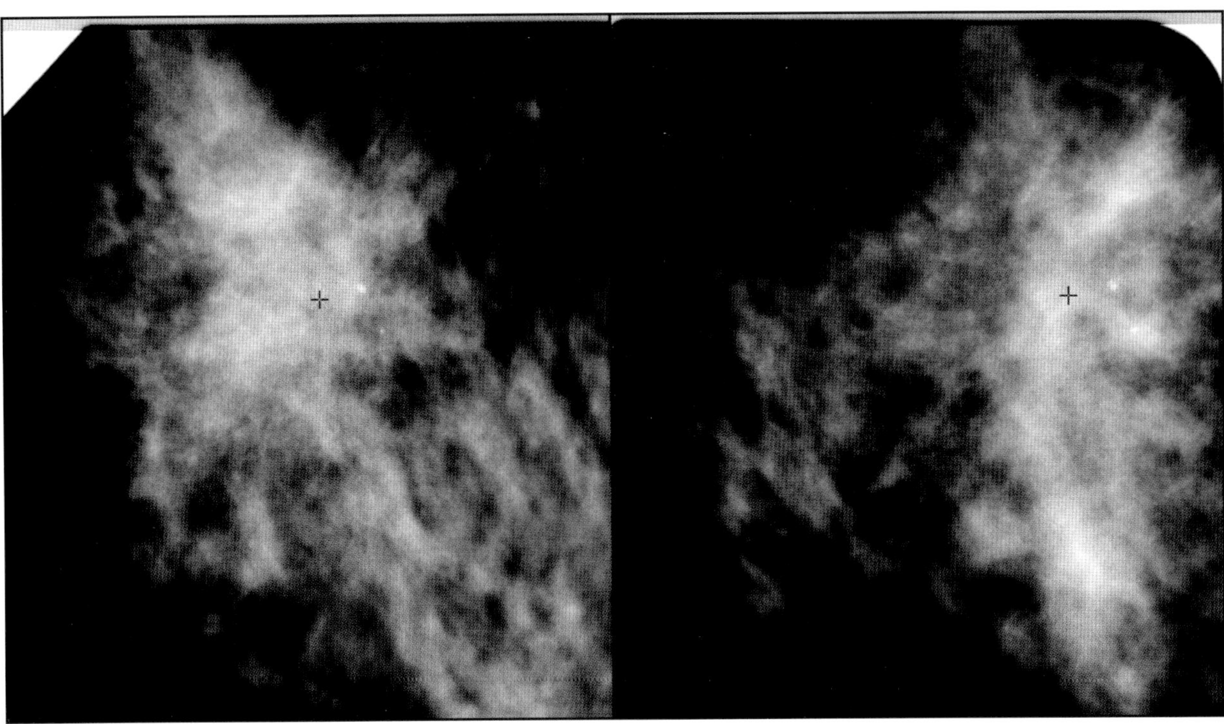

Figure 3.1b. Diffuse Abnormalities. The abnormality was difficult to perceive in the digital images. The core biopsy was read as negative, and subsequent open biopsy showed a small focus of lobular carcinoma in situ (probably an incidental finding).

Patient Expectations

Some patients have unrealistic expectations for procedures such as stereotactic biopsies. They may feel that a benign result from a core biopsy is the definitive last word, which is clearly not the case. Or, conversely, they may feel that any margin of error is intolerable, and would only trust the "gold standard" of surgery. Honest and supportive discussion about the procedure may help allay some patients' fears. However, clinicians should be careful not to be too strong an advocate for the procedure, even if in their judgment the procedure would be of great benefit to the patient. *The patient must feel that she has come to her own conclusion*, or she may blame the physician personally for a less than perfect outcome. Reassuring patients that open surgical biopsies can be easily done following a core procedure, if needed or desired, helps many patients accept the relatively low false negative biopsy rate for cores. Patients with true misgivings about the procedure should be encouraged to seek surgical consultation, and their feelings should be respected and validated. (Type I)

Practice Variations

Often, the clinician performing a stereotactic biopsy does not perform the mammographic screening or work-up exams. Consequently, the clinician may, upon review of the case, disagree with the decision to biopsy, or with the type of biopsy selected. This situation also occurs for other breast procedures, such as needle localization for open biopsy. The desire to "correct" the recommendation must be carefully balanced with the anxiety of the patient, which would naturally be heightened as a result of contradictory advice from her imaging consultants. The level of expertise of both the first and second reader should be taken into consideration.

Many, if not all, of these situations can be avoided if there is supportive and effective communication among the diagnostic team. An established policy to review as a group all requests for procedures, or to have them all reviewed by one member of the group, can reduce conflicts. Such cases could be divided into "judgment calls" or "mistakes." For those cases involving merely a difference in clinical judgment, mammographers can proceed with a biopsy or needle localization. On the other hand, if the mammographer perceives a new mammographic feature (or discovers a previously unknown part of the patient's history), the clinician may consider acting on his or her own judgment. In this case, the mammographer assumes that the first clinician would most likely revise his or her initial opinion when they share the new observation. For example, several biopsies have been canceled as a result of detecting milk-of-calcium menisci characterizing a cluster of calcifications. (Type I)

Stereotactic Errors

A number of pitfalls exist that can lead to inaccurate three-dimensional localization. Many of these errors may be detected upon reviewing the pre- or postfire stereo pair. If the clinician can determine a specific cause for the error, correction is possible. If the needle is near the abnormality, take an offset core sample (also referred to as multiple sampling). Offset cores are needed for the periphery of abnormalities to reduce sampling error. Taking cores while adjusting coordinates to hit the center of an abnormality increases efficiency.

Never trust the position coordinates without doing a "reality check." Make sure the abnormality is in the upper, medial corner of the scout image, as indicated in the calculated coordinates. This review is more straightforward with Cartesian positioning systems than with polar coordinates, but is possible with either system. If there is a significant discrepancy between the coordinates and the prediction, try calculating the position again, or repeat the localization stereo pair. The depth of the abnormality should be no more than *half* the actual compressed width of the breast (not including the thickness of the compression plate), if the shortest path to the abnormality has been properly chosen. For this reason, *do not accept Z dimensions greater than half the total compression width.*

Also, when localizing multiple targets, such as distinct calcifications, check the Z coordinates to make sure that the calcifications are truly a single cluster, and not just artifactually projecting over the same region **(Figures 3.2 a and b)**.

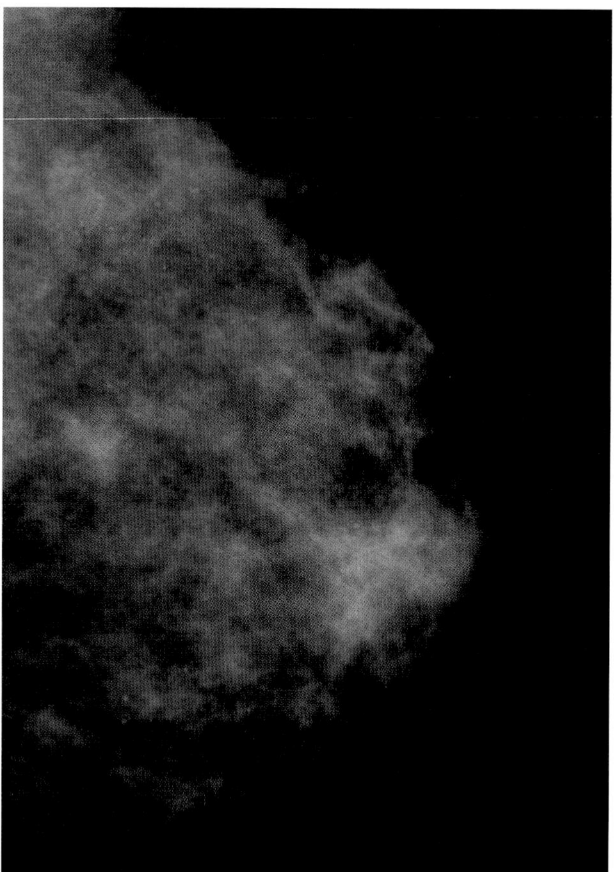

Figure 3.2 a. Multiple Targets. A relatively small breast with innumerable calcifications.

Improper Calibration

The calibration of the stereotactic unit must be checked regularly, usually before each case. Individual needles may vary in length, and the needle holders may have been misaligned during the previous procedure. Calibration is not merely an exercise. During one difficult case, some torque was inadvertently applied to the distal needle support. It was not realized until later that the needle tip moved up toward the table as the support arm was slid out to the skin surface, indicating that the arm had slipped slightly down as a result. To compensate during that procedure, the coordinates were adjusted down a few millimeters, and the unit was later realigned by a service call. Again, these real-time adjustments are more easily performed with Cartesian positioning systems. (Type I)

The biopsy gun must be properly seated in its holder on the unit, or the needle will not reach the Z value **(Figures 3.3 a and b)**. Always check that the gun has been slid against the stop at the patient end of the gun holder. Quickly check the depth of the needle by targeting over the needle tip on the prefire stereo pair. (Type I)

Patient Motion

The localization procedure assumes that the patient (and the abnormality) have not moved between the localization stereo pair and the subsequent needle placement. Involuntary

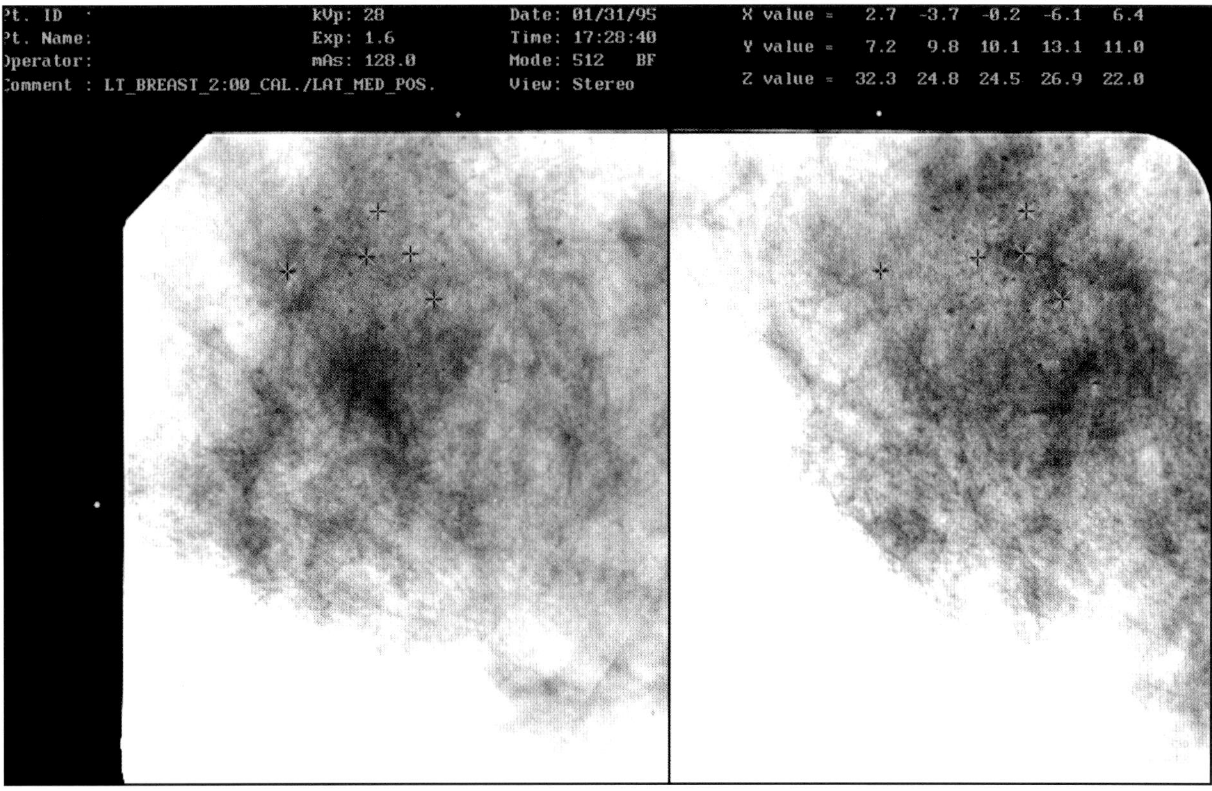

Figure 3.2b. Multiple Targets. When individual calcifications were localized, a wide range of Z values were determined, indicating a widely scattered distribution. The calcifications were seen on the specimen images, and proved beign at pathology in the setting of fibrocystic changes.

movements, such as coughs, tremors, or laughs may shift the position of the breast, even though it is fixed to some extent by compression. If gross motion is noticed, repeat the localization procedure, after trying to reduce the likelihood of additional movement. Because subtle displacement may be hard to detect, *place a small localization dot in one corner of the biopsy field.* Small displacements would then be easily seen as the dot moves away from the corner, or is hidden behind the paddle. The dot also allows quick repositioning if necessary. Although most clinicians do not think it is necessary to premedicate patients to reduce anxiety and resultant motion, premedication is used in a few centers with reportedly good results.

Mammographers have less motion problems if they perform the procedure as quickly and safely as possible. Prepare for needle placement before the localization stereo pair, with the syringe for local anesthesia, povidone-iodine solution and alcohol, and biopsy needle ready to use, so that the needle may be positioned as quickly as possible. Have an assistant operate the stereo computer unit under the clinician's supervision, so that he or she can remain in sterile gloves and quickly use the derived coordinates. With practice, the mammographer should be able to reduce the time between the localization stereo pair and the prefire stereo pair to 60 seconds for a digital imaging unit. (Type I)

Abnormality Motion from Anesthesia

Parker described a case in which an abnormality was displaced by the installation of local anesthetic immediately adjacent to the target abnormality, deep along the biopsy needle tract[1]. It was felt initially that such deep installation would reduce the discomfort of the procedure, especially with the introduction of the larger 14-gauge core needles. However, 14-gauge needles are usually well-tolerated without such a deep installation. There is a variable amount of discomfort reported by patients, often varying from sample to sample, but is usually described as minor or very brief. In addition to possibly displacing abnormalities, deep anesthetic may mask abnormalities by silhouetting their borders, as a pneumonia may silhouette the diaphragm. We recommend the use of subcutaneous local anesthesia only, for most core biopsies. (Type I)

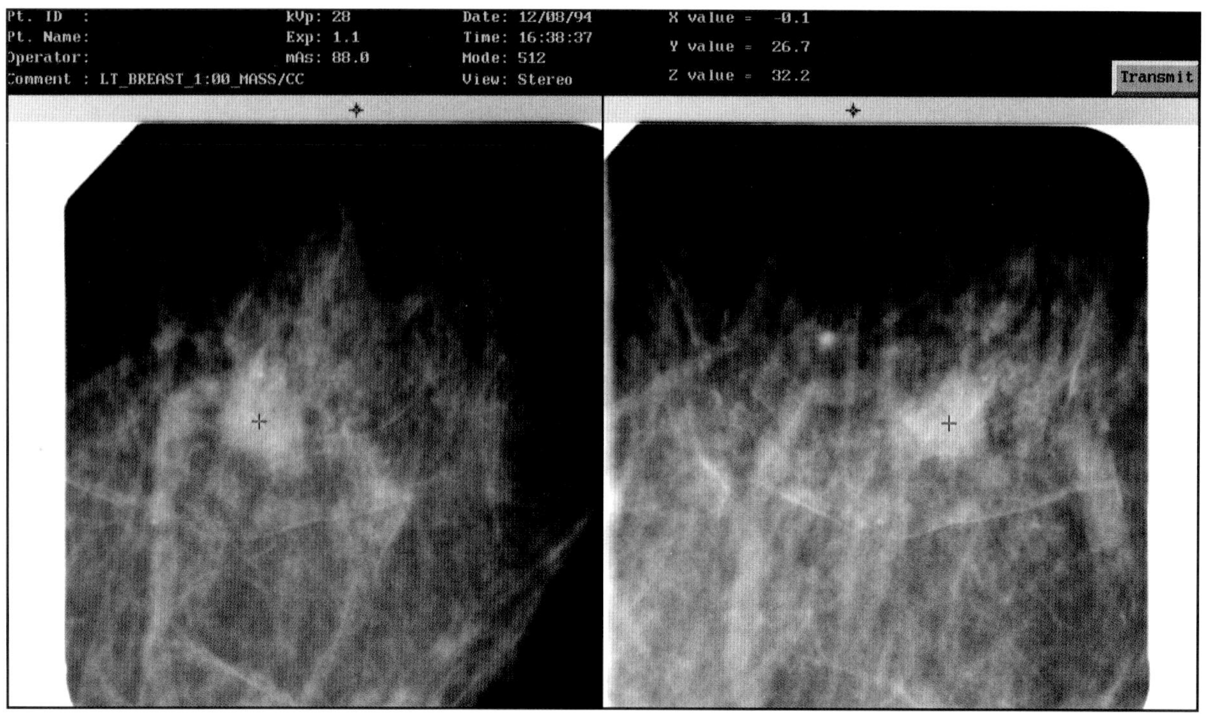

(a)

Figure 3.3 a and b. Biopsy Instrument Placement. An abnormality was localized to a depth of 32.2 mm **(a)**. When the needle was positioned, another stereo pair was obtained, and the tip depth was measured at 15.9 mm **(b)**. The biopsy gun had not been completely pushed into place in the holder. Note also that the abnormality, which was clearly seen on the localizing images, is partially obscured by hematoma after the needle placement **(b)**. In review of the scout image (not shown), a large vessel was seen passing the biopsy field; try to avoid vessels, if possible.

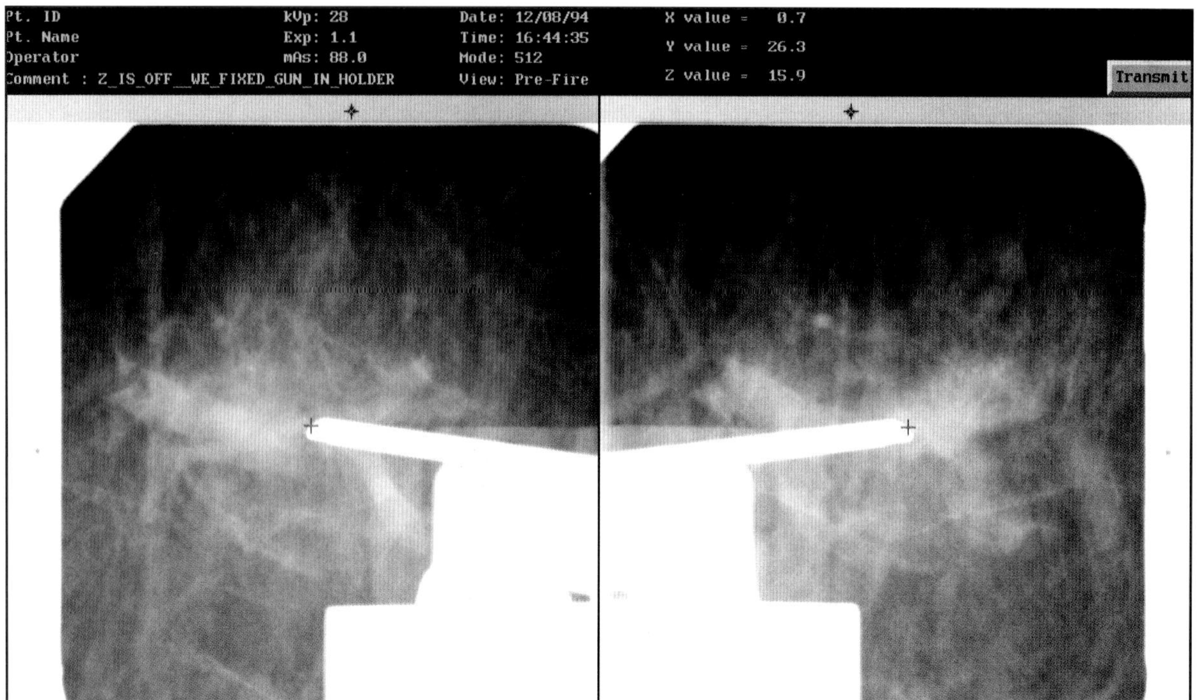

(b)

Abnormality Motion from the Needle

Certain abnormalities may resist smooth penetration by the biopsy needle because they are very firm or elastic **(Figure 3.4)**. Many fibroadenomas fall into this category, as well as some firm breast cancers. The localization coordinates may have been accurate initially, but the prefire image shows that the needle tip is proximal to its intended location, or is no longer in line with the abnormality. The needle may have been positioned with great accuracy but as a result of its insertion, the abnormality shifted away from the original targeted position.

There are several ways to adjust for this complication. First, the abnormality will shift less if compression is increased, fixing the whole breast more firmly. Explain the shift to the patient, and determine if she can tolerate a greater degree of compression.

A second technique relies on the core needle design, which samples tissue from the side of the needle tract, not the tip. Thus, the clinician can create a tract to accommodate the throw of the needle manually, and then fire the gun through this tract. Simply align the needle over the abnormality, and slowly advance the needle through the abnormality. Check with a stereo pair that the needle has gone through the abnormality after the needle's deepest excursion. If successful, retract the needle to its usual prefire position 5 mm proximal to the abnormality center.

A third technique suggests retracting the needle tip a few more millimeters, for example, 7-8 mm proximal to the abnormality, then firing. The abnormality will initially be less displaced by the needle, and the quick action of the gun may overcome the elastic resistance of the abnormality and the surrounding breast tissue. Given a throw of 23 mm, there is leeway in the depth dimension (up to perhaps one-half the stated throw) that allows for such an adjustment. (Type I)

Inability to See Abnormality on Stereo Pair

Subtle abnormalities seen on a screening or diagnostic mammogram may be difficult to see with the stereotactic biopsy unit. The first reason is that the breast tissue in the biopsy window is not directly compressed; it is pulled into compression by the surrounding breast tissue, which is directly compressed by the margin of the biopsy paddle. This reduced degree of compression results in some imaging degradation, especially as a result of superimposed parenchymal elements. (Similarly, the images obtained during a needle localization in the compression paddle window are less sharp than the fully compressed work-up images.)

Second, it is sometimes difficult to compare a screen-film image from the abnormality work-up with a digital image because of inherent differences in imaging characteristics. For example, a histogram equalization filter typically produces a digital image with greater contrast than the corresponding screen-film image. Also, the screen-film image usually has only a small, stable degree of magnification, whereas the digital image as displayed on a monitor may demonstrate variable degrees of magnification. Thus, it may be more difficult to identify corresponding structures between digital and screen-film images.

Third, the abnormality may be obscured by a hematoma at the biopsy site (Figure 3.3b). Finally, only a relatively small portion of the central breast is imaged through the biopsy window, so peripheral clues for image orientation, such as the nipple, skin, and chest wall are not usually seen on digital images.

If an abnormality is fairly conspicuous on a work-up image, such as a definite mass or an easily perceived cluster of calcifications, and is not seen on the initial scout digital image, the window was probably not positioned properly over the abnormality. It may be difficult to "hunt" for the abnormality if landmarks are absent or ambiguous, especially in a large breast. To avoid this situation, begin the exam on a standard mammography unit with the needle localization in place. Place a skin marker over the abnormality, using the same orientation as planned in the stereotactic biopsy. Then transfer the patient to the stereotactic table and have the technologist center the marker in the biopsy window. With this approach, the clinician can usually image the abnormality on the first attempt. Some stereotactic models now allow a screen-film cassette to be placed in front of the digital detector array, allowing this localization to be performed without moving the patient.

More subtle abnormalities lead to additional considerations, especially in a large breast. The work-up may have identified a "pseudo-abnormality" that is transient, or is a variant of the underlying parenchymal pattern. The abnormality may also be hard to find in a large breast. In either of these cases, taking repeat images with a mammography unit, and marking the skin over the abnormality if it is seen, may help solve the problem. In some stereotactic units, a spot compression device may be fitted into the biopsy window to improve the image quality and reduce parenchymal overlap and scatter. This may help identify and properly locate faint abnormalities.

Most units also allow for digital image processing, such as sharpening and smoothing filters, black-white inversion, and window and level adjustments (see chapter 5). Keep in mind that such image manipulation can render many image fea-

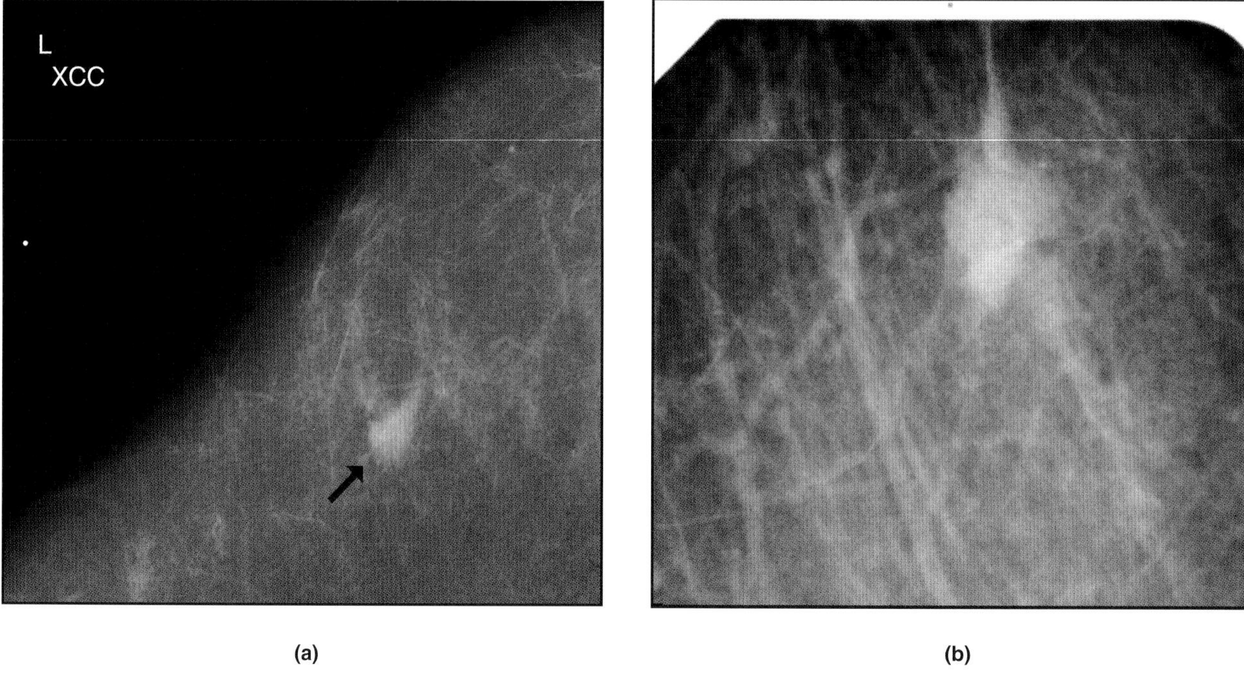

(a) (b)

Figure 3.4 a-c. Abnormality Motion. A small, firm abnormality within an overall fatty breast, as seen on the XCC view **(a) (arrow)**. The stereo scout thus easily shows the abnormality **(b)**. After positioning the needle, the abnormality has been clearly displaced **(c) (arrows)**. Pathologic review of the cores failed to make the diagnosis of ductal carcinoma in situ that was found on open biopsy.

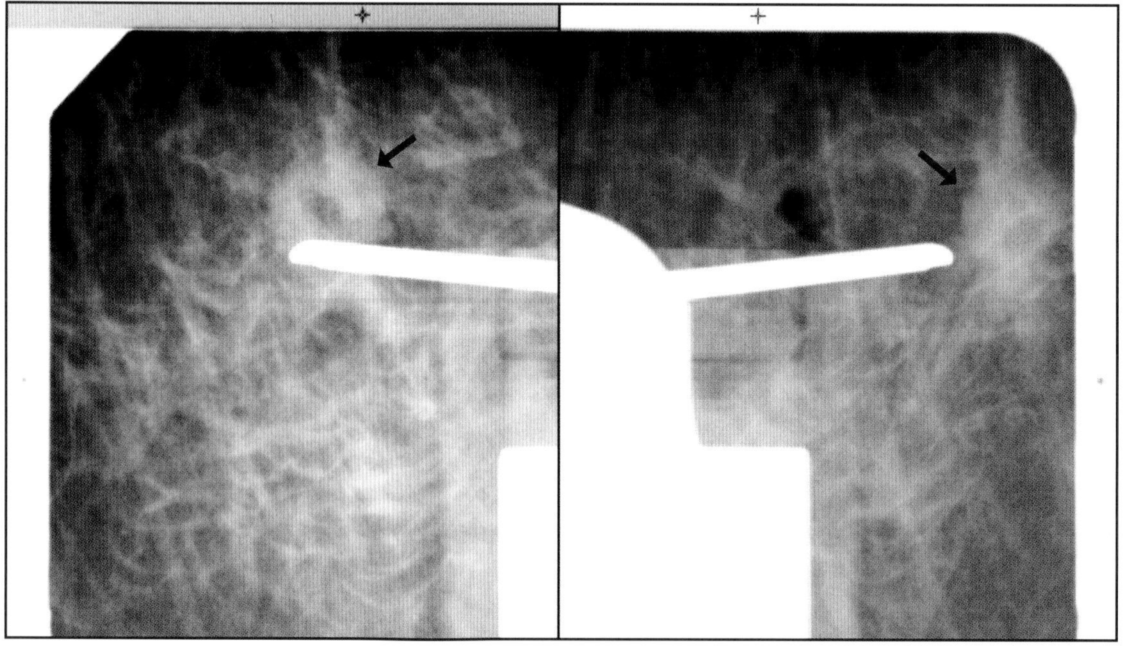

(c)

tures, such as scattered parenchyma or artifacts, into the appearance of an abnormality. A good strategy for its use is to process images to find areas of interest. However, always return to the unprocessed image to review those areas, and then make a clinical judgment.

Sometimes an abnormality can be seen only on one of the two stereo images. This may be due to adjacent parenchyma, which silhouettes the abnormality from one perspective. In that case, release the breast and reposition it. After repositioning, the obscuring parenchyma may be in a slightly shifted position. Occasionally, a small degree of obliquity may be added to the view to discern the abnormality from surrounding structures. Finally, if the abnormality can be reasonably approached from a different perspective, it may offer a clear view of the abnormality on both stereo images. For example, if an abnormality is in the upper outer quadrant, both the superior or the lateral approach may be acceptable; the shortest biopsy path is usually tried first but often the path lengths are approximately the same from both directions.

If the abnormality is seen only on one of the stereo images but is not obscured by breast structures, it probably projects off the lateral edge of the image. Based on other structures and previous images, the direction in which the abnormality moves in that image should be predictable. Abnormalities may be at any height on the stereo pair, since the height does not change with stereo angulation. But *the abnormality must be fairly well-centered in the left-right axis* because the abnormalities will shift along that axis on the angled views, and may "march off" the imaging field. The technologist may correct this difficulty by recentering the abnormality in the left-right axis within the biopsy window.

Never try to "guess" where the abnormality is in the stereo pair. If, despite all attempts, an abnormality can be imaged only on one of the stereo images, it is best to cancel the biopsy. (Type I) This situation must not be confused with the more common clinical problem of abnormalities that can be seen only on one projection during standard screen-film mammography. In this case, a stereotactic biopsy may be possible from one projection, if the abnormality can be seen with both 15°-angled views, and the biopsy path length is appropriate.

Deviation of the Biopsy Needle

The 14-gauge needle in use at most centers for core biopsy is fairly rigid, especially with its cannula in place. However, some breasts contain very dense fibrous stroma, and some cancers are exceedingly firm (partially from a reactive desmoplastic fibrosis induced by the neoplasm). Some surgical scars are also quite firm. These tough tissues may deflect the needle tip, or even grossly arc the needle away from its intended path.

The needle is supported at its proximal end in the gun on a movable distal support arm. The movable arm can only move up to the skin surface, so the whole distal portion of the needle in the breast is fixed only on one end. The working end of the biopsy needle has the least support with deep abnormalities in large breasts. This is another reason that the shortest path to the abnormality should be chosen, in most cases. Whenever the needle is advanced within the breast during needle positioning and gun firing, the movable distal support arm should extend out as far as possible.

The biopsy needle may also be deflected postfire when the stroke margin is small. This occurs because the tip approaches the tough dermal and subdermal tissue on the distal side of the breast **(Figure 3.5)**.

The tip of the stylet has an asymmetric wedge shape, to drive it down as it is fired out of its cutting sheath (cannula). When the more rigid sheath follows an instant later, it straightens the stylet, optimally filling the sample notch with tissue. Thus, the needle normally will follow a slight arc downward, most commonly in dense tissue. If the prefire images are well-aligned in the vertical axis but consistent vertical error is evident in the postfire images, consider this downward arcing as a possible cause, and compensate manually by adjusting the coordinates based on the needle position. Parker suggests prebending the stylet in this direction to increase sample size[1]. However, the resultant deviation may reduce the accuracy of the sampling localization. (Type II)

In one case, a patient had a focal area of distortion with calcifications. Repeated attempts to position a biopsy needle failed (despite clearly seeing the abnormality on the stereo pair) because the needle was grossly deflected by the abnormality. The clinician was not able to get any closer than 15 mm from the periphery, but took a few samples without much hope for a diagnostic result. Each of the samples demonstrated invasive ductal cancer, which was later confirmed on lumpectomy. Two lessons can be learned from this case. First, if a firm breast abnormality can grossly deflect a rigid biopsy needle, this must be occurring to a lesser extent on other moderately firm abnormalities. Second, it is best to take samples even when it is not possible to achieve a satisfactory needle position. The value of a positive result will not be diminished in such cases (of course, a negative result would not be credible in such a situation). (Type III)

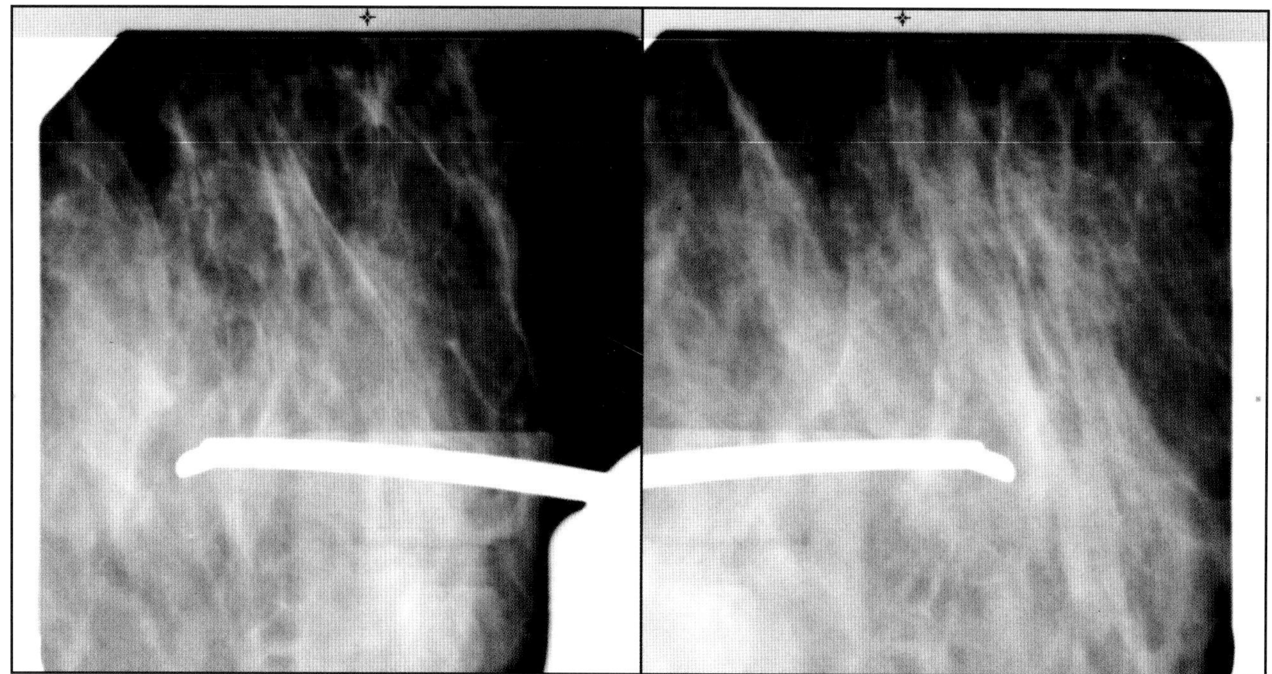

Figure 3.5. Needle Deflection. Even though the stroke margin was positive in this case, the tough distal tissue bent the stylet significantly. In this extreme example, the stylet was bent so severely that it was "stuck," and the needle had to be removed from the gun and rotated to retract it.

Multiple Findings

There are two types of multiple findings that can complicate a core biopsy procedure. The first involves multiple similar findings, such as multiple, similarly sized masses, or multiple groups of calcifications. These may be difficult to identify uniquely on the localization stereo pair images. Care must be taken to ensure that the same abnormality is localized within both of the stereo pair images, or the coordinates will be incorrect. There are several methods of determining if the correct abnormality has been selected within each of the stereo pair images. On some units, an intermediate offset angle (7.5° to each side) may be selected; a stereo pair with this reduced angulation should help identify which abnormality on the fully angled stereo pair goes with the abnormality on the straight scout image. However, targeting should never take place on the reduced angle views.

Second, abnormalities will move only in the left-right axis, not toward or away from the chest wall, so the height of the abnormality may help distinguish it. Do not rely solely on abnormality size, unless it is significantly different from other abnormalities, because abnormalities are somewhat asymmetrical in three-dimensional space. Therefore, asymmetric abnormalities may project different apparent sizes from different projections. For the same reason, abnormalities may look spherical on one view and ovoid on another, so do not rely on shape alone. However, the height of an abnormality should be constant (see chapter 2). (Type I)

Another situation involving multiple findings occurs when two findings appear to be related to a single abnormality, but in reality merely project over one another **(Figure 3.6 a and b)**. For example, if a mass is seen with some central calcifications, check orthogonal views from the screening or work-up screen-film image to ensure that the calcifications project within the mass on all views. If it is assumed that they are at the same locus, the clinician may be unpleasantly surprised upon attempting to localize the findings on stereo pair images. (Type I)

Inaccurate Estimation of the Center of Masses

Masses are localized with reference to their estimated center. Highly irregular masses, or masses with very unclear margins, may reduce the clinician's confidence in selecting an estimated center. Because abnormalities may have asymmetrical projections with different apparent shapes on each

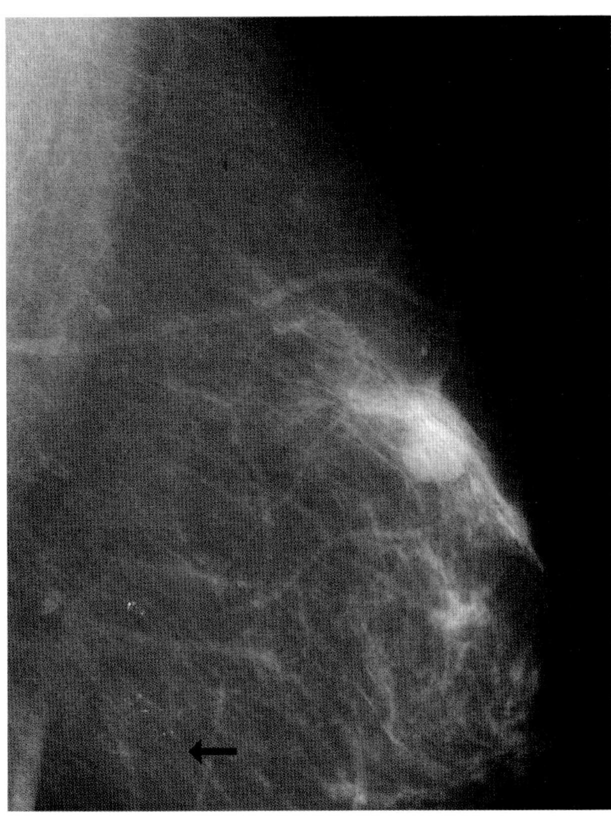

(a)

of the stereo pair images, the accuracy of center estimation is again reduced. In most cases, sufficient accuracy can be achieved to obtain reliable biopsy samples. First, as mentioned previously, the height of the abnormalities should remain constant, so only the left-right axis and the depth axis are subject to this imprecision. Second, small abnormalities are intrinsically focal because there is very little distance between their "center" and their periphery. Thus, the derived coordinates remain useful. Large abnormalities, however, are large targets and are more likely to be successfully biopsied, even if a center estimation error is present. A center estimation error may be only, at most, a small fraction of the radius of an abnormality. Furthermore, since biopsy passes with offsets of the same magnitude are taken in all directions, the center estimation error can be considered statistically equivalent to measurement noise, without a dramatic degradation in localization accuracy. (Type III, not clinically significant)

Selecting Different Calcifications from a Stereo Pair

When localizing a cluster of calcifications, spatial accuracy is best when one individual calcification can be identified on each of the stereo images. The largest error would result if the two different calcifications selected are in reality at opposite sides of the cluster, appearing to be adjacent to each

Figure 3.6 a and b. Multiple Findings. A large "cluster" of calcifications were seen inferiorly on the MLO view **(a) (arrow)**. The CC view demonstrates that there are two distinct clusters of calcifications **(b) (arrows)**. Always check the work-up images carefully before performing the stereotactic biopsy.

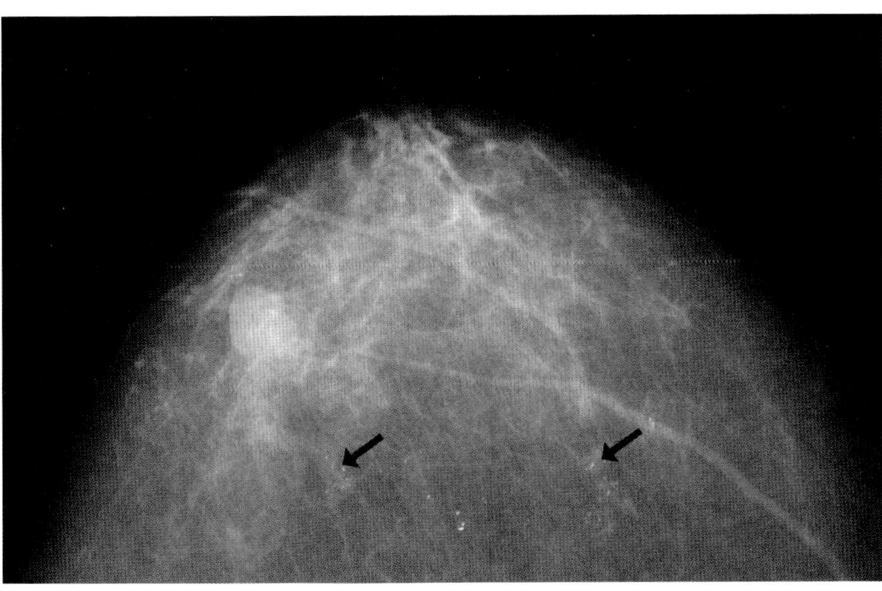

(b)

other only by projection. Conceivably, a very distant calcification, such as a solitary dermal calcification or secretory calcification, may project over a true cluster and, if selected from a stereo pair, would generate useless coordinates. Try to select calcifications that are distinct enough to identify uniquely on each view, but also try to select calcifications with typical morphologies for its cluster. If one calcification has a very different morphology than the other elements of the group, carefully inspect the screening and work-up mammographic images to ensure that it does not lie at a distance from the group, such as in the dermis. (Type I)

Incorrect Reference Points

Each image in a stereo pair must have a reference point marked, so that the localization algorithm can calculate meaningful coordinates. On some units, the point is detected automatically from the digital display. However, this detection feature may incorrectly identify the reference point, which would totally invalidate its results. Consequently, the reference point selection must be checked by the team doing the stereotactic biopsy. At some window and level settings, the reference point may be difficult or impossible to see. When this occurs, adjust the settings until you can confirm its proper selection.

The most common cause for errors in reference point selection is chest or abdominal wall tissue that drapes down from the side of the table opening, obscuring the point and often the top of the biopsy window as well. This can usually be easily corrected by repositioning the patient on the table, or using some firm cardboard or plastic over the side of the table opening to hold the loose tissue above the imaging plane.

Keep in mind that in rare cases with a high degree of compression, the bending of the biopsy/compression plate may move the reference point above the receptor field. Also, the density of the underlying breast in the area of the reference point may be so high or low that the reference point cannot be seen at the standard window and level settings. This, of course, may be easily corrected by manually adjusting the display parameters. (Type I)

Incorrect Angulation

On some units, the x-ray tube may be angulated to several positions, one of which is the proper 15° setting for localization purposes. If an incorrect angulation is selected for calibration or clinical localization, results will be significantly in error. Thus, if calibrations are way off, or localizations far off the mark, try obtaining the offset images again. In some cases, a clinician may want to recreate the discrepant calibration results by deliberately choosing an incorrect offset. (Type I)

Reversed Film on Localizer

Most stereotactic units have a localization viewbox to obtain coordinates from screen-film offset images. The film must be placed on the viewbox in the correct orientation, or the localization algorithms will calculate incorrect coordinates. For each type of unit, the proper position and orientation of the film must be known and, if localization errors are noted, the film's orientation should be checked. (Type 1)

Reversed Order of Digital Imaging

On some units, there is a mandatory order in obtaining the two digital offset images. Obtaining the images in the incorrect order results in a significant error in coordinate calculation, similar to the error from reversing of the film on the screen-film localization viewbox. As in that case, if the calibration or clinical images are way off, repeat the images while paying close attention to the offset order. This error is easily preventable if the directions for offsets are clearly marked on the unit's housing. (Type 1)

Sampling Errors

Many malignant tumors of the breast demonstrate a varied microscopic appearance from location to location within a given abnormality. This heterogeneity is evident in the pathology reports from breast biopsies, with many different hyperplasias, atypias, and malignancies often reported from the same sample. The surgical biopsy specimen is usually sectioned, with representative slices from a number of distinct sites, to try to discover the full range of histology. The report is typically summarized by the most malignant component found.

Core biopsy specimens preserve the local histology of that portion of a breast abnormality, but cannot offer any information about adjacent areas or the degree of heterogeneity in the abnormality as a whole. This is the primary reason that multiple core biopsies are obtained for each abnormality, including a series with an arbitrary offset so that the peripheral portions of an abnormality are included. These peripheral cores often contain the most aggressive cellular elements. Multiple passes with offsets also increase the probability of hitting an abnormality. However, if this was the only reason for multiple passes, we could conclude the procedure when we knew the biopsy pass was successful, such as through an easily seen mass or target microcalcifications in the core specimen. Multiple passes are equivalent to multiple snapshots of the abnormality; there may be important nests of cells that by chance are not sampled. The more passes performed, the more complete the picture of the abnormality. This need to reduce sampling error must be balanced with the length of the procedure, the probability that important new information will be obtained, and extra patient discomfort. In recent literature, 5 passes offer a good trade-off between sampling completeness and procedural efficiency, in many cases.

Insufficient Number of Passes

Some procedures must be terminated in midstream for many reasons, including the inability of the patient to continue, running out of a stock item needed for the procedure, etc. If some specimens are obtained, they should be sent for analysis, remembering that a positive pathologic report is very reliable. As discussed later in the analysis errors section, confidence in a negative report should be adjusted down to some degree in these cases. (Type III)

No Calcifications in the Core Specimens

When a cluster of calcifications is the target abnormality, it is very helpful to obtain an image of the core specimens to prove that the targets have been sampled **(Figure 3.7)**. If after 5 passes, no target calcifications are seen, carefully check the stereo pair images again to make sure that the target coordinates remain properly aligned. Then perform an additional 4 passes with slightly different offsets. This second set of specimens is also imaged, but the biopsy is often ended at this point, with or without specimen calcifications seen. Very cooperative patients who would like to maximize the yield of the core biopsy (and reduce the need for open biopsy to follow) may be willing to undergo a third set of offset core biopsies. Also check that the calcifications in the core specimens have the same morphology and size as the targets, so that an adjacent benign microcalcification is not mistaken for the targeted abnormality. (Type II)

Radial Scars

In addition to its heterogeneous cellular makeup, radial scars display a macroscopic gradient of findings from their periphery to the center, which the pathologist cannot assess from disparate core specimens. Thus, it may not be wise to rely on a diagnosis involving radial scars using core biopsy. If a mammographic abnormality has hallmarks of a radial scar (a lucent center, asymmetrically "bundled" spicules, very slow growth), the clinician might consider opting for open biopsy. Another option is to perform stereotactic biopsy, only to establish a malignant diagnosis, following with an open biopsy if no malignancy is detected. Some investigators believe that once a frank malignancy has been essentially ruled out with a core biopsy **(Figure 3.8 a and b)**, these abnormalities can be safely watched with short interval follow-up mammography. (Type I)

Phyllodes Tumors

Phyllodes tumors, which often present as large tumors in relatively young women, often display a variable histologic pattern in different regions of the tumor. Since all of these tumors must be excised to prevent local (or occasionally distant) recurrence, the utility of stereotactic biopsy is limited. If the surgeon prefers to know a diagnosis before excision to help plan the procedure, a core biopsy may assist the workup. However, the aggressiveness of the tumor (and thus the prognosis for recurrence) is not reliably estimated by the limited sampling from the core biopsies. (Type II)

Insufficient Samples

Unlike the variable yield of fine needle aspiration cytology, large 14-gauge core biopsy passes routinely obtain an intact cylindrical core of tissue with a minimum of artifact. There are cases, however, in which the yield is visibly low, with an empty or almost empty sample notch after each pass.

Adipose Tissue

Adipose tissue is soft and easily compressible. These characteristics can lead to scanty sample volumes. Adipose tissue itself is almost never the target of the biopsy but comes from surrounding fatty replaced breast parenchyma. Occasionally, fat may be sampled within a hamartoma (also called a fibroadenolipoma), or within a lymph node. The soft milieu of a fatty replaced breast may allow the target to be more easily displaced by needle placement or firing. This can be partially compensated for by increasing the compression of the breast, as mentioned earlier. (Type I)

Stylet Flexibility

Parker[1] suggests that gently bending the stylet at the proximal end of its sample notch may increase yield. This increases the downward deflection of the stylet as it shoots forward and thus theoretically increases the filling pressure of tissue into the notch as the stiffer outer sheath (cannula) is pro-

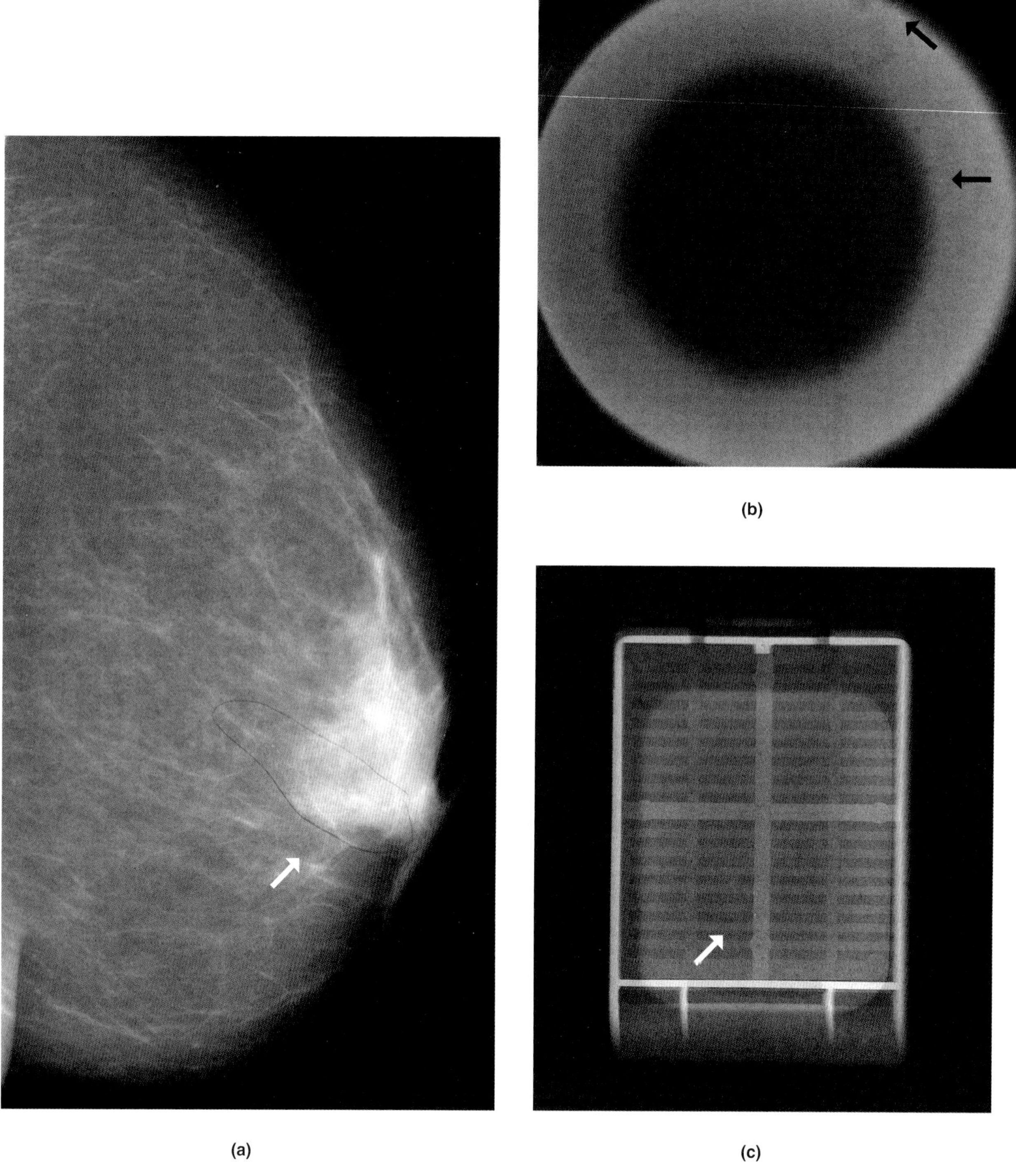

Figure 3.7 a-c. Specimen Radiography. The initial reading of the core biopsy on these calcifications was benign **(a) (arrow)**. However, the core specimen film showed that target calcifications were present in the cores **(b) (arrows)**. Open biopsy showed DCIS. An image of the remaining block **(c)** from the core tissue showed many more calcifications **(arrow)**, and deeper cuts showed DCIS. Just as there is sampling error from needle placement, the pathologist samples only a small portion of any biopsy sample.

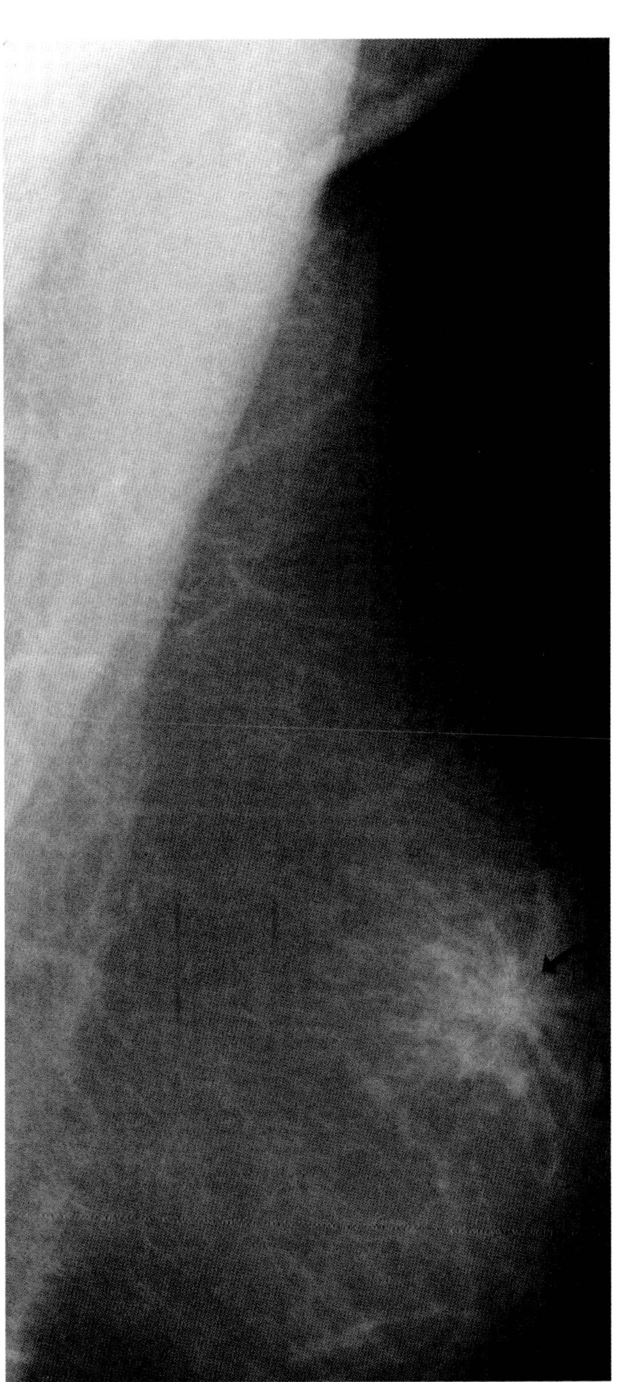

Figure 3.8a. Radial Scars.This abnormality **(arrow)**, which was followed for a number of years before this biopsy, has many of the classic mammographic features of a radial scar.

pelled at the next instant. This does not necessarily greatly increase the sample yield and may have several disadvantages. For example, the tip could deflect downward, reducing the predictability of the sampling localization. Metal fatigue could also be induced at the bent stylet sample notch end. Thus, this technique should be used with caution, if at all. (Type II)

Cutting Edge at/or Proximal to Dermis

The cutting edge that cleanly slices the sampled core is at the distal end of the outer sheath, and is seen 7-9 mm proximal to the stylet tip in both pre- and postfire configurations. This edge should be placed completely through the skin nick before firing, if possible, because the edge can hit very tough tissue in the dermis and can be slowed down or even stopped before a good sample has been obtained. When this occurs, the operator may hear a dull thud, rather than the usual crisp snapping sound of the needle as it is fired into the abnormality. This is most often a problem when sampling superficial abnormalities because the tip is placed 5 mm proximal to the abnormality center, so that the cutting edge lies 12-14 mm proximal to the abnormality. There are several ways to compensate for this.

First, use a slightly smaller gap between the tip and the abnormality center. With a 23-mm throw gun, a reasonable sample can usually be obtained with the tip 2 mm proximal to an abnormality. For large masses, the operator can eliminate the gap entirely, if necessary.

Second, the abnormality may be obliqued slightly to increase the apparent depth of the abnormality **(Figure 3.9)**. This maneuver also reduces the distance behind the abnormality, so it works best with larger breasts.

Third, the needle may be positioned distal to the abnormality and slowly retracted into position. The skin may be pulled outward with the motion of the sheath and may remain proximal to the cutting edge **(Figure 3.10)**. Finally, the clinician can widen the incision, so that the edges of the skin incision are loose and cannot be easily caught by the needle's cutting edge. The incision can be widened by a cross incision with the scalpel, that is, two passes at right angles to each other **(Figure 3.11)**. (Type I)

Short-Throw Gun

Twelve-millimeter throw guns consistently produce small, scanty samples. Given the mechanism of action of the inner stylet and outer cutting sheath, it is not surprising that samples are significantly smaller. The sample notch is only partially uncovered with the short throw and has less of a chance to deflect down to fill its notch with tissue (see

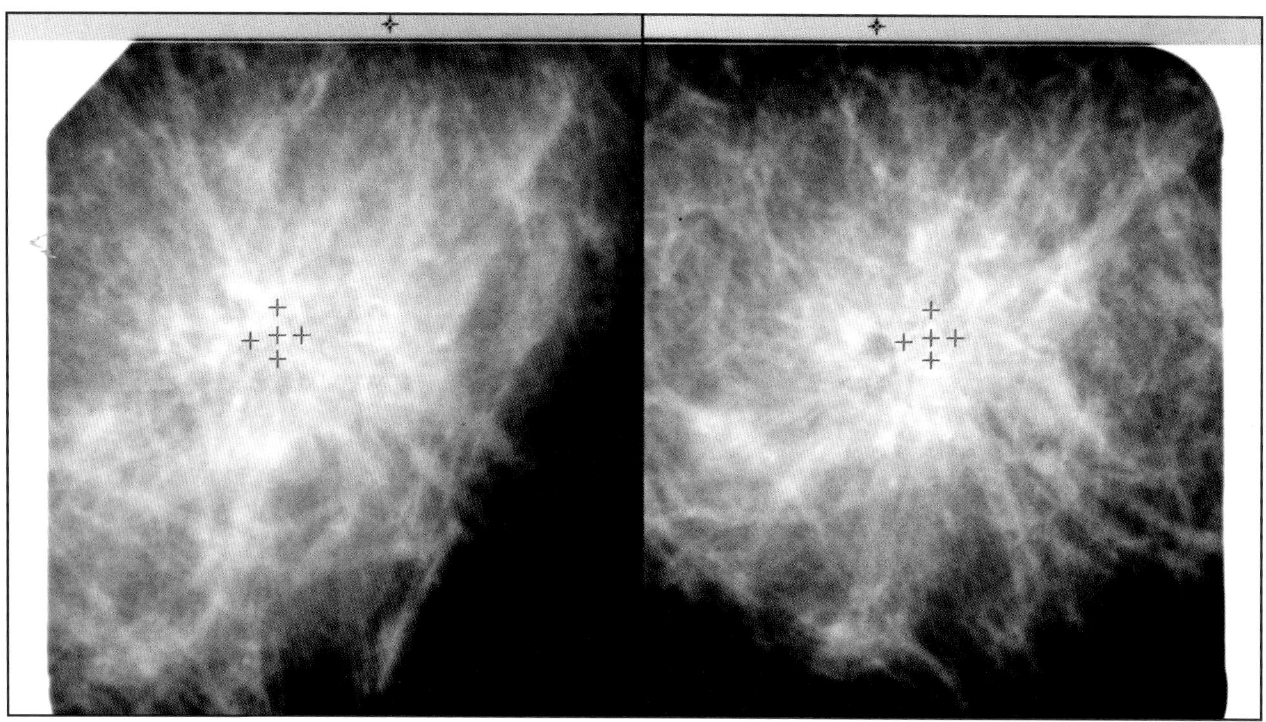

Figure 3.8b. Radial Scars. The core biopsy was read as a radial scar, showing that, in some cases, this entity can be reliably identified from cores.

chapter 2). Often, the tissue that is obtained consists of a few separate fragments, rather than a coherent core of tissue. It is best to use short or variable-throw guns only when necessary, such as in a small breast or in the retroareolar region. (Type I)

Analysis Errors

After the procedure, the biopsy results must be reviewed to arrive at recommendations for the patient and her referring physician. These recommendations must take into consideration the prebiopsy estimated probability of malignancy, the biopsy results, the confidence estimate about the procedure, and the patient's preferences. It is very helpful to construct an outcomes table **(Figure 3.12,)** to create a rational basis for such recommendations, and to help patients (and referring doctors) understand the various outcome options.

The ACR grades mammographic findings on a scale of 1-5. Usually, only abnormalities in the 3-5 range are biopsied. Type 3 abnormalities are probably benign but have a known (small) probability of malignancy, such as well-circumscribed growing masses. Type 4 abnormalities have approximately a 50% chance of malignancy, such as a cluster of indeterminate calcifications in an older woman. Type 5 abnormalities are probably malignant, such as spiculated masses.

There are also three possible pathology results. A reading of a carcinoma is reliable, since we know of almost no false positives in this setting. There are two types of benign readings: *specific benign*, in which the result corresponds and accounts for the mammographic finding, and *nonspecific benign*, in which normal breast tissue only is seen.

If the target is a well-circumscribed mass, and the pathologist reads the sample as a fibroadenoma, the clinician can confidently assume that the mammographic abnormality was "hit" and properly identified with a specific benign diagnosis. If, for a different case, no target calcifications were noted in a set of specimens, which demonstrated only adipose tissue and normal gland tissue, the benign result is nonspecific.

This table offers a structured, consistent approach, but must be adjusted by two other relevant factors: confidence

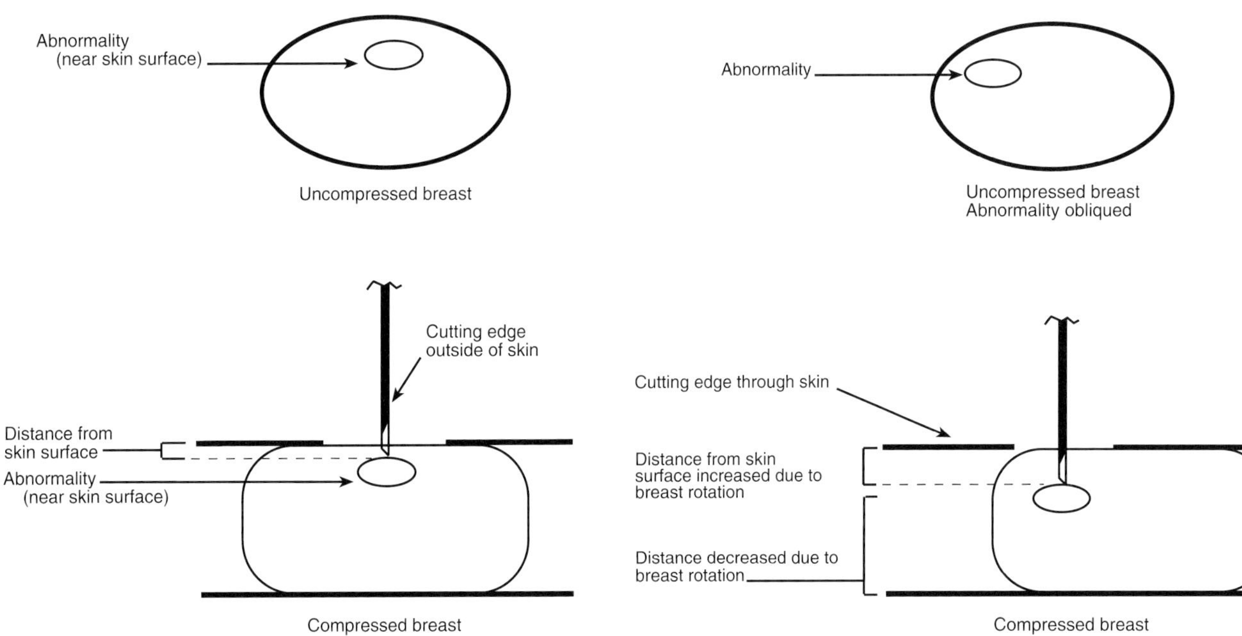

Figure 3.9. Cutting Edge Proximal to Dermis. Oblique positioning may help biopsy superficial abnormalities in the larger breast. Using a small degree of obliquity increases the path length before the abnormality, but reduces the postabnormality distance that must accommodate the throw of the gun.

in the procedure and patient preference. Thus, the table offers a starting point for the clinician who performs the biopsy, and should not be followed rigidly. The table also should be developed with local experience and preferences. As more data on the sensitivity and specificity of the procedure is published in the literature, we can expect to see further adjustments.

Atypia

In most studies of stereotactic biopsy, severe atypia is treated aggressively, usually with a recommendation for surgical biopsy for confirmation. The concern is that undersampled heterogeneous abnormalities may hide nests of invasive cells, and the atypia may be the only clue to their presence. It will take a few more years before clinicians learn whether the present practice of 5 or more core biopsy passes sufficiently covers this situation. There have been some cases in which atypia alone was seen on core biopsy, with a malignancy seen on open biopsy. As long as clinicians consider atypia as "malignant" in this context, it will keep sensitivity high. We will later learn whether it is safe to increase specificity by treating some atypia (perhaps low-grade) conservatively. (Type II)

Unexpected Pathologic Results

Not infrequently, we will obtain a pathology report from the core procedure that does not directly correspond to the prebiopsy impressions. For example, one might occasionally find "fibroadenoma" in cases with a small group of calcifications with no apparent mass, or lobular calcifications are noted when none are seen in mammography, even in retrospect. Do not consider such findings as a specific benign result because of the lack of correlation with the image. They may be "innocent bystanders" that are serendipitously caught in the sampling notch, and may indicate that the sampling needle placement was less precise than optimal. (Type I)

Also remember that the pathologists review only a few selected sections from core specimens, so that they also are subject to sampling errors (Figure 3.7). If you are surprised by a diagnosis, consider asking the pathologist to review the

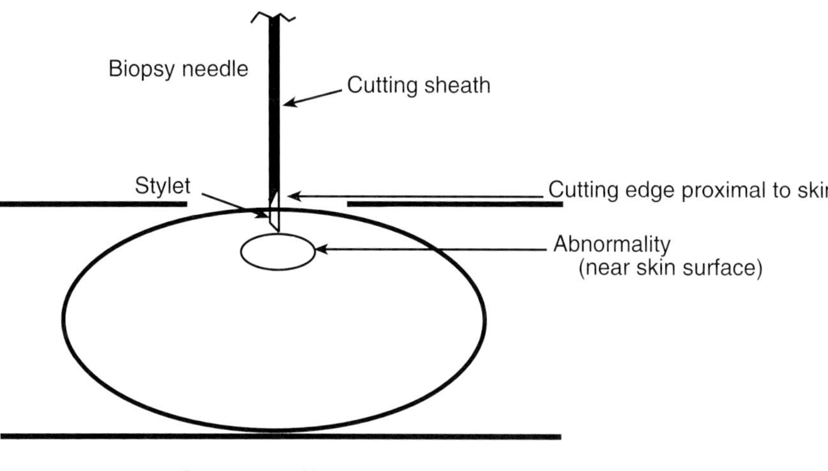

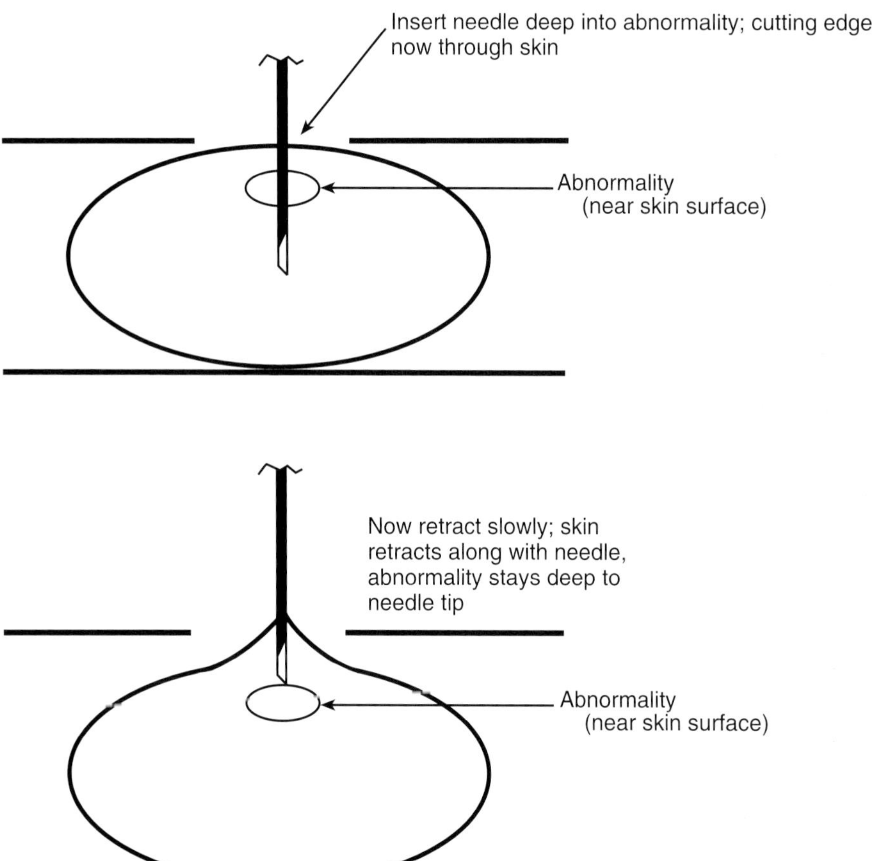

Figure 3.10. Tenting the Skin. Another technique for superficial abnormalities requires a small skin nick, so that the needle "tents" the skin. Place the needle deep to the abnormality and slowly retract, "tenting" the skin proximally. Check with a stereo pair that the abnormality remains fixed in the deeper breast tissue.

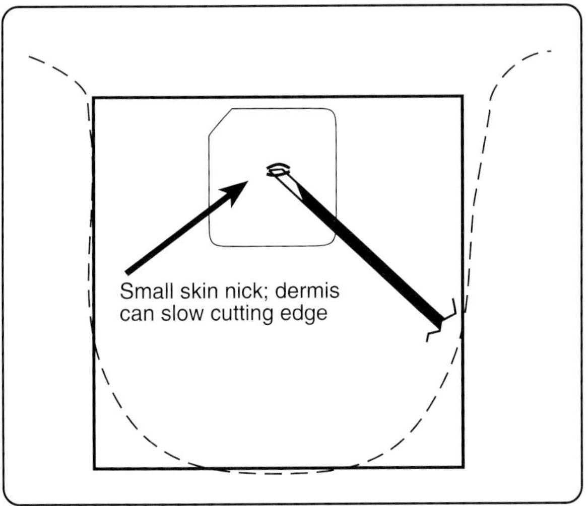

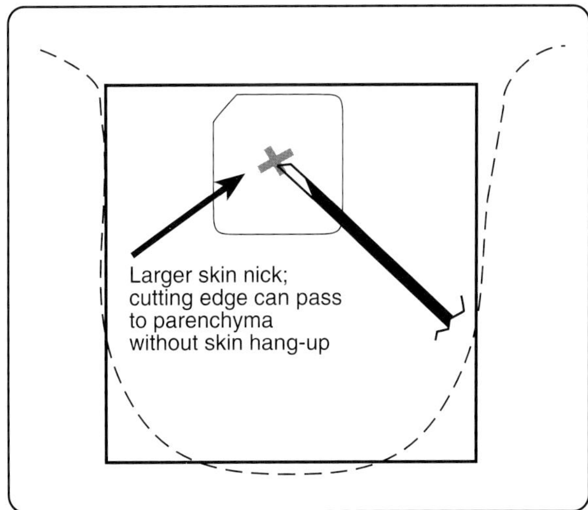

Figure 3.11. Cross Incision. Another approach to superficial abnormalites involves making a more generous incision, so that the cutting edge will not be impeded. Make a cross-incision by making two bisecting perpendicular cuts.

blocks, and take a specimen film of the block if the targets were calcifications. (Type I)

Confidence Level Concerning the Biopsy Procedure

Some biopsies will proceed very smoothly, and the clinician can feel very confident about the accuracy of the results, for example, when target calcifications are definitely in multiple cores. However, we will always have some more problematic cases in which some coordinates had to be "fudged" a little, or the patient seemed to be moving a bit. In those cases, record the difficulties and, when reviewing the results, lower the confidence in benign results, accordingly. Some clinicians feel that a specific benign diagnosis is still fairly reliable, but others may want to build confidence in the procedure as they begin by handling these aggressively at first. Of course, if a clinician recommends biopsy for many borderline cases, the referring physicians may rightfully wonder about the cost-effectiveness of core biopsy; therefore, try to balance the need for feedback with their concerns. (Type II)

Communication Failures

As in much of modern medicine, many problems arise when there is insufficient or incorrect communication. The clinician performing the biopsy procedure should tell the patient about the procedure and its risks and benefits, and clearly state how the results will be sent to her. Mammography sites

		ACR Grade 3	ACR Grade 4	ACR Grade 5
Biopsy results	**Cancer**	Treat	Treat	Treat
	Specific benign	Screening	6-month follow-up	Rebiopsy
	Nonspecific benign	6-month follow-up	Rebiopsy	Rebiopsy

Figure 3.12. Sample Management Protocol.

are legally responsible for communicating results to the appropriate person (either to the patient herself or to her physician) in a timely manner. Understandably, patients often do not remember what they are told while they are in an anxious state, and clinicians may have time pressures at work that rush them along. A simply worded printed description of the procedure can save time for both the clinician and the patient, and reduce errors. Reports and recommendations to physicians should be sent in as timely and safe a manner as possible. Some sites fax all their biopsy reports as soon as they are prepared. (Type I)

Follow-up

Centers that perform stereotactic biopsies should establish an ongoing database in which biopsy and surgical results, as well as long-term follow-up, are recorded. Tracking such data will quickly illustrate problems, such as one physician with a remarkably different biopsy rate. The local data can be used as a marketing tool to convince patients and referring physicians of the safety and accuracy of core biopsies at their center. The data can also be used as an index of quality for medicolegal disputes, just as mammographic audit data can be used to defend against a malpractice suit. (Type I)

References

1. Parker, S.H., Jobe, W.E. 1993. *Percutaneous Breast Biopsy* 71. New York: Raven Press.

Equipment Design and Selection

Kathleen M. Willison
Robert J. Pizzutiello

4

Introduction

This chapter focuses on both the design and selection of equipment for stereotactic breast biopsy, with an emphasis on stereotactic core biopsy. The design section details the technical components of a stereotactic breast biopsy unit. The section on selection of equipment provides a guide to understanding the various issues in equipment purchase and application.

There are two types of stereotactic breast biopsy equipment currently available — the "add-on" upright unit that attaches to an existing dedicated mammography unit **(Figure 4.1)**, and the dedicated prone position stereotactic table **(Figure 4.2)**. The components of both systems serve the following functions:

- Patient support and immobilization
- Breast positioning
- Imaging (scout and stereo projections)
- Targeting of the abnormality
- Coordinate calculation
- Needle guidance and sampling
- Patient safety

It is useful to have an overview of both system types to fully understand the imaging and stereotactic issues discussed later in this chapter.

Prone Units

The components of a prone SBB system include:

- Pedestal for support of the unit
- Patient support table with aperture for the dependent breast
- Breast support
- Compression arm
- Biopsy/compression plate
- Needle guidance system
- Computer for targeting and coordinate calculation
- C-arm and generator for producing x rays

Prone units are self-supported by a pedestal in the rear of, or beneath, the patient support table. Unlike add-on devices that must attach to an existing mammography unit, the prone table design includes the necessary components to provide x rays for imaging the breast. Beneath the table, a horizontal c-arm receives the dependent breast for imaging. The x-ray tube is at one end of the c-arm and the image receptor is at the opposite end. The c-arm also houses the breast support, the compression arm that supports the biopsy/compression plate, and the needle guidance system. The biopsy/compression plate typically consists of a paddle (of varying size) with an open window of about 50 mm x 50 mm to allow needle access. The biopsy team works seated below the table, which is adjustable in height. The sole purpose of the system is to perform stereotactic localization and needle biopsy. Prone units are not designed for routine mammography.

Patient Support and Immobilization

The examination table provides support and effective immobilization of the patient in the prone position. The breast support and biopsy/compression plate, along with motorized or manual compression, provide immobilization of the breast. Manufacturers of prone units typically recommend restricting patient weight to no more than three hundred pounds.

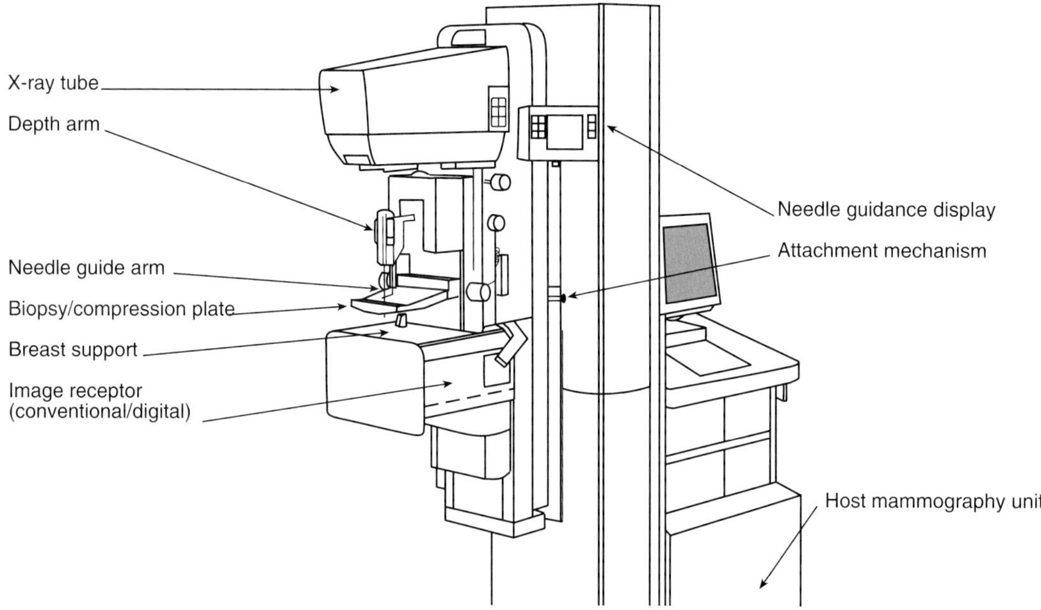
X-ray tube
Depth arm
Needle guide arm
Biopsy/compression plate
Breast support
Image receptor
(conventional/digital)
Needle guidance display
Attachment mechanism
Host mammography unit

Figure 4.1. Add-on SBB System.

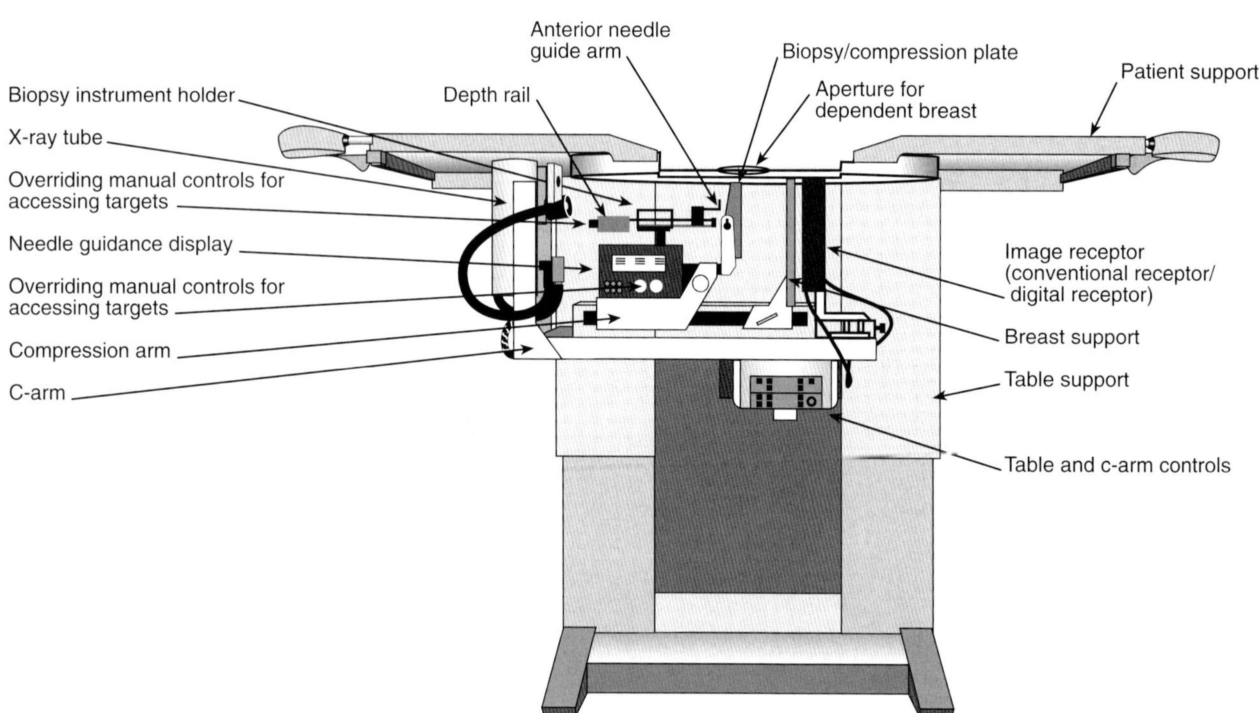
Anterior needle
guide arm
Biopsy/compression plate
Patient support
Biopsy instrument holder
Depth rail
Aperture for
dependent breast
X-ray tube
Overriding manual controls for
accessing targets
Needle guidance display
Overriding manual controls for
accessing targets
Compression arm
C-arm
Image receptor
(conventional receptor/
digital receptor)
Breast support
Table support
Table and c-arm controls

Figure 4.2. Dedicated Prone SBB System.

Breast Positioning

The patient support and c-arm apparatus provide the means to position the breast. The support table allows for the prone position of the patient with the ipsilateral breast dependent through an aperture in the table **(Figure 4.3)**. The location of the aperture may be at the center of the table or offset to one end. The table aperture should be wide enough to allow the maximum amount of breast tissue to be available for positioning. The c-arm apparatus rotates simultaneously with the breast support and image receptor at least 180° to provide the entry position for biopsy **(Figure 4.4)**. One unit has a center aperture design, providing continuous 360° access around the breast. The center aperture design allows positioning of the patient at either end of the table, and combined with c-arm rotation, provides 360° access **(Figure 4.5)**. The c-arm design also allows the x-ray tube to angle independent of the breast support, providing for stereo acquistion. Motorized compression, an inherent part of the compression arm, allows the technologist to have both hands free for positioning.

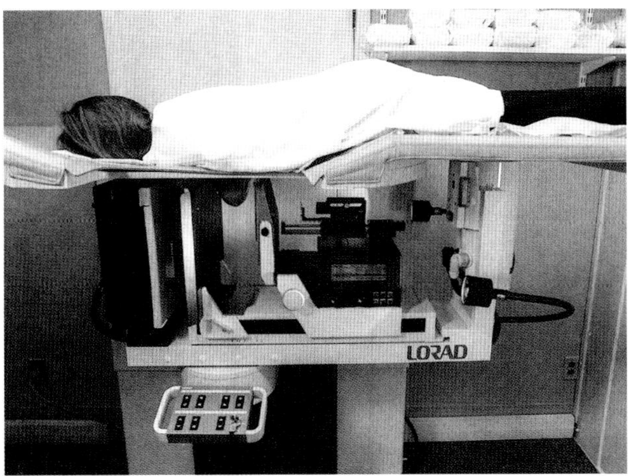

Figure 4.3. Positioning with a Prone Table. The patient is prone with the ipsilateral breast dependent through an aperture in the table.

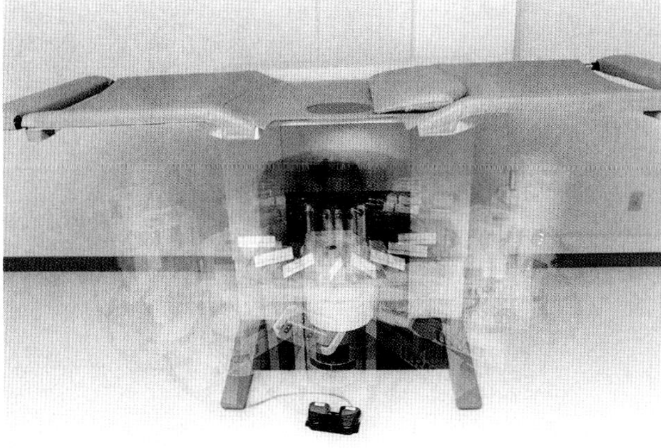

Figure 4.4. Continuous 180° Rotation. The c-arm should provide 180° rotation around the breast.

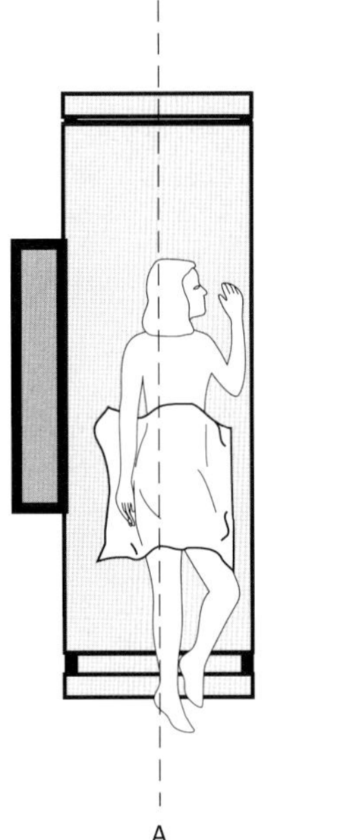

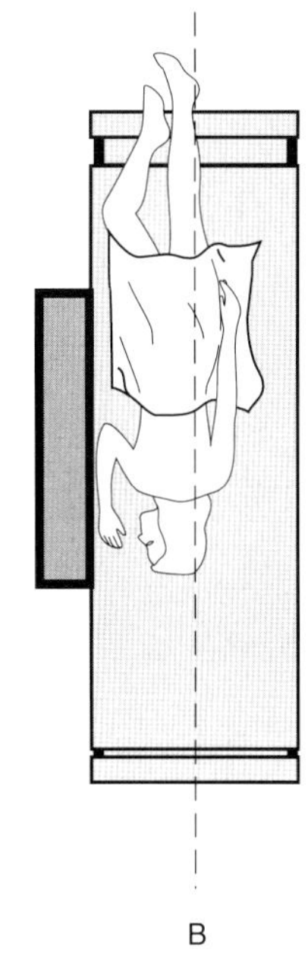

Figure 4.5. Center Aperture Table Design. The center aperture design allows positioning at either end of the table, and with 180° rotation, permits 360° access to the breast.

Accessories

The system should include a number of compression plates to accommodate the positioning process. A perforated scout paddle **(Figure 4.6)**, with matching aperture, allows the technologist to "scout" a larger area for abnormalities that are difficult to find. When employing a digital receptor, a cassette holder that fits over the digital box is necessary to achieve the scout.

Add-on Upright Units

The components of an upright SBB unit include:

- Apparatus for attachment to the host mammography unit
- Breast support/cassette tunnel
- Compression arm

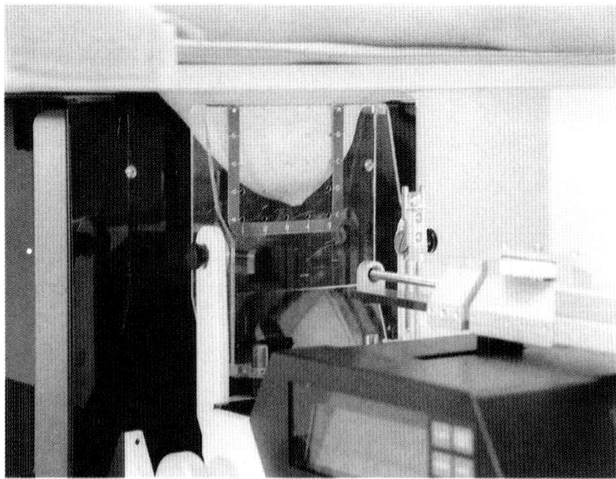

Figure 4.6. Perforated Scout Paddle. A larger perforated compression paddle allows the technologist to scout and mark a larger area when scouting for low-density abnormalities.

- Biopsy/compression plate
- Needle guidance system
- Computer for targeting and coordinate calculation

The upright add-on stereotactic unit receives support from the c-arm or pivot collar of the host mammography system. The host system provides imaging capabilities necessary for the procedure. Add-on equipment provides stereotactic localization and needle biopsy with the patient in an upright position. The unit is put into place for biopsy and removed after completion. Installation and removal should be relatively simple, requiring a minimal amount of time. The system, including the mammography unit, must provide for stability of the stereotactic device, as calculations for localization require a 1 millimeter tolerance. Working space between the tube head and the breast support should be adequate to allow the biopsy team to perform tasks easily. The distance between the tube head and the breast support should also accommodate the needle guidance system and biopsy instrument assembly, allowing for stereo acquisition.

Patient Support and Immobilization

The patient is seated or semirecumbent and must support herself in the necessary biopsy position. The breast support/cassette tunnel supports the breast. The biopsy/compression plate along with the compression arm immobilizes the breast. There are no weight restrictions for add-on units.

Breast Positioning

The c-arm of the host mammography system can rotate simultaneously with the stereotactic device to provide the positional approach for biopsy. Ideally, the c-arm should allow 360° access to the breast. Most upright mammographic units allow the c-arm to rotate close to 360°. However, when using the stereotactic biopsy system, the same range may not be feasible or available. Restrictions may result from mechanical constraints, or because of the patient's proximity to the unit. The body may interfere with the x-ray beam, c-arm rotation for stereo images, or with cassette placement and removal. With most add-on units, the compression arm of the stereotactic unit is independent of the host unit's compression arm and controls; thus, compression is usually manual.

Design of Stereotactic Equipment

Awareness of equipment design can ensure proper use of equipment and foster an understanding of equipment potential and limitations. The essential purpose of stereotactic breast biopsy equipment is to accurately localize and sample a breast abnormality of questionable nature. However, imaging and stereotactic properties often pose conflicting demands. The balance a unit achieves between these two sets of demands determines how efficiently the unit will perform over a wide range of patient and abnormality types. A good system addresses the issues in a way that promotes the desired end result of safe, effective, and accurate biopsies. The design of an SBB system focuses on three separate areas: imaging, stereo acquisition and localization, as discussed below.

Design Components of Imaging

Imaging needs for the SBB procedure include a *scout image*, acquired with the c-arm perpendicular to the breast support, and *multiple stereo pairs*. The key imaging requirement of a stereotactic breast biopsy system is to visualize the abnormality with sufficient clarity to distinguish it from background tissues, thereby allowing targeting, localization, and sampling with a biopsy needle. This task is quite different from the imaging requirements of mammography, which are detection and characterization. Although these differences allow some flexibility in the acceptable appearance of the abnormality for stereotactic biopsy, the biopsy procedure places unique demands on imaging design.

Mammography Versus SBB

The application of optimal technical factors in diagnostic mammography provide the image quality necessary to detect and characterize an abnormality. The design of the dedicated mammography unit takes into consideration the focal spot size, the source-image receptor distance (SID), the object-image receptor distance (OID), and other geometric factors. The technologist positions the breast on a breast support equipped with a Bucky and applies vigorous compression with optimal technical factors, using a high-resolution, high-contrast screen-film combination. Optimal film processing produces the final image to reveal the abnormality.

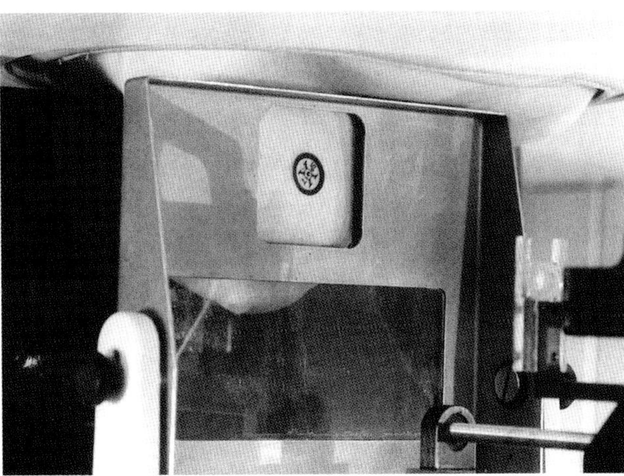

Figure 4.7. Open Biopsy Window of the SBB System. The open biopsy window reduces compression over the area of interest, thereby increasing the object-to-image receptor distance.

In contrast, the conditions of stereotactic biopsy negatively affect two image quality factors. The necessary positioning of the abnormality close to the compression surface (for safety and accuracy) and away from the image receptor increases the OID. Furthermore, SBB results in reduced compression over the area of interest (increasing the OID) due to the open biopsy window **(Figure 4.7)**. The combination of the increased OID and reduced compression *increases geometric blur and degrades visibility of detail*, thereby reducing visibility, or effectively eliminating the visualization of some abnormalities. As a result, other imaging properties become more significant in meeting the imaging requirements for the biopsy procedure. It is especially important that further image degradation be kept to a minimum, a factor with add-on units. The imaging properties of both the prone and add-on SBB systems are discussed later in this chapter in the section entitled *Geometric Considerations*.

Imaging Field

With stereotactic breast biopsy, the localized area of concern requires only a small imaging field, usually about 6 cm square (or less). Limiting the field size avoids exposure to the remaining portion of the breast and limits scatter. A digital receptor will further limit the size of the imaging field to an area of approximately 50 mm x 50 mm (see chapter 5).

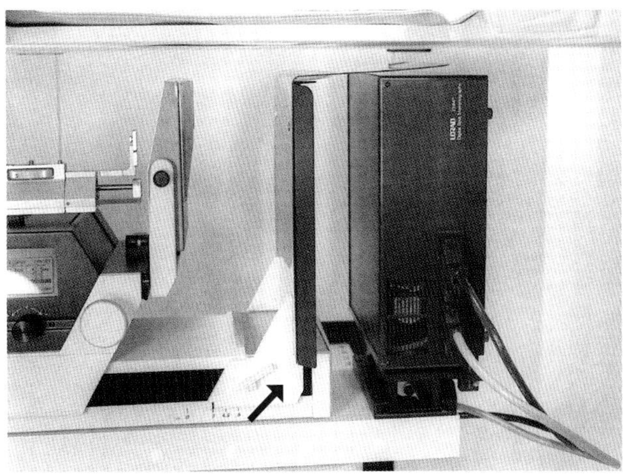

Figure 4.8. Independent Breast Support. In this design, the breast support **(arrow)** is independent of the image receptor, maintaining abnormality visualization on the stereo pair with increasing compression thickness. The independent support also provides an air gap for scatter control.

Breast Support

With some SBB units, the image receptor, or cassette tunnel, will also function as the breast support. One unit design provides an independent breast support **(Figure 4.8)**. This latter design allows for abnormality visualization with stereo shift in those breasts with increased (6 cm and up) compression thickness (see later discussion under *Shift and Visualization*).

Image Receptors

The image receptor rests at one end of the c-arm opposite the x-ray tube. The receptor can act as the breast support, or be independent of the support. The former design fixes the receptor in place, *prohibiting movement with the tube head*

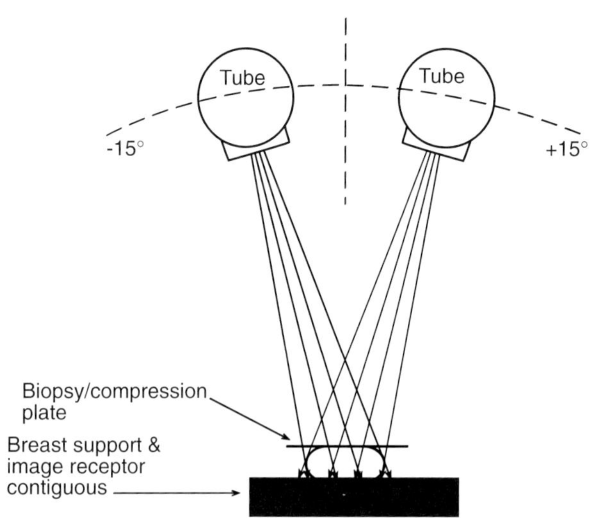

Figure 4.9. Fixed Image Receptor. The x-ray beam will form a 15° angle with stereo rotation, contributing to shape distortion and image blur.

for stereo imaging. This causes the x-ray beam to form a 15° angle with the fixed image receptor upon stereo rotation **(Figure 4.9)**, contributing to shape distortion. The beam will also traverse the image receptor at an oblique angle, contributing to image blur. This stationary design, found on some prone and all upright units, does not allow the use of a Bucky for scatter reduction.

The later design allows the image receptor to be independent of the breast support **(Figure 4.10)**, enabling the image receptor to *rotate with the tube head* upon stereo rotation. An independent receptor also allows the use of a Bucky and provides an air gap to diminish scatter. In this design, the x-ray beam remains perpendicular to the image receptor during stereo rotation. This eliminates shape distortion, minimizes geometric blur, and enhances the visibility of detail.

Conventional screen-film systems are used with SBB equipment for both prone and upright units. Digital image receptors are currently available for prone tables and some upright units (see chapter 5).

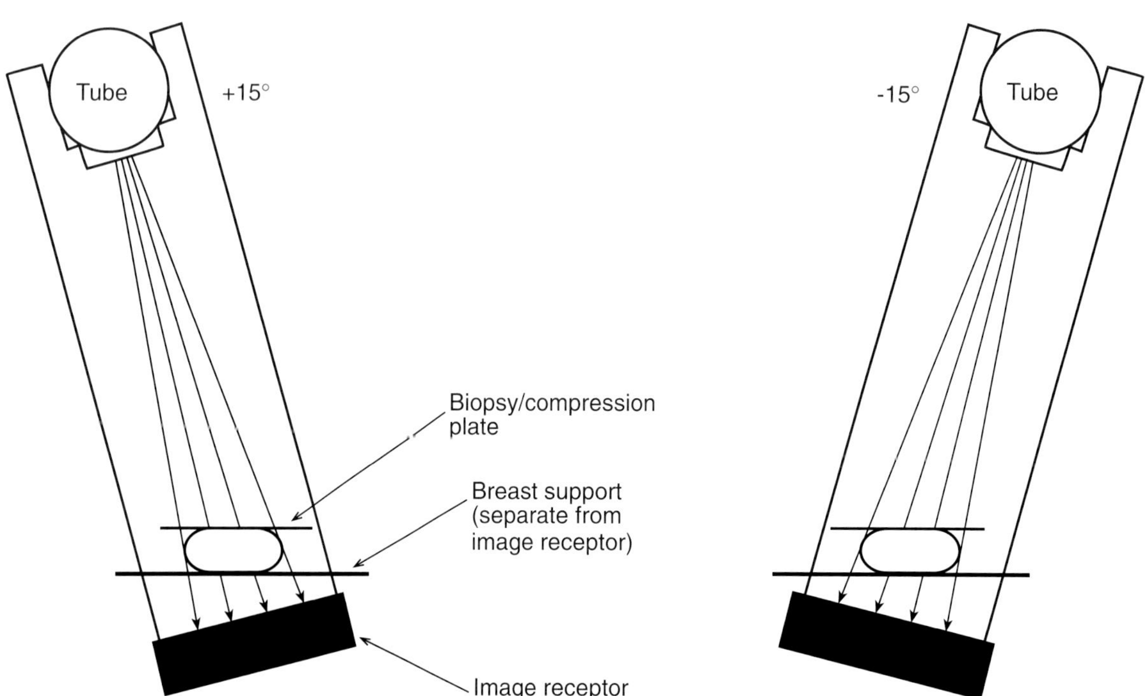

Figure 4.10. Independent Image Receptor. The x-ray beam remains perpendicular to the image receptor, prohibiting shape distortion and blur at the intensifying screen. This also allows the use of a Bucky and provides an air gap for scatter control.

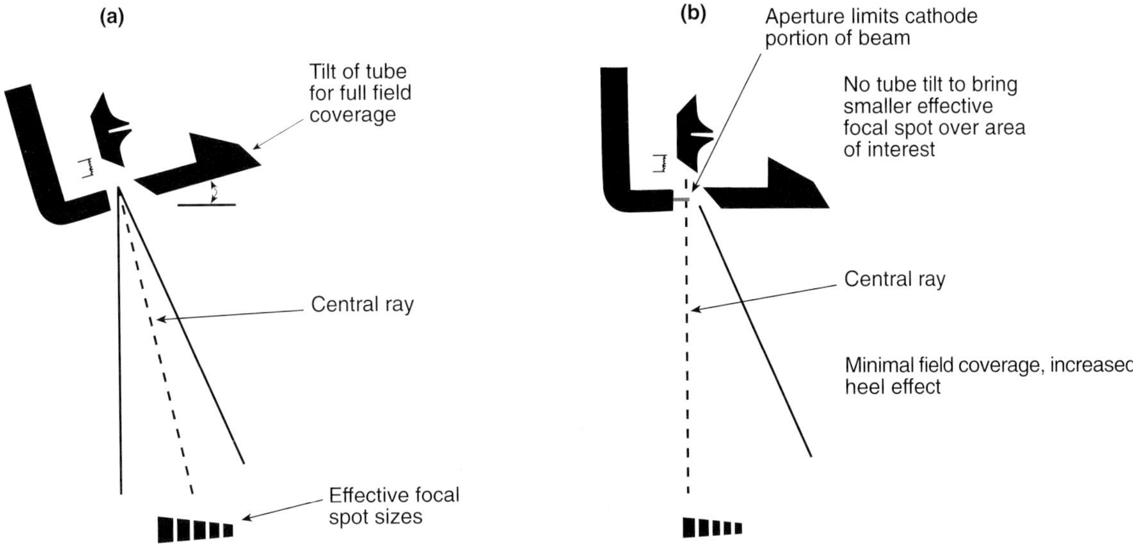

Figure 4.11a and b. X-ray Tube Tilt. For dedicated prone SBB equipment, the x-ray tube does not have to be tilted for field coverage as in routine mammography **(a)**. This allows a smaller effective focal spot over the area of interest **(b)**.

Scatter Reduction

The presence of scatter in any image will reduce subject contrast and visibility of detail. As mentioned earlier, the open biopsy window and the requirements for patient comfort for the duration of the procedure make it difficult to achieve the vigorous compression that is used to effectively reduce scatter in diagnostic mammography.

In screen-film SBB, scatter reduction is best accomplished with the use of a grid. A moving grid is preferable to a stationary grid, which produces grid lines that may interfere with the visibility of detail. However, because of grid cutoff with stereo angles, an upright system and some prone units *cannot* use a grid. In those cases, the combination of suboptimal scatter control and minimal compression may diminish the visibility of detail, resulting in the inability of the system to image some minute or low-density abnormalities.

Utilizing the air-gap technique for SBB is beneficial for conventional screen-film systems. However, in digital systems — where conventional grids are not usable due to *moiré* patterns produced from the combination of the grid lines and pixels — the air gap is an invaluable technique to reduce scatter. Although postprocessing of a digital system allows adjustment of contrast, it cannot improve the subject contrast, that is, the information content of the image in space. Providing an air gap reduces scatter and improves

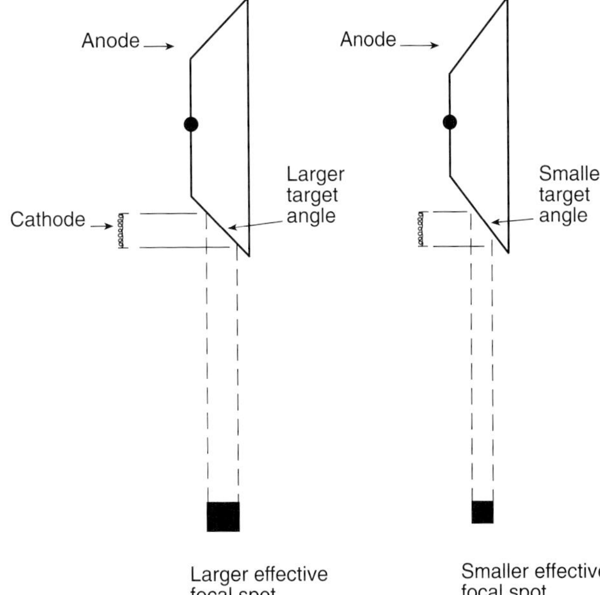

Figure 4.12. Target Angle. A smaller effective focal spot is obtainable with decreased target angle. Although this increases the heel effect, the small field in use for SBB is not affected.

image quality, as long as the increase in OID is in balance with the geometry of the unit and does not introduce objectionable geometric blur.

Geometric Considerations of Imaging

Prone units—Since the field coverage of a prone unit is designed to be limited to a small area for biopsy, the x-ray tube does not have to be tilted to provide coverage for a large field, as in routine mammography. This results in a smaller effective focal spot over the area of biopsy (**Figure 4.11**).

Smaller effective focal spot sizes are also obtainable by decreasing the target angle (**Figure 4.12**). Although this approach increases the heel effect, it will not significantly affect the biopsy field in conventional imaging systems. A digital image receptor requires the electronics of image processing to correct for nonuniformities in the x-ray beam, through a technique called "flat fielding"[1].

Increasing the SID will also reduce the effective focal spot size; however, this must be in balance with dose and exposure time to avoid motion blur. Balancing these factors minimizes the effective focal spot size without significantly increasing heat load on the target, because the actual focal spot size does not change.

Upright add-on units—Because an add-on unit has to fit into an "existing" geometry, the SID is not always optimum. In fact, the placement of the stereotactic unit above the original film plane can reduce the SID by as much as 20 cm. This diminishes the effective focal spot size and increases geometric blur. The combination of blur with suboptimal scatter control, minimal compression, and shape distortion may eliminate many abnormalities from visualization.

Design Components of Stereo Acquisition

The most important design consideration of an SBB system is its ability to provide the two perspectives that constitute the stereo pair. The stereo pair is acquired with the x-ray source at two different positions. The design of prone or upright stereotactic systems allows the c-arm to rotate independent of the breast support to provide the necessary views. The cassette tunnel or Bucky allows the shift of the cassette to prevent overlap of the stereo images with screen-film systems, whereas image overlap is not a problem with digital receptors.

Angle of Stereo Acquisition

To acquire stereo images, the x-ray tube must be capable of providing two different perspectives of the area of interest[2-4]. In most other stereoradiography, a lateral shift of the x-ray tube in the horizontal or vertical direction provides the two perspectives. As a result of this lateral shift, different portions of the x-ray beam are used to image the area of interest, possibly resulting in loss of image quality. In contrast, the design of an SBB system allows the technologist to *rotate* the x-ray tube in the horizontal axis only to achieve the two perspectives. This system feature allows the use of a more restricted beam, and maintains the smallest focal spot possible over the area of interest to maintain image quality.

The angle of acquisition for stereotactic analysis of the

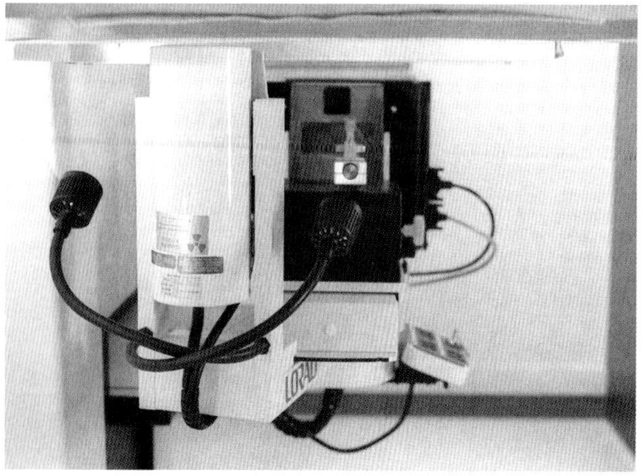

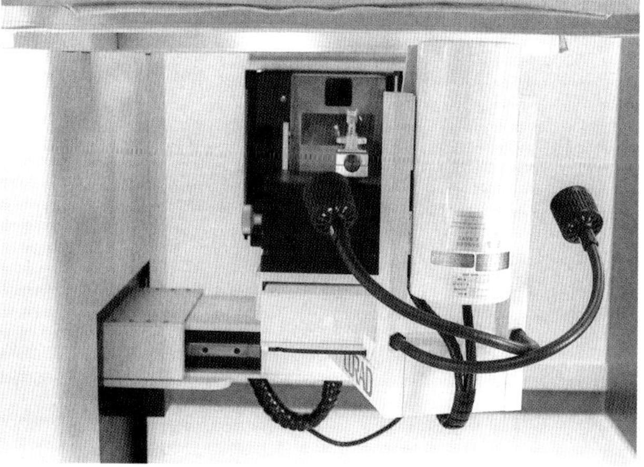

Figure 4.13. Angle of Stereo Acquisition. The angle of acquisition for stereo analysis is most often, but not exclusively, +/- 15° from the normal position of the x-ray tube. Ultimately, the degree of angle is a compromise between accuracy, identification, and logistics.

breast is most often, but not exclusively, +/- 15° from the normal position of the x-ray tube **(Figure 4.13)**. The degree of angulation is not arbitrary but a compromise between accuracy, identification, and logistics. To achieve accuracy, *the angles of stereo acquisition must be great enough to provide the most accurate depth coordinate.* The most precise approach would be to image the stereo pair 90° apart. However, this is impractical because of dose, geometric unsharpness, and other design considerations. Furthermore, the clinician must be able to identify the abnormality on both stereo images to target it for localization.

The greater the stereo angle, the more difficult it will be to maintain identification of the target abnormality. Ideally, the smallest shift from normal would be best. However, accuracy requires a compromise with identification because the accuracy of the depth calculation decreases as the angle diminishes[5,6]. Finally, the logistics of space and practicality for tube rotation require the angle to be kept to a minimum. *Angles of +/- 15° provide 1 millimeter precision in coordinate determination,* without excessively altering the projection of the abnormality.

With add-on units (where the breast support of the SBB system is separate from the original c-arm configuration of the mammographic unit), the rotational pivot point of the c-arm defines the angle of the x-ray beam relative to the breast support of the stereo unit. For example, if the pivot of the c-arm is not isocentric, then the angle of the c-arm may be +/- 22° for stereo acquisition. However, the incident angle at the breast support of the stereo unit is still +/- 15°. Another scenario may have the angle of the c-arm at 15°, but the incident angle at the breast support may be less, having an impact on the accuracy of the depth coordinate.

Shift and Visualization

In most cases, the abnormality will shift from its original scout position in the imaging field on both stereo images (see chapter 2). Maintaining visualization with increasing compression thickness can be a problem if the system design for stereo acquisition does not adjust for shift and compression thickness. Shift and nonvisualization are especially critical with the current field size of digital receptors (50 mm x 50 mm). Suboptimal design of the beam-limiting device **(Figure 4.14)** and the breast support contribute to nonvisualization.

Nonvisualization occurs with greater breast thickness, usually 6 cm and up, depending on the geometry of the unit and the depth of the abnormality. An adjustable breast support, independent of the image receptor, can accommodate varying breast thicknesses **(Figure 4.15)** when utilizing a digital receptor.

Nonvisualization is more likely to occur if an SBB system permits the more proximal abnormality (closer to the compression plate) to shift a greater distance than a distal abnormality (closer to the breast support); see chapter 2. This becomes more problematic if the unit does not have an adjustable breast support. If both planar images do not demonstrate the abnormality, or the same portion of the abnormality, then accurate targeting is not possible.

Allowable Compression Widths

The short distance between the tube head and breast support of some add-on units may limit the vertical distance of the compression arm. This constraint limits patient acceptance based on breast thickness.

Design Components of Localization

In addition to the stereo images, the SBB equipment must provide for localization of the abnormality. An SBB system uses a computer system to perform this critical function. The computer system must have a user interface that facilitates identification and targeting of the abnormality for three-dimensional coordinate determination. In addition to the stereo pair, the necessary components for three-dimensional localization include:

- Reference point(s)
- Targeting device
- Computer

The Reference

The equipment manufacturer determines the location of the reference point(s) to calculate coordinates. The method of display of the stereo pair, and shift of the abnormality in relation to this reference, will determine the exact three-dimensional position to within 1 mm. For some units, the location of the reference is on the biopsy/compression plate, proximal to the compressed breast. Other manufacturers locate the reference point(s) on the breast support, distal to the compressed breast. This reference is part of the stereo pair, even if it is absent on the resultant images (in some digital units the references are an inherent part of the algorithm for localization). Knowledge of the location of the reference point(s) is helpful to correlate with the given calculated coordinates (see chapter 2).

Coordinate Calculation Device

A computer performs coordinate calculation. In screen-film systems, a back-lighted digitizing tablet **(Figure 4.16)** and a mouse with a targeting device electronically record the

(a)

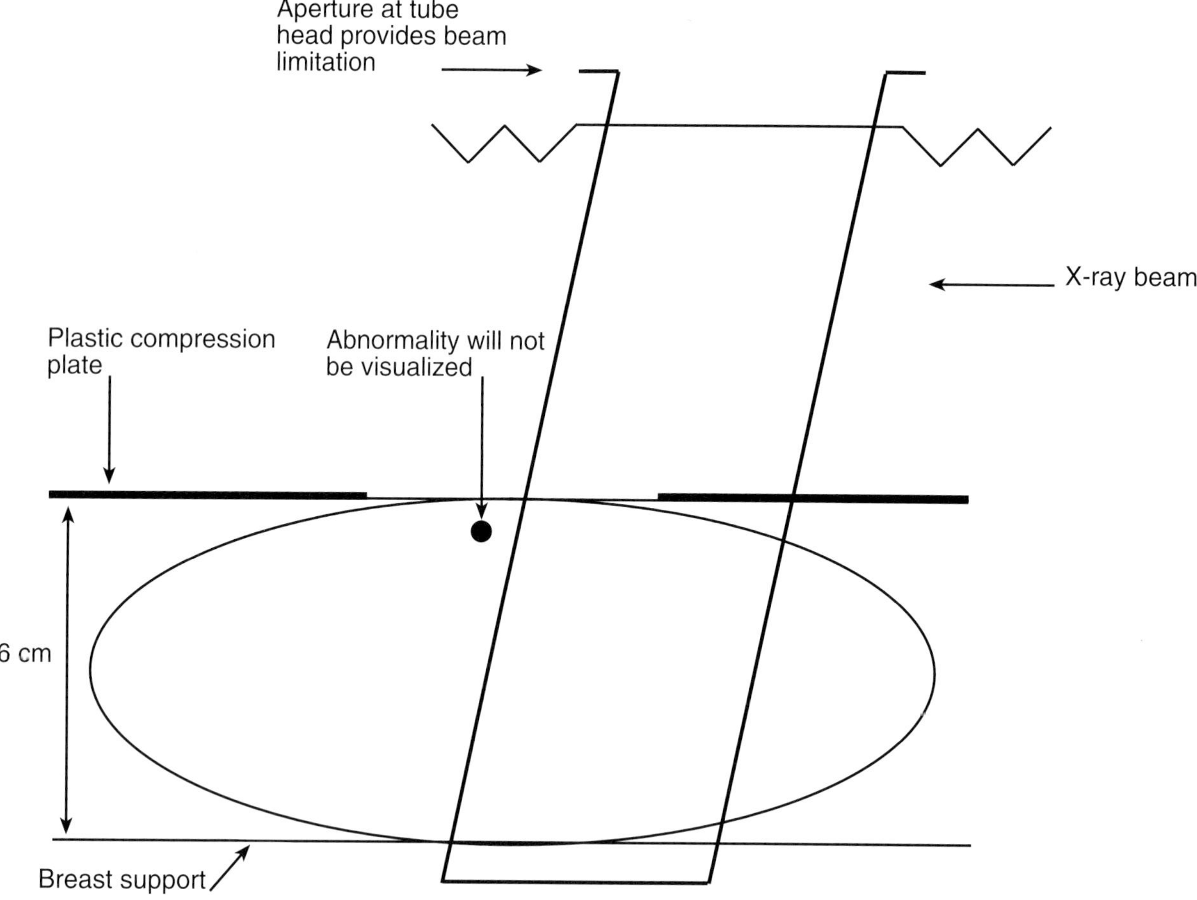

Figure 4.14 a and b. Beam Limitation and Visualization with Stereo Shift. When beam limitation occurs at the tube head **(a)**, the imaging area decreases as breast thickness increases. This design may eliminate the more proximal abnormality from the imaging field with increasing breast thickness. Beam limitation at the biopsy/compression plate **(b)** provides a wider imaging field at the proximal surface, which will maintain visualization (in most cases) with increasing breast thickness.

(b)

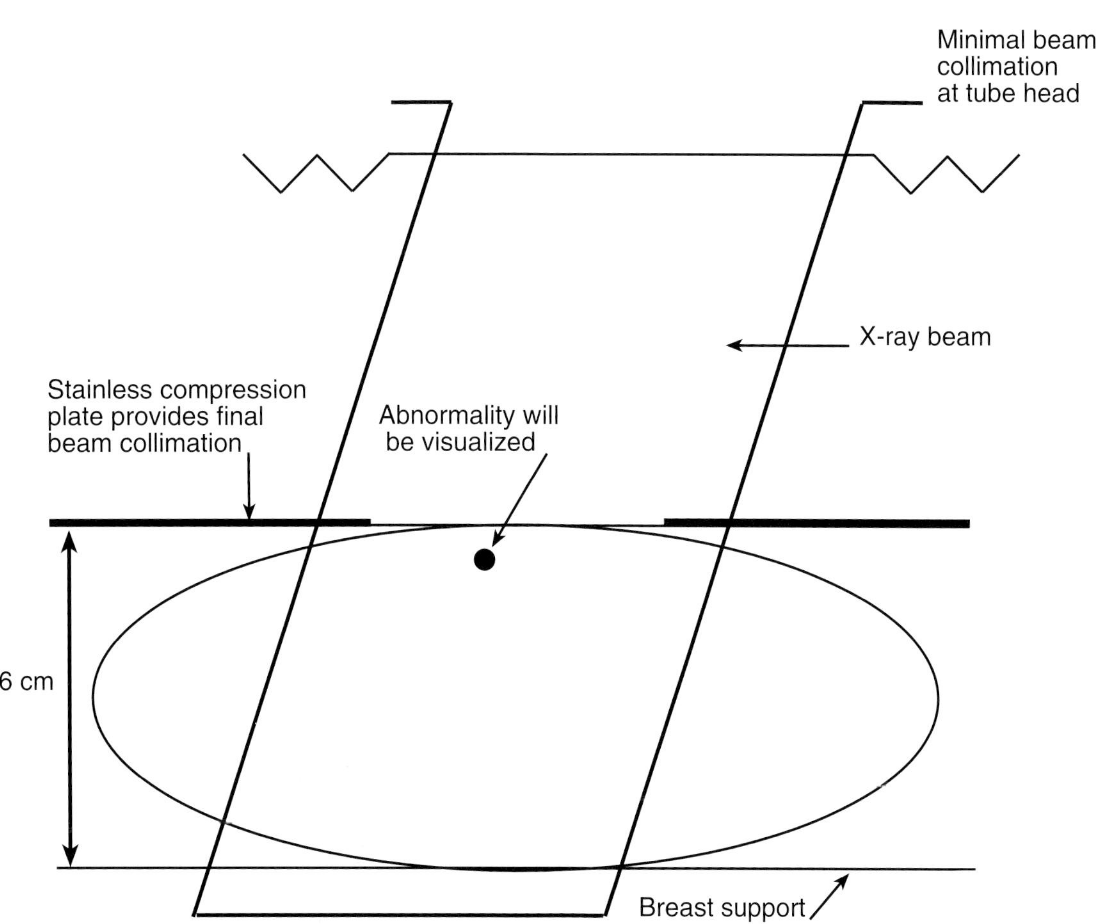
Minimal beam
collimation
at tube head
X-ray beam
Stainless compression
plate provides final
beam collimation
Abnormality will
be visualized
6 cm
Breast support

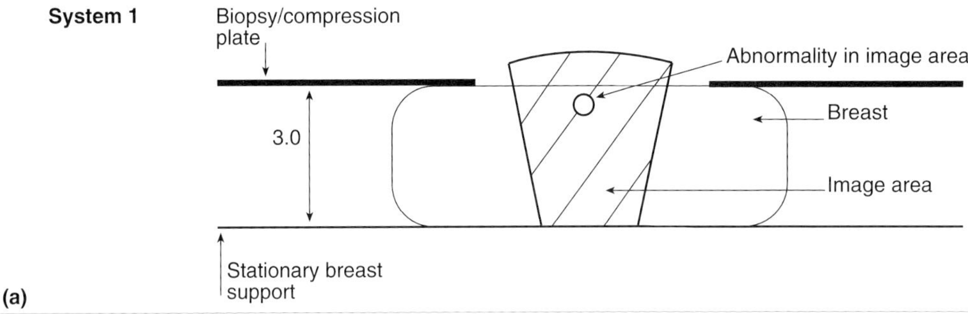

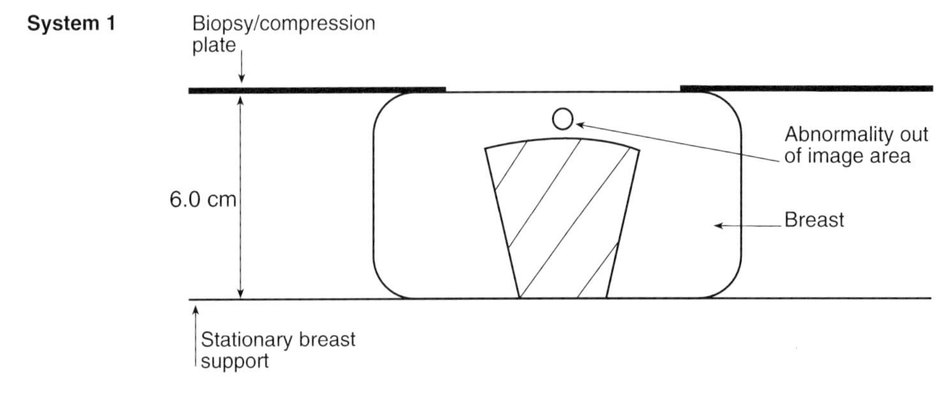

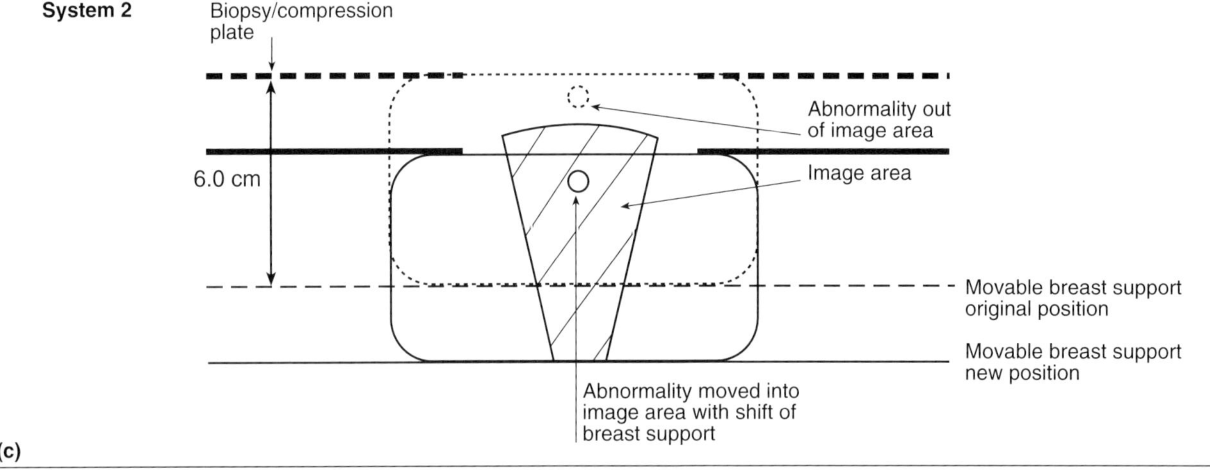

Figure 4.15. Adjustable Breast Support and Visualization with Increasing Breast Thickness. In System 1**(a)**, with a stationary breast support, abnormality visualization is possible with thinner (less than approx. 6 cm) compression; however, with greater compression widths **(b)**, the abnormality is outside the field of view. In System 2, with a movable breast support **(c)**, visualization of the abnormality is maintained by moving the breast support, thereby moving the abnormality into the field of view.

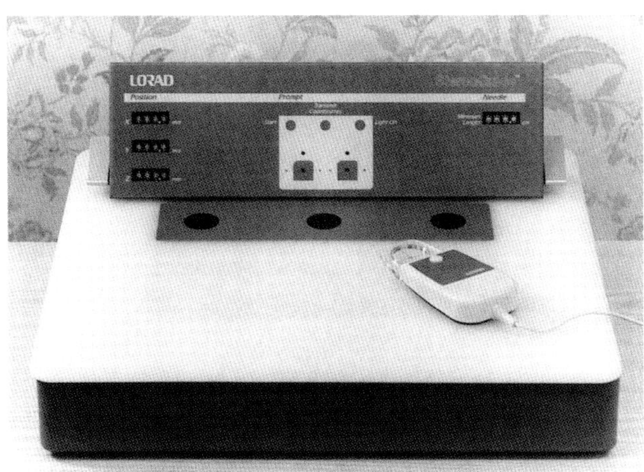

Figure 4.16. Digitizing Tablet. A back-lighted digitizing tablet and a targeting "mouse" provide the means for coordinate calculation with screen-film systems.

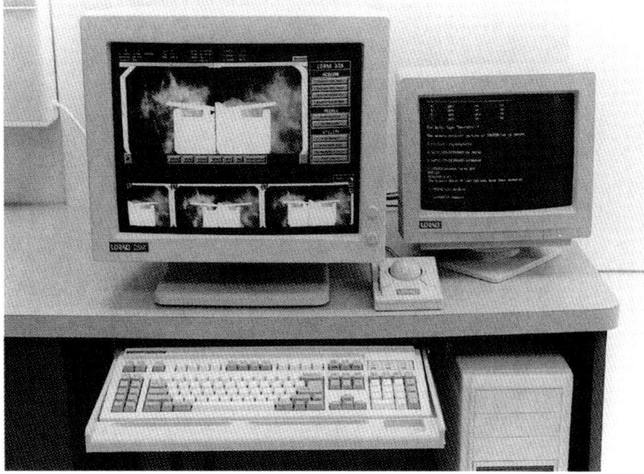

Figure 4.17. Targeting with a Digital System. When using a digital system, the trackball and monitor allow the user to target the abnormality on both stereo images.

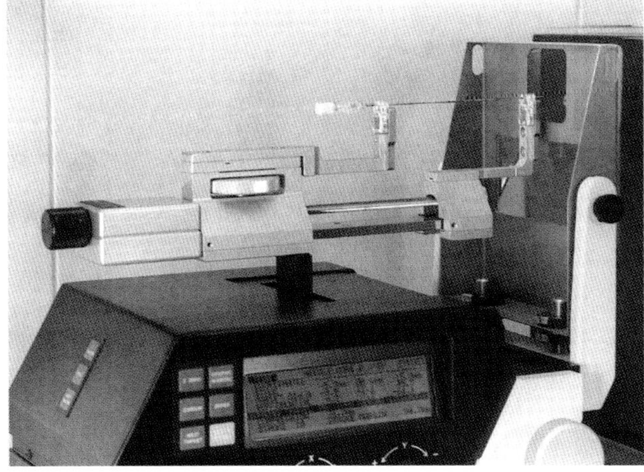

Figure 4.18. Needle Guide Arm and Needle Guides. Needle guide mounting arms provide support for the needle guides, which maintain accurate needle placement.

selected points for abnormality localization. With a digital image receptor, the system computer provides the means for targeting the abnormality. A trackball moves a cursor on the monitor, allowing the user to mark the reference point(s) and target the abnormality on both stereo images **(Figure 4.17)**. The system should include software that maintains sequencing of target points to ensure accuracy. Targeting and calculations (excluding the identification of the abnormality) should take no more than a few seconds. The electronic transfer of coordinates to the needle guidance system is available on some units to ensure accurate coordinate transfer. The computer or microprocessor may also determine minimum needle length in the case of fine needle aspiration or needle localization.

Needle Guidance System

The needle guidance system includes:

- Depth axis that provides mounting for the biopsy instrument and needles
- Coordinate markings, or LCD panel read-outs
- Manual or motorized guidance of coordinate controls
- Needle guide arms/needle guides
- Mounts for the biopsy instrument and needles

The needle guidance system maintains stability and accuracy for needle placement. A permanently fixed system, rather than a removable system, provides for accuracy and efficiency. Needle guide mounting arms provide support for the needle guides and should be easy to install. Needle guides fit onto the mounting arms to provide accurate needle movement into the breast **(Figure 4.18)**. The needle guides should be stable but easy to remove with unexpected patient movement **(Figure 4.19)**, restricting the amount of injury to the breast. A detachable cradle or holder for the biopsy instrument secures the gun in place to prevent movement when firing **(Figure 4.20)**.

The needle guidance system provides readily visible coordinate markings, or digital read-outs, **(Figure 4.21)** that illustrate the horizontal (X or H), vertical (Y or V), and depth

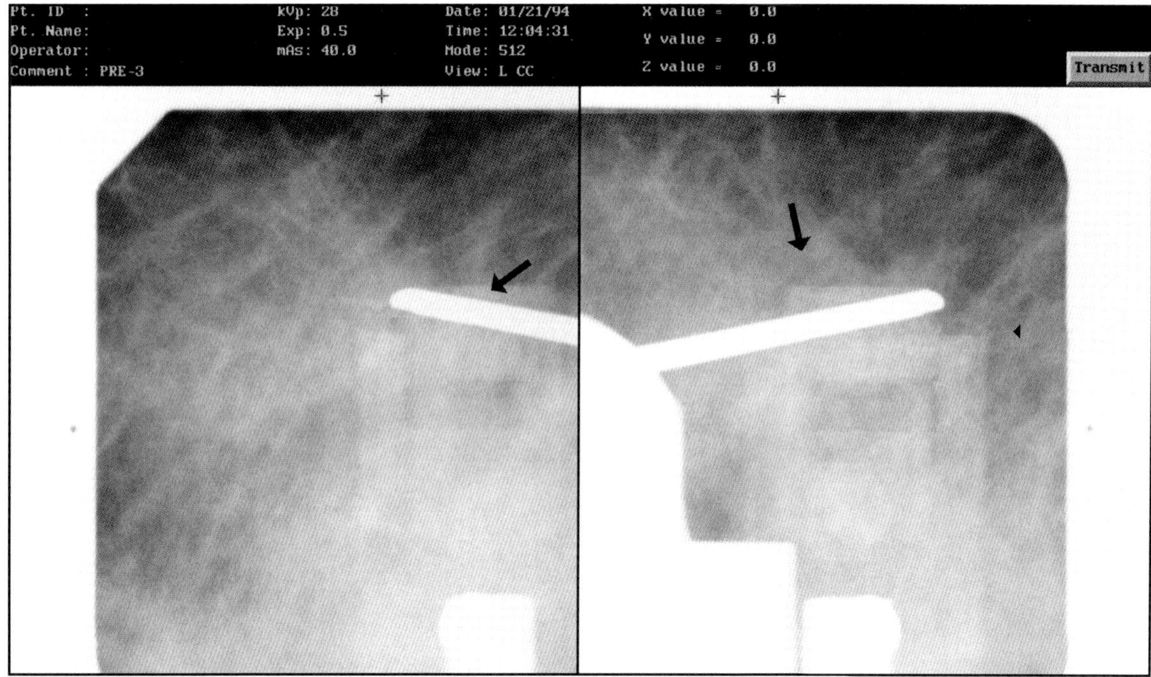

Figure 4.19. Removable Needle Guide. Despite restraint, this patient moved upwards off the table, pulling on the biopsy system. Injury to her breast was minimal because the needle guide "popped off," as demonstrated on these stereo images **(arrows)**, preventing the tearing of skin and breast tissue. The needle guides are normally seated evenly with the holder **(arrowhead)**.

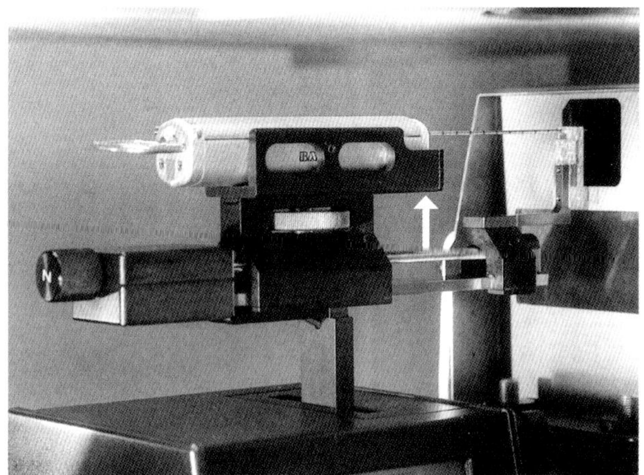

Figure 4.20. Biopsy Instrument Holder. A detachable cradle or holder **(arrow)** secures the gun in place to prevent movement upon firing.

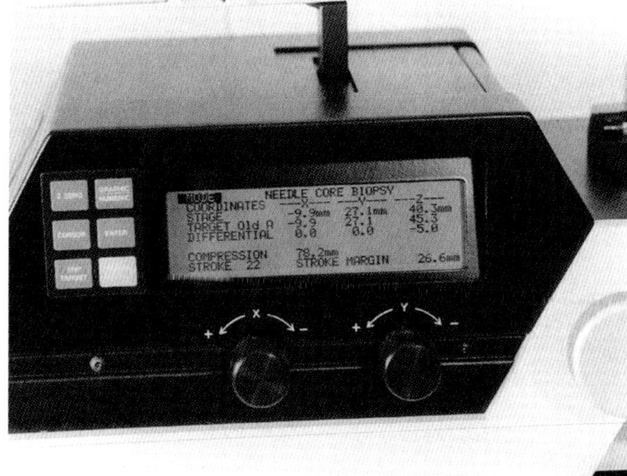

Figure 4.21. LCD Display. An LCD display, or similar display, shows the coordinates of the target abnormality and the position of the stage.

coordinates (Z or D). Rotating coordinate controls allow smooth and accurate movement of the guidance system to the abnormality position. This is especially useful for the depth coordinate. A rotating control will allow steady, consistent pressure for needle insertion.

Motorized Versus Nonmotorized Guidance Systems

Motorized movement of the needle guidance system assists the clinician in the biopsy process. While automation is a desirable feature, it is not a prerequisite to perform biopsy. It is important, however, to also have manual control over the needle guidance stage. The nonuniformity of breast tissue and the instability of abnormalities create opportunities for abnormality movement. Correcting errors is a simple task if the guidance system has a manual adjustment. In fact, it can prevent the reacquisition of stereo images, thereby decreasing exam time and reducing patient exposure. A motorized device should move the needle in the horizontal (X) and vertical (Y) directions only. A fail-safe device to prevent further horizontal and vertical needle movement, once the needle has entered the skin surface, will add to the unit's safety.

Needle Calibration and Stroke Margin

The guidance stage and computer should provide for the calibration of needle length or needle/biopsy instrument length. Automated calculation of stroke margin should be inherent in the system. Visual indicators or audible alarms that indicate available space for needle excursion are also extremely helpful to the biopsy team.

Selection of Equipment

Choosing equipment with knowledge of its capabilities and limitations is crucial to the success of a breast biopsy program. The equipment should provide the means to perform needle biopsy efficiently and accurately. Ideally, the unit should be capable of performing the procedure on a wide range of patients and abnormalities, with minimal restrictions. The unit should also be comfortable for patient and convenient for operators.

The first equipment decision involves the selection of a prone or upright unit. Cost is usually the most influential factor. A prone system is about twice the cost of an upright unit (for an already existing mammography unit). Space allowance is a secondary consideration. Unlike an add-on unit, a prone unit requires its own suite. Although cost and space are important considerations, decision makers should consider all the ramifications associated with equipment selection.

For example, the prone table is designed solely to perform needle biopsy. In contrast, the combination of an add-on device with the existing mammography unit does not always provide the best biopsy environment, which may limit patient acceptance for SBB and thereby affect the success of the biopsy program. This is not to say that add-on equipment cannot be used successfully[7]. Ultimately, the biopsy team must weigh program goals and equipment features and benefits against the financial investment. The biopsy team should consider the following significant issues:

- Patient tolerance
- Patient acceptance
- Stereotactic properties
- Accuracy
- Digital image receptors
- Patient safety
- Operator access
- Proficiency, ease-of-use, and time
- Service

Patient Tolerance

The breast biopsy program will meet greater success with greater patient tolerance of the procedure. This can be enhanced with an equipment design that provides maximum patient comfort. Comfort translates to the patient's ability to remain immobile for the required time, a critical issue for successful procedures. Comfort will also enhance the patient's perception of a successful procedure. Comfort, however, is not simply a matter of patient convenience, but a significant quality of care issue. The decision to use add-on equipment over prone equipment should be based on numerous considerations, as described below.

The breast must be immobile during the entire procedure, which can be as brief as 20 minutes or as long as an hour or more. If the patient moves even a few millimeters at any time after obtaining the initial stereo images, it may be necessary to retake the stereo images, retarget, and/or reposition, and repeat all subsequent steps. This can add considerable time to the procedure, and additional fatigue, which in turn reduces the patient's ability to remain motionless.

If the patient can see the needle and apparatus, fear-induced vaso-vagal reactions and vaso-vagal syncope become an additional issue in maintaining immobility[8]. Patient motion, vaso-vagal reactions, and vaso-vagal syncope may complicate or terminate the procedure. Thus, diagnostic mammography units equipped with add-on devices are at a distinct disadvantage. The patient is upright, or semi-recumbent, and self-supporting, all of which contribute to fatigue and motion. She may have full view of the needle guidance apparatus, which can lead to anxiety and fear and therefore vaso-vagal reaction or vaso-vagal syncope. Add-on units may also limit available approaches to the breast, resulting in awkward positions that contribute to patient discomfort and motion.

The recumbent position made possible by dedicated prone biopsy units eliminates the need for self-support. Furthermore, the patient does not have direct view of the biopsy needle and apparatus. These attributes have a positive influence on the patient's ability to remain immobile, thereby reducing procedure time. In addition, vaso-vagal reactions and vaso-vagal syncope are unusual in the recumbent position[8]. For these reasons, the prone system allows the biopsy team to focus on completing the exam expediently.

Patient Acceptance

The stereotactic unit should provide for a wide range of patient and abnormality types, allowing for the greatest latitude in patient acceptance. Although 100% acceptance is not possible with any unit, the equipment should not be the limiting factor in the majority of cases.

Body Habitus

The unit should be capable of comfortably supporting patients of any body habitus, including those who are tall or obese. Prone tables have a recommended weight limit of 300 pounds. Upright units have no weight restrictions, however, patient proximity to the unit may eliminate access to the abnormality. For prone positioning, the patient must also be able to lie recumbent for the required period of time. Patients with severe arthritis or back trouble may be unable to hold a prone position for any length of time and may be more tolerant to an upright position.

Abnormality Access

The design of the patient support and c-arm apparatus should allow access to all areas of the breast, including posterior and inferior abnormalities and those in the axilla. In some cases, the breast abnormality can be accessed in the mammographic projection in which it was optimally visualized. Alternatively, other projections have to be available to provide a better approach when necessary. Preferably, the equipment should allow for continuous 360° access around the breast to facilitate biopsy from any approach. The 360° approach not only allows access to 6:00 abnormalities, but also provides many other inferior approaches to the breast. Continuous 360° rotation is also advantageous in maximizing access to posterior and chest wall abnormalities (see chapter 6).

Visibility of the Abnormality

As explained earlier in the design section, a number of important technical factors are necessary to successfully image a wide range of abnormalities. Add-on units have significant technical limitations, especially for low-density masses and microcalcifications. This is primarily due to the absence of a Bucky and increased geometric distortion. Furthermore, visibility of an abnormality must be maintained in both the scout and stereo images. Nonvisualization is not only a function of technical factors but also a consequence of overlapping structures. Superimposition of structures on either stereo image can obscure the breast abnormality and prohibit targeting. Thus, the unit should provide a wide range of approaches to better position the abnormality free of superimposition (see chapter 6).

Stroke Margin

Patient acceptance for core biopsy depends on breast positioning that provides adequate positive stroke margin. A system with continous 360° access provides the widest range of biopsy approaches, increasing the number of patients who can undergo this procedure.

Compression Thickness

The stereotactic unit should be suitable for all breast sizes. Upright units may have limitations regarding the possible range of breast thickness that the system design can accommodate between the compression plate and the breast support. In addition, with greater compression thickness, the geometry of some upright and prone units may allow an abnormality to shift outside the field of view of the image receptor. This type of design will inhibit visualization on one or both stereo images, possibly eliminating these patients from stereotactic biopsy.

Stereotactic Properties

The angle of stereo acquisition and abnormality visualization with stereo shift are critical issues. How well the unit functions in this respect will determine accuracy and patient acceptance.

Accuracy

While theoretically there is no difference in accuracy between prone and upright equipment, issues of accuracy can arise as a result of other contributing factors, such as patient stability. The removal and placement of the stereotactic device can also contribute to inaccuracy with add-on units.

Both Cartesian and polar coordinate systems are utilized in SBB (see chapter 2). No scientific proof exists that demonstrates that one coordinate system is more accurate than the other.

Digital Image Receptors

Early acceptance of stereotactic core biopsy met resistance because of the duration of the SBB procedure. The use of conventional screen-film imaging systems adds a minimum of fifteen minutes of processing time to the 30-45 minutes of procedure time. Exam duration could also increase to as much as 90 minutes or more because of extended processing, multiple scouts, and repeat stereo images resulting from procedural difficulties. This not only limits the number of patients who can tolerate the exam, it also prohibits some sites from using this modality due to time and cost per procedure. Digital imaging provides near real-time imaging, producing images in 4-16 seconds.

In addition, digital systems provide postacquisition image manipulation, allowing for enhanced contrast discrimination over a wide range of exposures. A reduction in dose and overall procedural cost may also be realized in most cases[9].

The use of a digital system in conjunction with an add-on unit can make this equipment more attractive, as it reduces the procedure time, thereby decreasing some of the undesirable effects that result from fatigue and motion. A digital system may also enhance image quality for these systems.

The image quality of a digital receptor system is also important. The elements defining the image quality of a digital system are discussed in chapter 5.

System speed is another important consideration, especially access to image processing after acquiring the image. Ideally, image manipulation, such as window, level, and edge enhancement should be instantaneous.

The archiving of images should not require a great amount of time. An *auto save* from the random access memory (RAM) to the hard drive, automatic down-loading to optical disk, and automatic "dumping" from the hard drive to create space all save procedural time, as well as the time spent to archive poststudy images.

Patient Safety

The stereotactic unit should provide for maximum patient safety. Specifically, determining stroke margin should be an inherent part of the unit's calculations. Very few upright units have this feature, requiring manual calculation of the stroke margin.

Prone tables should provide adjustable table heights that allow the patient to get on and off the table safely. The stability of the patient in the recumbent position should also be a prerequisite in the design of the biopsy table.

Motorized devices that control the needle guidance system should have a built in fail-safe that prohibits motorized movement once the needle has advanced through the skin into the breast. Without this fail-safe, it is possible to injure the breast if the motorized device accidentally moves the needle once it has passed through the skin.

With the angulation of polar coordinate systems, it is possible that the needle can move beyond the imaging field. This is most likely to occur after the excursion of the biopsy needle, as seen on postfire images. The clinician has little reassurance that the needle has remained within the confines of the breast. This may be a critical issue with extremely posterior abnormalities that are close to the chest wall.

Operator Access

SBB equipment should provide for the comfort and convenience of system operators. The clinician and technologist should have ample space and access to the breast, the biopsy instrument, and the needle transport system. Dedicated prone biopsy units offer significant advantages over upright units, as upright units allow limited space between the stereo apparatus and the x-ray tube head. Positioning of the breast must also permit easy access by the biopsy team. While visualization of the abnormality may be possible using a particular projection, the same projection may limit the biopsy team's working space, restricting the number of approaches for biopsy.

For prone units, the technologist should have visual contact and fingertip control of the table or c-arm controls **(Figure 4.22)**. Controls should be accessible, easy to use, and out of patient reach.

Positioning requires the technologist to accurately center the abnormality in the biopsy window. The unit should provide for gross as well as fine movement of the patient's breast. Prone units provide this flexibility of movement with a panning c-arm apparatus, or floating table support. However, the technologist will have more control over movement with a movable c-arm apparatus than with a floating table design. In a floating table design, the table carries the patient weight, making small adjustments difficult. Upright units require the technologist to move the patient to appropriately center the abnormality for imaging. Motorized foot control for compression, available on most prone systems, allows the technologist to have both hands free for positioning. This feature allows the technologist to make minor centering adjustments while holding the breast in place.

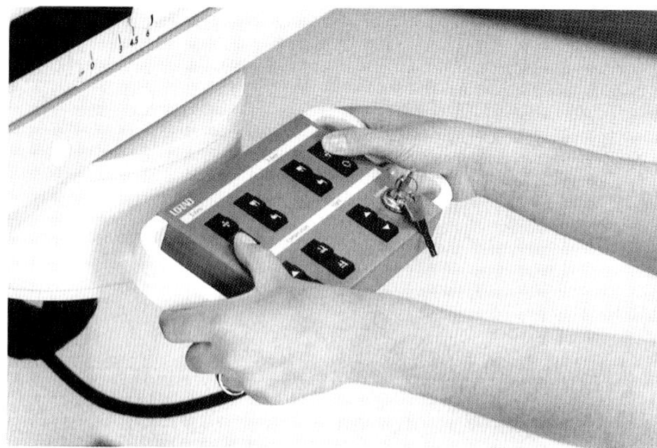

Figure 4.22. Table Controls. Fingertip controls allow for smooth movement of the table or c-arm for positioning.

Proficiency, Ease-of-Use, and Time Investment

Besides the technical differences between the prone and upright units, proficiency is a critical issue The ease with which the biopsy team can utilize a modality is an important factor in equipment choice and its ultimate usefulness. In terms of proficiency and ease-of-use, dedicated prone biopsy tables provide advantages over the upright add-on units. Using an upright unit is more labor intensive for the technologist. Because the patient is sitting, the technologist must physically move her, rather than adjust the equipment. Equipment must also be applied and removed as needed.

Upright units are often chosen over prone tables based on the assumption that there will be a small number of biopsies. While upright equipment costs less, it is more time consuming to use, more labor intensive, and requires more manual steps. Furthermore, with low volumes, the team is less likely to be comfortable with the equipment and the tasks associated with the procedure. Low volumes would lessen the desire to use the equipment, especially those cases that are perceived to be other than just "average," which would narrow patient acceptance.

The investment in time required by the technologist and clinician to perform procedures is critical to weigh against the initial investment. If the equipment adds an excessive amount of time to complete the procedure, it will most certainly be used less. Upright units entail more time in equipment setup, patient positioning, and execution of the procedure — usually one hour (minimum) to 90 minutes or more. Prone units require a minimum of one half-hour to one hour or more. The use of a digital receptor with prone or add-on units also reduces procedural time, thereby increasing system use.

The use of upright units also affects the normal mammography schedule. Even with appropriate scheduling for stereotactic work, complications that increase procedural time are difficult to predict consistently in advance.

Service

Service is a significant issue in equipment purchase. If a malfunction occurs that requires service, it is important to know that service will be timely. The proximity of experienced service engineers, their service territory, and back-up plans are important service considerations.

References

1. Roehrig, H., Fajardo, L., Yu, T. 1993. Digital X-ray Cameras for Real-time Stereotactic Breast Needle Biopsy. *Physics of Medical Imaging* SPIE Volume 1896:213-224.

2. Nordenstrom, B. 1975. New Instrument for Biopsy. *Radiology* 17:474.

3. Bolmgren, J., Jacobson, B., Nordenstrom, B. 1977. Stereotactic Instrument for Needle Biopsy of the Mamma. *American Journal Roentgenology*.

4. Nordenstrom, B., Zajicek, J. 1977. Stereotaxic Needle Biopsy and Preoperative Indication of Non-palpable Mammary Lesions. *Acta Cytologica*.

5. Price, J.L. and Butler, P.D. 1971. Stereoscopic Measurement in Mammography. *British Journal of Radiology* 901.

6. Chen, H., Bernstein, J., Paige, M., Cramptom, A. 1989. Needle Localization of Non-palpable Breast Lesions with a Portable Dual-Grid Compression System. *Radiology* 170:687-690.

7. Fajardo, L.L. 1990. Stereotactic Breast Biopsy with Add-on Units, In Parker, S.H. & Jobe, W.E. *Percutaneous Breast Biopsy* New York: Raven Press.

8. Helvie, M., Ikeda, D., Adler, D. 1991. Localization and Needle Aspiration of Breast Lesions: Complications in 370 Cases. *American Journal of Roentgenology* (October) 157.

9. Dershaw, D.D., Fleischman, R.C., Liberman, L., Deutch, B., Abramson, A.F., Hann, L. 1993. Use of Digital Mammography in Needle Localization. *American Journal of Roentgenology* 161:559-562.

Digital Imaging: Elements and Application for Stereotactic Biopsy

Kathleen M. Willison
Richard Van Metter, Ph.D.

5

Introduction

Digital imaging is not new to radiology[1], however, its clinical use in imaging the breast is relatively recent. Currently, there are two types of digital systems in use for breast imaging[2-6]. One technology acquires an image conventionally using *screen-film image receptors*, then digitizes the information through scanning methods. The second type uses a digital image receptor to acquire the image electronically. Stereotactic breast biopsy utilizes the latter method.

For most mammographers, stereotactic breast biopsy may be the first contact with a digital modality. The imaging chain and the imaging characteristics of electronic acquisition are significantly different from conventional systems to warrant a description and explanation of this modality. This chapter will focus on *electronic acquisition* and discuss the components and characteristics of digital imaging and its application in stereotactic breast biopsy procedures.

Currently, the field of view for direct electronic acquisition in breast imaging is approximately 50 mm x 50 mm (see later discussion of CCDs). In the meantime, ongoing research and development is seeking solutions that apply electronic acquisition to full field diagnostic imaging as a tool for detection, characterization, and diagnosis of breast abnormalities. However, such capabilities are not yet adequate for clinical applications[2,7,8]. But as a tool to *identify* previously detected, characterized abnormalities, electronic acquisition has superior qualities for the purpose of stereotactic localization and biopsy that make it an effective alternative to conventional screen-film imaging systems. The field of view currently possible with electronic acquisition rarely limits the biopsy team when examining the small region of the breast required for biopsy.

Definition of Terms

Before discussing the digital imaging chain and its characteristics, it is helpful to understand the following terms and their role in digital image quality.

Signal

We define signal as the useful information coming into the imaging system carried by the modulation of exposure caused by the patient (**Figure 5.1**). Signal increases in proportion to the amount of exposure to an anatomical part. This signal propagates through each stage of the imaging chain and is finally displayed. Signal can be lost or distorted at each step of the digital imaging chain. A digital imaging system may have excellent spatial and contrast resolution capabilities but if there is insufficient signal emerging from the imaging chain, image quality may be inadequate.

Noise

Image noise obstructs our ability to "see" faint signals. Noise appears as random variations in the displayed image that are *unrelated* to, not a result of, patient anatomy. There are several sources of noise. One fundamental source of noise is *quantum mottle* caused by random variation of the finite number of x-rays used to take an image; this noise is proportional to the square root of the exposure. Other sources of noise include the intensifying screen, the CCD, the display monitor, and intervening electronics.

Signal-to-Noise Ratio

Signal-to-noise ratio (SNR) describes the amount of useful information captured by an imaging system compared with

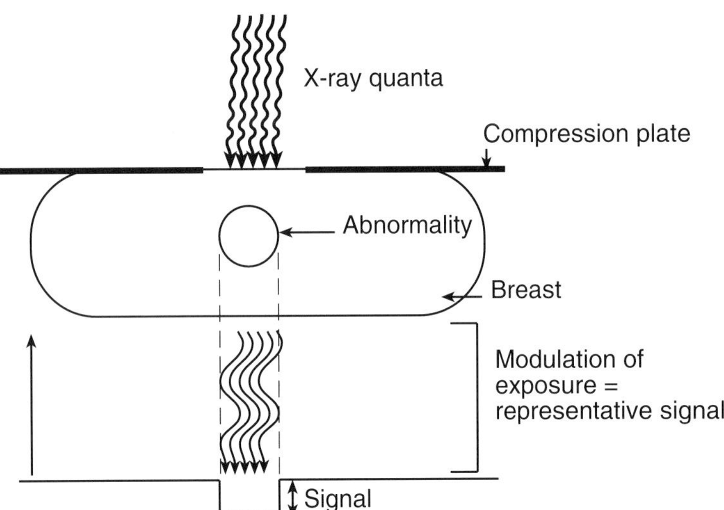

Figure 5.1. Modulation and Signal. The x-ray beam is attenuated by changes corresponding to the anatomy with which it interacts. This *modulation* results in representative signal.

the level of noise. Signal-to-noise ratio generally increases with increasing exposure. *Greater* signal-to-noise ratio allows improvement in the ability to visualize small faint signals. As a result of postacquisition image manipulation (see later discussion), digital systems do not depend on a preset exposure range, rather, *signal-to-noise ratio is a determining factor in abnormality visualization* **(Figure 5.2)**.

Characteristics of a Digital Receptor

Procedural Time

Perhaps the greatest advantage of digital imaging for stereotactic localization and biopsy is near real-time imaging for abnormality positioning and needle placement. When compared with conventional imaging methods, the digital modality reduces total procedure time by one-half, producing images within *4-16 seconds*, rather than the 2-3 minutes of processing time per film necessary for conventional imaging methods.

Improved Imaging Environment

A digital receptor generally provides a more optimal environment than conventional systems to record, store, and display images. The most distinguishing feature of the digital system is the capture or detection of an image *separate* from display, providing a wide range of features beneficial to stereotactic breast biopsy.

Flexible Exposure Range

With conventional methods, the characteristics of a screen-film system limit the usable density range to a portion of the D log E curve. For mammography, the most useful optical density range is about 1.05-1.6. If the density falls outside this range, there may be little or no usable image, as discrimination of adjacent structures is greatly hindered. A digital imaging system provides good imaging efficiency over a wide range of exposures, *relying on exposure to provide adequate signal-to-noise ratio, rather than a preset optical density range* **(Figure 5.3)**. The digital recording device is sensitive to minute changes in x-ray absorption over a wide range of exposures, providing abnormality visualization even at reduced exposures. For SBB, technique and dose can be reduced, if the reduced exposure provides adequate visualization of the abnormality.

Linear Response

Unlike a conventional screen-film system whose exposure

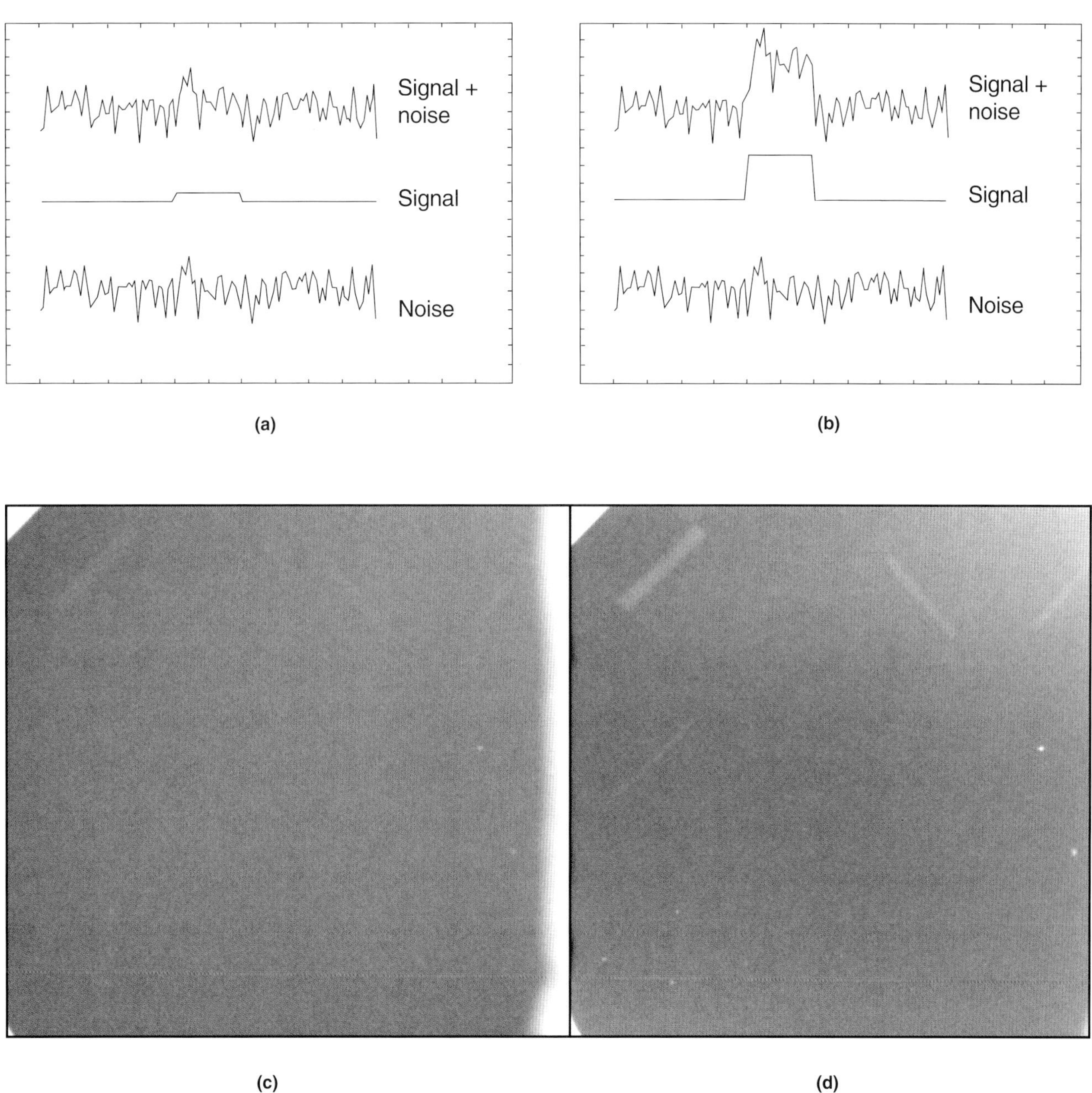

Figure 5.2 a-d. Signal-to-Noise Ratio. **Figure 5.2a** illustrates the noise level, faint signal, and finally signal-to-noise ratio. The noise interferes with visualizing the faint signal. **Figure 5.2c** of the familiar ACR phantom illustrates low SNR, resulting in faint visualization of the first 3 fibrils but not the fifth fibril on the second line. **Figure 5.2b** illustrates the same noise level, however, the signal is increased to overcome the noise, resulting in visualization. **Figure 5.2d** illustrates the same portion of the ACR phantom; the increased SNR results in visualizing the fifth fibril, as well as better delineation of the first three fibrils (note the visualization of the specs in both images).

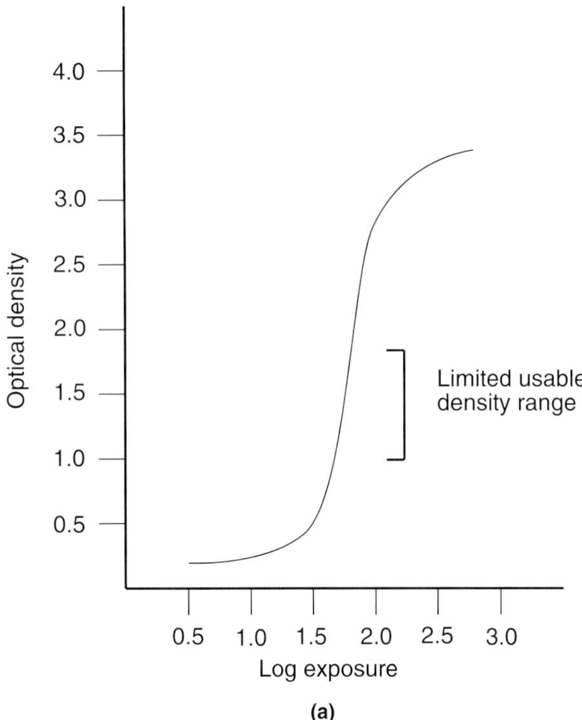

response is nonlinear, the detectors used in digital systems are linear. In addition, reciprocity failure, a phenomenon of conventional screen-film systems, does not occur with digital receptors. Therefore, while it can be expected that doubling exposure will not necessarily result in a doubling of density in a screen-film system, *doubling exposure in a digital system will always double signal.*

Postacquisition Image Manipulation

The recording of an image with conventional methods is determined by the screen-film combination, processing, and technical factors, such as, kVp and mAs, without the ability to alter or enhance the results during display. After exposure and processing, the density range of the mammogram may not be optimal for demonstrating the pathology of interest.

Through image processing capabilities, a digital system provides the ability to *manipulate* the image postacquisition during display. This creates an imaging environment less sensitive to over- or underexposure for more clinically useful results. Most important, postacquisition manipulation allows the user to alter the density and contrast of a specific area, and to bring out subtle changes in contrast without per-

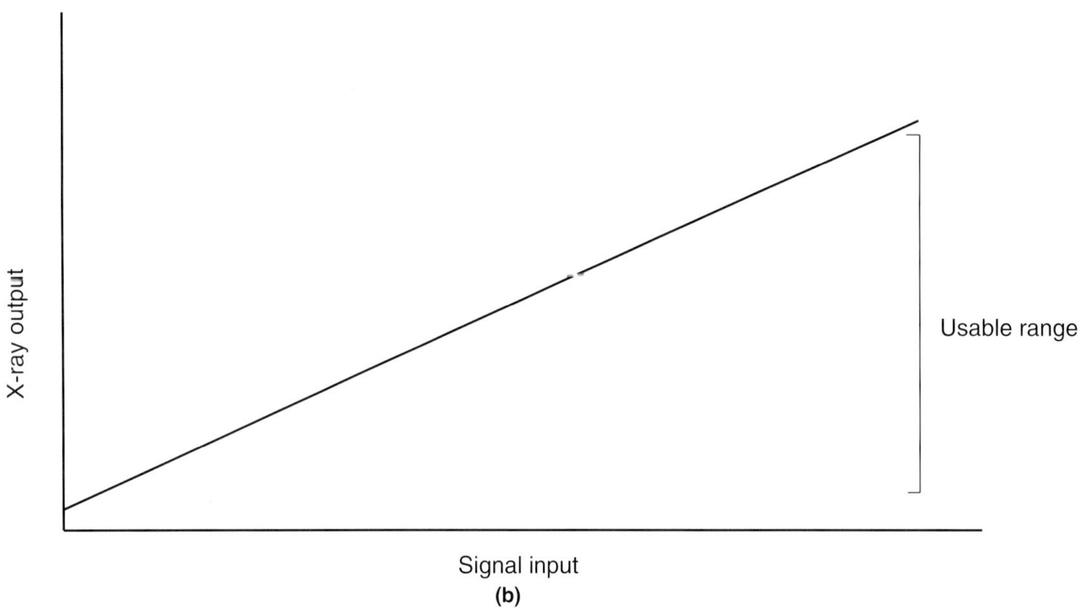

Figure 5.3 a and b. Response Curves. **Figure 5.3a** illustrates the D log E curve of a screen-film system; only a portion of the curve results in usab information. **Figure 5.3b** illustrates the response curve of a digital system, which is less limited in exposure range for a usable image.

manent degradation of the remainder of the image (**Figure 5.4**). Postacquisition image manipulation is by far the most significant feature of a digital system.

Contrast Resolution

Digital systems appreciably increase the range of exposure values over which high-contrast sensitivity can be obtained. The ability of a digital system to detect small changes in exposure difference in adjacent areas enables the visualization of most abnormalities. Image processing capabilities (such as window and level) allow the display of selected exposure ranges at high contrast. For this reason, poor subject contrast of breast pathology against glandular structures, and contrast and detail degradation resulting from other characteristic conditions of the SBB procedure, become less important. The sensitivity of the digital system also creates a more scatter-tolerant environment.

Contrast resolution is a measure of the system's ability to visualize, for practicable purposes, a detail of particular size and shape. Even though contrast resolution may be greater with digital imaging, *spatial resolution (which is a measurement of detail/blur)* is generally more limited. Screen-film systems provide a spatial resolution of about 16-20 lp/mm[9]. Currently available digital systems provide about 8-10 lp/mm[10].

Spatial resolution is normally measured with high-contrast bar patterns. However, the ability to discern small objects in practice (such as microcalcifications, the borders of low-density masses, and the fine lines of architectural distortion) can depend on contrast resolution as well as spatial resolution, and will be influenced by noise. Thus, it is entirely possible for a system to have *high spatial resolution but poor visibility of detail as a result of insufficient contrast resolution.*

Imaging developments in mammography have always strived to achieve a balance between spatial resolution and the need for higher contrast, while maintaining low dose and adequate exposure latitude. For example, the change from a direct x-ray film system to a screen-film combination demonstrated that increasing contrast could compensate for the loss of spatial resolution by improving visibility of detail. This phenomenon is again demonstrated with a digital imaging system. In most cases, *the increase in contrast resolution with a digital system largely compensates for the loss in spatial resolution*. Although spatial resolution will need to

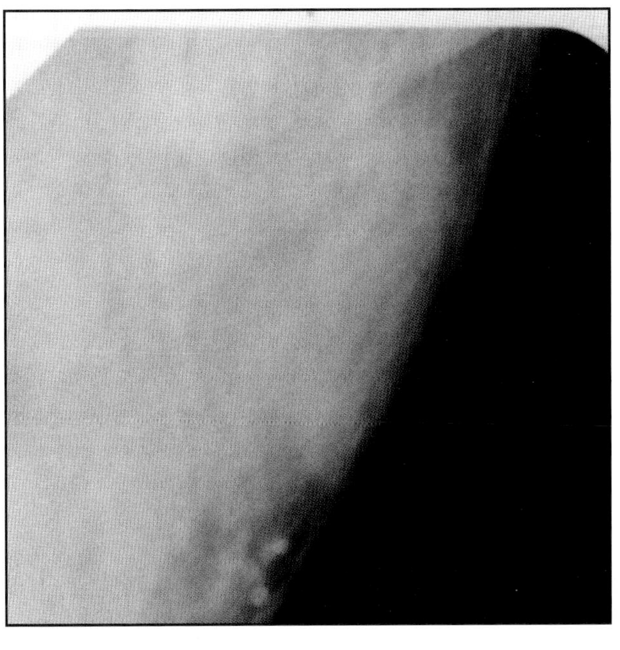

(a)

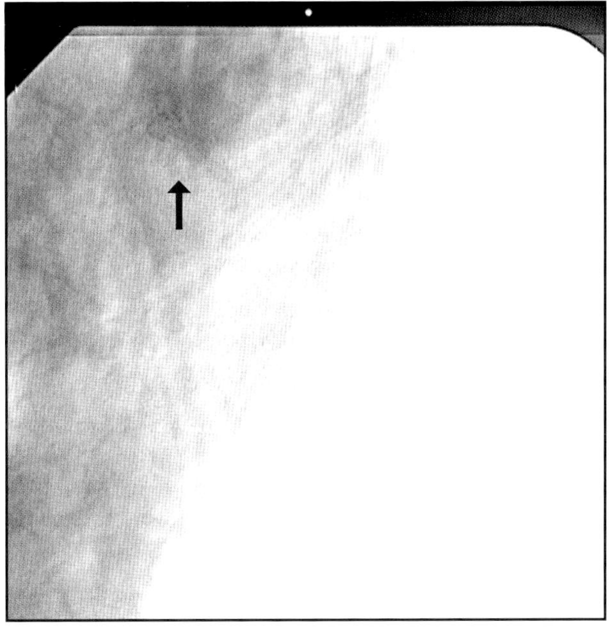

(b)

Figure 5.4 a and b. Postacquisition Image Manipulation. The initial display image is not permanent **(a)**. Image manipulation allows the user to bring out subtle changes in contrast without permanent image degradation **(b) (arrow)**.

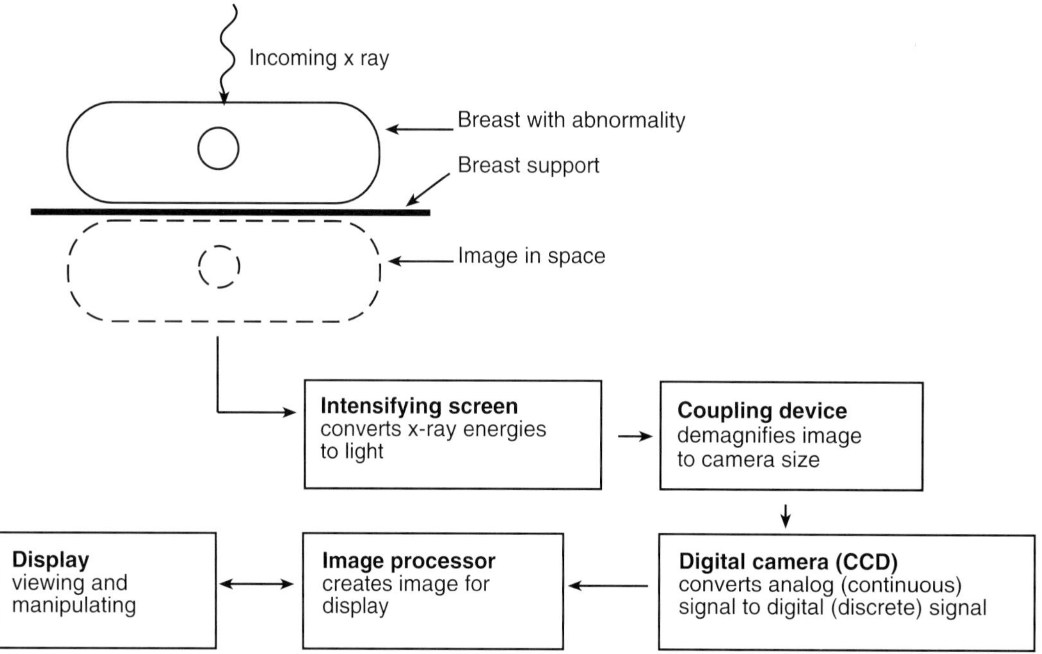

Figure 5.5. Production of a Digital Image.

improve for diagnostic full breast digital imaging[2], currently available resolution is adequate for the SBB procedure, where *identification* and not characterization of the abnormality is the imaging goal. Clinical studies will eventually determine the appropriate balance of contrast resolution and spatial resolution for each digital imaging application.

Digital Imaging Systems

System Performance

Optimal system performance requires an understanding of the image acquisition process and the factors that contribute to image quality. This understanding should be as complete as our comprehension of screen-film image production. Technical application with a digital system can become as second nature as it is with conventional imaging, if the user understands the factors that contribute to digital image acquisition and display.

Overview of Digital Image Acquisition

The *production* of a digital image **(Figure 5.5)** for SBB is initiated in the same manner as that for a conventional image, by first creating an image in space (aerial image). An intensifying screen produces a visible image by converting x-ray photons to light photons. The resulting image undergoes demagnification through a light-coupling device, and is focused on the digital camera. The digital camera, which includes the charge-coupled device (CCD), records the analog (continuous) signal, quickly scanning and converting it to digital (discrete components) signals through the analog-to-digital converter. The information is then processed and displayed on a monitor. Once displayed, the image can be manipulated through the system's image processing algorithms.

Digital Systems for SBB

Currently, there are two types of digital systems in use with SBB: the lens-coupled system† and the fiber optic-coupled system††.

† LORAD®, a division of Trex Medical Corporation, a Thermo Electron Company.
†† Fisher Imaging Corporation.

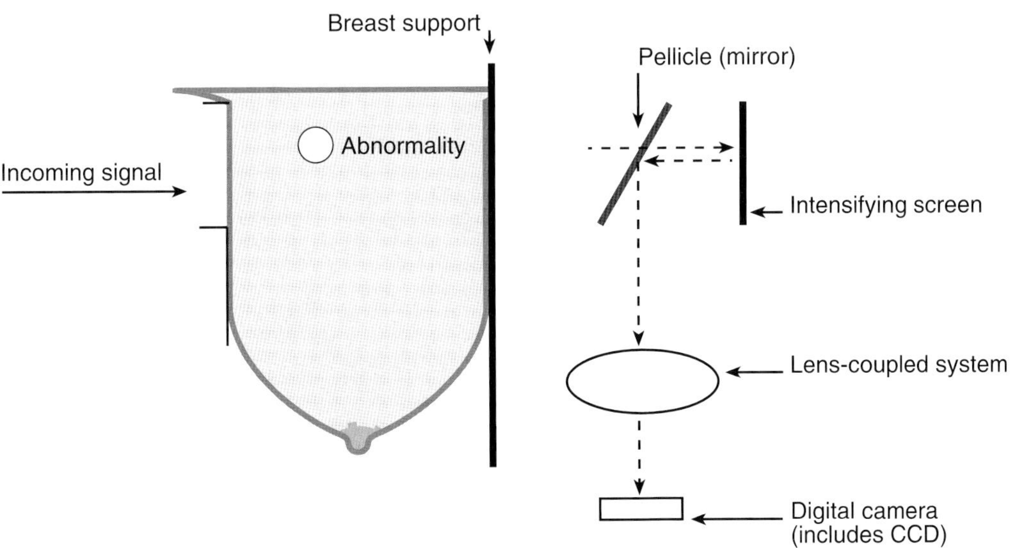

Figure 5.6. Lens-Coupled System. This digital system produces an image by illuminating the intensifying screen; this image is reflected by a very thin mirror and demagnified by a lens. The image is then captured by the digital camera.

Lens-Coupled System—Figure 5.6 illustrates a lens-based system. The x-ray quanta exiting the breast pass through an x-ray transparent pellicle (a thin mirror measuring 5-9 microns), irradiating the front surface of an intensifying screen. The light image emitted from the front of the screen is reflected by the pellicle and projected through the lens. The lens system demagnifies the image and focuses it onto the back side of a thinned silicone image sensor (CCD). The sensor is independent of the rest of the system, making it easy to upgrade and replace.

Fiber Optic-Coupled System—Figure 5.7 illustrates a fiber optic system. The x-ray quanta exiting from the breast illuminate the intensifying screen from the back surface. The light image is then emitted from the front surface of the screen through the fiber optic taper to the front of a silicone image sensor (CCD). The sensor is bonded to the fiber optic taper.

Both systems seek to achieve a balance among the many factors that contribute to image quality and to maintain low patient dose. The most significant differences between the two systems are the efficiency with which the coupling device collects light from the intensifying screen (the fiber optic system is more efficient) and the efficiency of light capture by the CCD (the lens system is more efficient)[8]. However, these and other differences reflect alternative approaches to achieving clinically useful system performance. These different approaches do not infer that one system is inherently better than the other. In practice, both systems have been shown to be effective for the purposes of SBB[8].

Elements of the Digital Imaging Chain

This section describes the components of a digital system and how each contributes to image formation and image quality. Image quality is determined by the "aggregate effects"[9] of contrast resolution, detail/blur, and noise. **Figure 5.8** summarizes the contribution to image quality of the following components of the digital imaging chain:

- Intensifying screen (or phosphor)
- Light-coupling device
- Digital camera
- Workstation

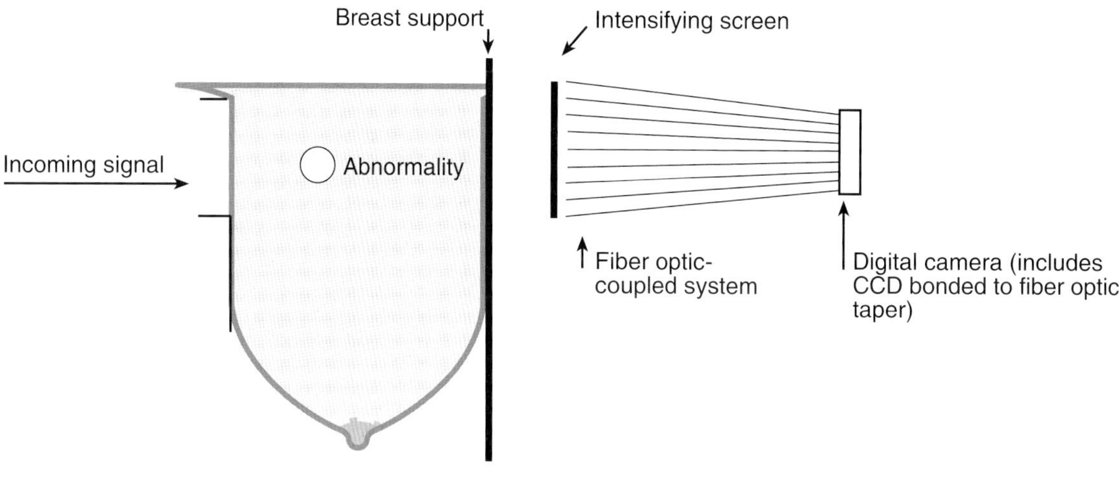

Figure 5.7. Fiber Optic-Coupled System. This digital system produces an image by illuminating the intensifying screen; the image is demagnified and transferred through a fiber optic taper to the digital camera.

Intensifying Screen (Phosphor)

The purpose of the intensifying screen in the SBB system is to provide a visible image in response to x-ray quanta, which is directed to the "face" of the charge-coupled device (CCD) for recording. To accomplish this, the phosphor in the intensifying screen absorbs x-ray quanta, producing light photons. In this sense, the intensifying screen is an "energy converter[11]." The contributions of the screen to loss of detail and noise are significant. However, contribution to loss of contrast resolution is minimal. How well the phosphor maintains the integrity of the image in space in the conversion process is determined by a number of factors.

The choice of screen *materials* as well as the screen *thickness* will influence the visibility of detail[11]. For example, other things being equal, thick screens are less sharp than thin screens. Screen material and thickness also determine the *x-ray quantum absorption* (how much of the x-ray beam is absorbed into the screen), and the *emission efficiency* of the screen (how well the screen emits light). In addition, the screen will not always produce the same intensity of light for a given energy of x-ray quanta, as a result of *conversion noise*. Ideally, a *screen* would absorb 100% of the incident x-ray quanta, fully converting this energy to corresponding energies of light. However, screens typically absorb 80-95% of the incident x-ray quanta[11]; of the absorbed energy, 5-20% will be converted to light. While these conversion efficiencies may seem low, the intensifying screen produces a sufficient number of light quanta per x-ray so that it is not the overall limiting component of a digital system.

The intensifying screens used in today's SBB digital systems are not specifically designed to work with a CCD as an image receptor. They are "adaptations" from conventional screen-film systems. The manufacturer's decision to use a particular intensifying screen has more to do with the design *requirements* of a digital system, than it does with its original intended use in a conventional screen-film system. For example, it may be more desirable for the phosphor to produce greater amounts of light, trading off some detail while providing increased signal-to-noise ratio[8]. This would necessitate a thicker screen than may normally be employed for mammography. Furthermore, a general radiography phosphor may have superior qualities useful for a specific SBB

Factors Affecting Digital Image Quality

	Image in Space	**Intensifying Screen**	**Light-Coupling Device**	**Charge-Coupled Device** (CCD) (Digital Camera)	**Display/Workstation**
Contrast Resolution	X-ray spectra Subject contrast Scatter	Not affected	Optic flare - reduces contrast similar to scatter	Bit depth	Setting of parameters Contrast and brightness settings Window and level Ambient light levels of viewing area Flare: light scattered back into screen
Detail/Blur	SID OID Effective focal spot Patient motion	Screen thickness Screen type	Optical unsharpness Lens or fiber optic system	Matrix size Pixel size	Spot size Spot shape Matrix size
Noise	Exposure level	Structure noise Conversion noise X-ray quantum absorption Emission efficiency	Coupling efficiency: no. of photons in > no. of photons out (efficiency of light transfer from phosphor to CCD)	Detective Quantum Efficiency (DQE) Electronic noise	Amplifier noise Phosphor grain noise Photon noise - emitted by monitor

Figure 5.8. Factors Affecting Digital Image Quality. This table summarizes the contributing factors to image quality at each stage of the digital imaging chain.

digital system, even though in a conventional screen-film system the screen is not designed for mammographic work.

Screen Orientation

The phosphor can be used as either a back screen or front screen. As a back screen, the screen is irradiated at the emitting (front) surface and the image recorded from the same surface (this is the orientation normally used for diagnostic mammography). As a front screen, the phosphor is irradiated at the back surface of the screen and recorded from the emitting (front) surface of the screen **(Figure 5.9)**.

The Light-Coupling Device

The light-coupling device provides a connection (thus, "coupling") from the phosphor to the digital image receptor. Current coupling devices are either lens or fiber optic (Figures 5.6 and 5.7). The coupling device is an important element in the digital system, providing both *demagnification* (minification) and *transmission* of the visible image from the intensifying screen. This device focuses the image on the charge-coupled device (CCD). The two coupling devices have different imaging characteristics. The manufacturer's choice to use one coupling device or the other depends on the design and goals of the system.

The coupling device is one of the critical factors in the image quality chain. CCD technology limits the size of the CCD, thus requiring demagnification of the image. The coupling device reduces by about one-half the 50 mm x 50 mm image produced by the intensifying screen (an important factor when considering pixel size).

Coupling efficiency, which describes the effectiveness of light transfer from the intensifying screen to the CCD, is critical. The greatest effect of the coupling device, whether lens or fiber optic, is the notable loss of signal (quantum sink), which can decrease signal-to-noise ratio and interfere with image quality [7,8,10].

Optical flare in the coupling device can also reduce contrast, which affects the image in much the same way as x-ray scatter. Optical unsharpness of the coupling device can also contribute to image degradation.

The Digital Camera

The purpose of the camera in the digital system is to *record* a visible image from the intensifying screen and to *convert*

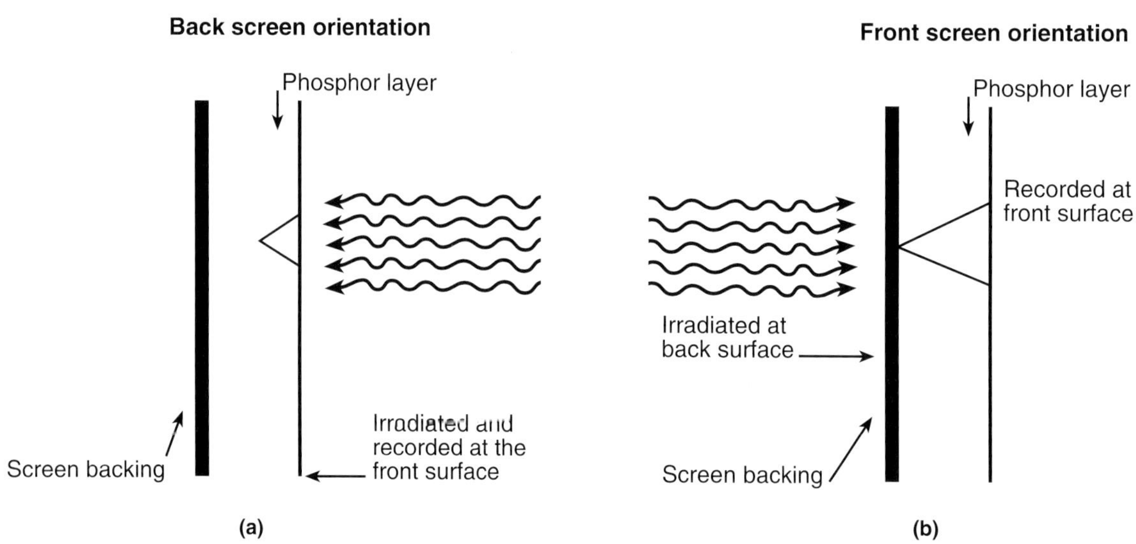

Figure 5.9 a and b. Intensifying Screen Orientation. **Figure 5.9a** illustrates an intensifying screen used as a back screen; the screen is illuminated and the image recorded from the front surface of the screen. This is the same orientation used in conventional mammography. **Figure 5.9b** illustrates an intensifying screen used as a front screen; the surface is illuminated from the back of the screen and recorded from the front of the screen.

that information to a digital image for storage, display, and manipulation. The camera includes three main elements: the charge-coupled device, the analog-to-digital converter, and a cooling system.

Charge-Coupled Device

A charge-coupled device, sometimes referred to as the matrix, array, or CCD, is the heart of the SBB digital system. The CCDs used in digital SBB systems are scientific grade and must be nearly flawless to perform the tasks of medical imaging and analysis. Current CCDs in use for SBB systems are small in size, measuring about 20 mm x 20 mm. Producing a larger CCD is not cost-effective due to the difficulty in maintaining a perfect CCD with increasing size[7].

The size of the CCD limits the digital system to a certain extent. Ideally, the recording device (CCD) should be in direct contact with the intensifying screen, just as in conventional screen-film systems. However, current CCD size would limit the imaging area to 20 mm x 20 mm, which is too small to be useful for SBB. To provide a larger and more useful imaging field (approximately 50 mm x 50 mm), a coupling device links the image to the CCD by demagnifying the image to the CCD's small size.

Effects on Image Quality—The CCD affects all aspects of the image, contributing to contrast and detail/blur (see *Image Matrix and Analog-to-Digital Converter*). The CCD also adds noise. Two factors influence the amount of noise added by the CCD. Electronic dark noise inherent in the CCD is one source (see *Cooling System*). The other source of noise arises from the limited number of light quanta detected by the CCD. This noise can be minimized by having a bright intensifying screen, efficient light coupling, and a CCD with high detective quantum efficiency (DQE).

CCD Performance—The CCD collects light from the coupling device and converts it to an electronic signal through a matrix of pixels (picture elements). The pixels are arranged on the face of the silicon chip **(Figure 5.10)** in a two-dimensional array. The pixels are photoconductive, that is, they respond to light by producing an electrical charge. Thus, when focusing an image on the matrix, electrons are produced in the pixels. The "intensity of the incident light"[12] from the phosphor determines the number of electrons at each pixel. It is helpful to think of the pixel as a "bucket" or "well" that "fills" with electrons, producing a charge level representative of the incident light **(Figure 5.11)**.

Image Matrix—The matrix describes pixel distribution, that is, how many square units or pixels the image will be divided into for sampling. The matrix has a height and width and is described by the number of pixels horizontally, times the number of pixels vertically. For example, if there are 16 individual pixels that define the character or anatomical part, four down and four across, then the matrix is 4 x 4 (Figure 5.10).

Currently, digital units for SBB use a 1024 x 1024 matrix (for a total of 1,048,576 pixels for sampling). One unit (manufactured by LORAD®) offers the choice of using the 1024 mode, but through a process called binning, the unit combines pixels to provide the user with a 512 x 512 matrix (for a total of 262,144 pixels for sampling).

The matrix size directly affects the maximum possible resolution of the image **(Figure 5.12)**. The larger the matrix, the greater the number of resultant samplings representing an anatomical part. It would seem that as many samplings as possible would provide more detail, however, this must be balanced with other factors. The number of pixels needed to represent an anatomical part is determined by both the size of the individual pixel and the size of the imaging field [13], as well as other factors that are explained below.

Size of Imaging Field and Effective Pixel Size—The size of the recorded image and the rate of demagnification determines the effective pixel size **(Figure 5.13)**. For example,

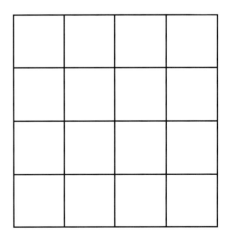

Figure 5.10. Matrix. Picture elements, or pixels, are arranged in a two-dimensional array and described as a matrix. This drawing illustrates a 4 x 4 matrix (a matrix is not always square).

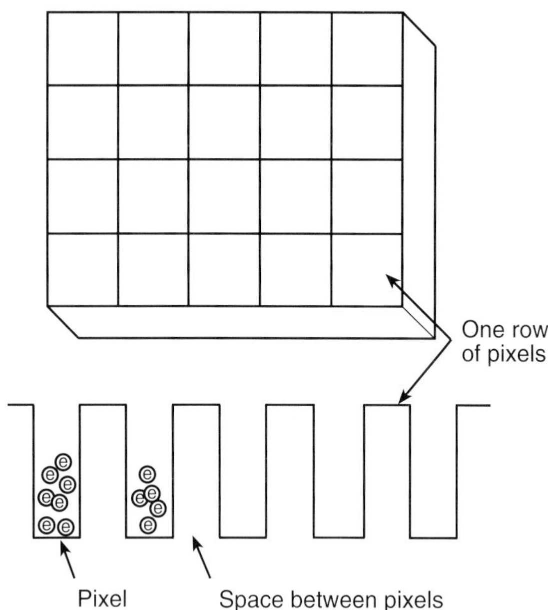

Figure 5.11. Pixels. It is helpful to think of the pixel as a "bucket" or a "well" that fills with electrons, producing a charge level representative of the incident light (note the space between the pixels).

for SBB, a 50 mm x 50 mm image produced at the intensifying screen is reduced (through the coupling device) to the approximate 25 mm x 25 mm CCD size. This means that the *pixel size* has to be small enough to image detail that has been demagnified to half its original size. The literature suggests that for SBB, available pixel size should be no greater than 50 microns[7,8,14], however, this resolution is not always required for the purposes of SBB. The effective pixel size for SBB is approximately 50 microns in the 1024 mode and 100 microns in the 512 mode.

Exposure (dose)—Matirx size also helps to determine technical factors and dose. A larger matrix (1024) with many more pixels requires greater exposure rates (or signal) than does a smaller matrix (512) with fewer pixels. Again, it is useful to remember the "well" comparison; 1,000,000 pixels in the 1024 mode require greater exposure than the 250,000 pixels in the 512 mode. In practice, the 1024 mode requires about twice the exposure of the 512 mode (using the same unit) to obtain comparable signal-to-noise ratios.

Resolution of the Underlying Image—The image projected from the coupling device has a certain degree of sharpness. The pixel size and the matrix size should be chosen to

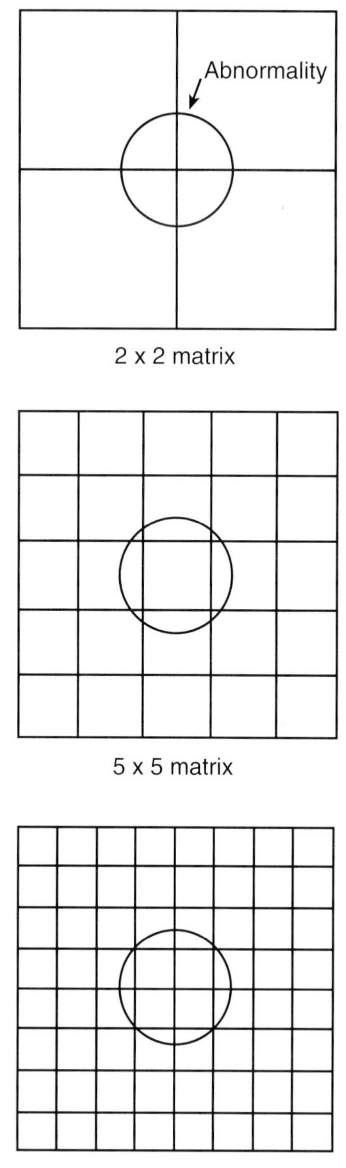

Figure 5.12. Matrix Size and Maximum Possible Resolution. The matrix size determines the maximum possible resolution. A greater matrix size results in a greater number of samplings. The 8 x 8 matrix will result in a greater number of samplings than the 2 x 2 or the 5 x 5 matrix. Matrix size, however, must be balanced with other factors, and should not exceed the resolution of the underlying image.

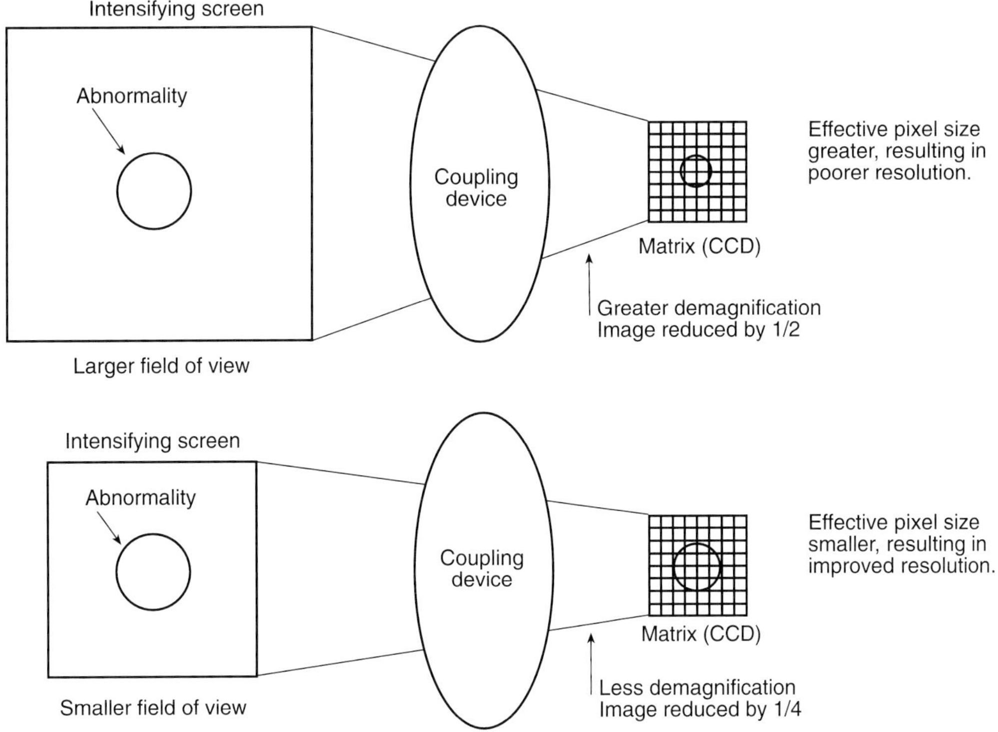

Figure 5.13. Effective Pixel Size. Given a certain size matrix, the rate of demagnification determines the effective pixel size at the intensifying screen. Illustrated here, the larger image has to be reduced to a smaller size for recording, resulting in a larger effective pixel size at the intensifying screen. Generally, the smaller the effective pixel size, the greater the resolution of the image. However, pixel size has to be balanced against other factors that limit resolution.

maintain this sharpness. Using a smaller pixel or larger matrix than necessary is impractical, as it increases dose without providing more information.

Processing Time and Archiving Space—Larger matrices require longer image processing time before display than do smaller matrices. The larger matrix also takes up more space, both on the hard drive and optical disk. For example, a 1024 x 1024 image with 2 bytes, or 16 bits per pixel (1 byte consists of 8 bits), requires a longer reconstruction time for its 2,000,000 bytes compared with the time a 512 x 512 image requires to reconstruct its 500,000 bytes.

Requirements of the Localization Procedure—Since the imaging goal of SBB is to identify abnormalities rather than characterize them, its matrix requirements are not as stringent as those of full breast diagnostic imaging. This is an important consideration when choosing a 512 matrix over a 1024 matrix. Well-defined abnormalities and most microcalcifications can be imaged with the use of a 512 matrix, which requires less exposure and procedure time (see *Technical Applications* section).

Analog-to-Digital Converter

The signal from each pixel is given a numerical value (or digital value) through the analog-to-digital converter. "Digitization" characterizes the signal by one of a discrete set of values **(Figure 5.14)**, that is, each digital system is limited to a certain number of values in which to describe incoming signal. Each pixel has a numerical value in the computer's storage, as determined by 1) the number of electrons produced in the pixel and, 2) the bit depth of the converter (discussed below). This numerical value is representative of the light level focused on an individual

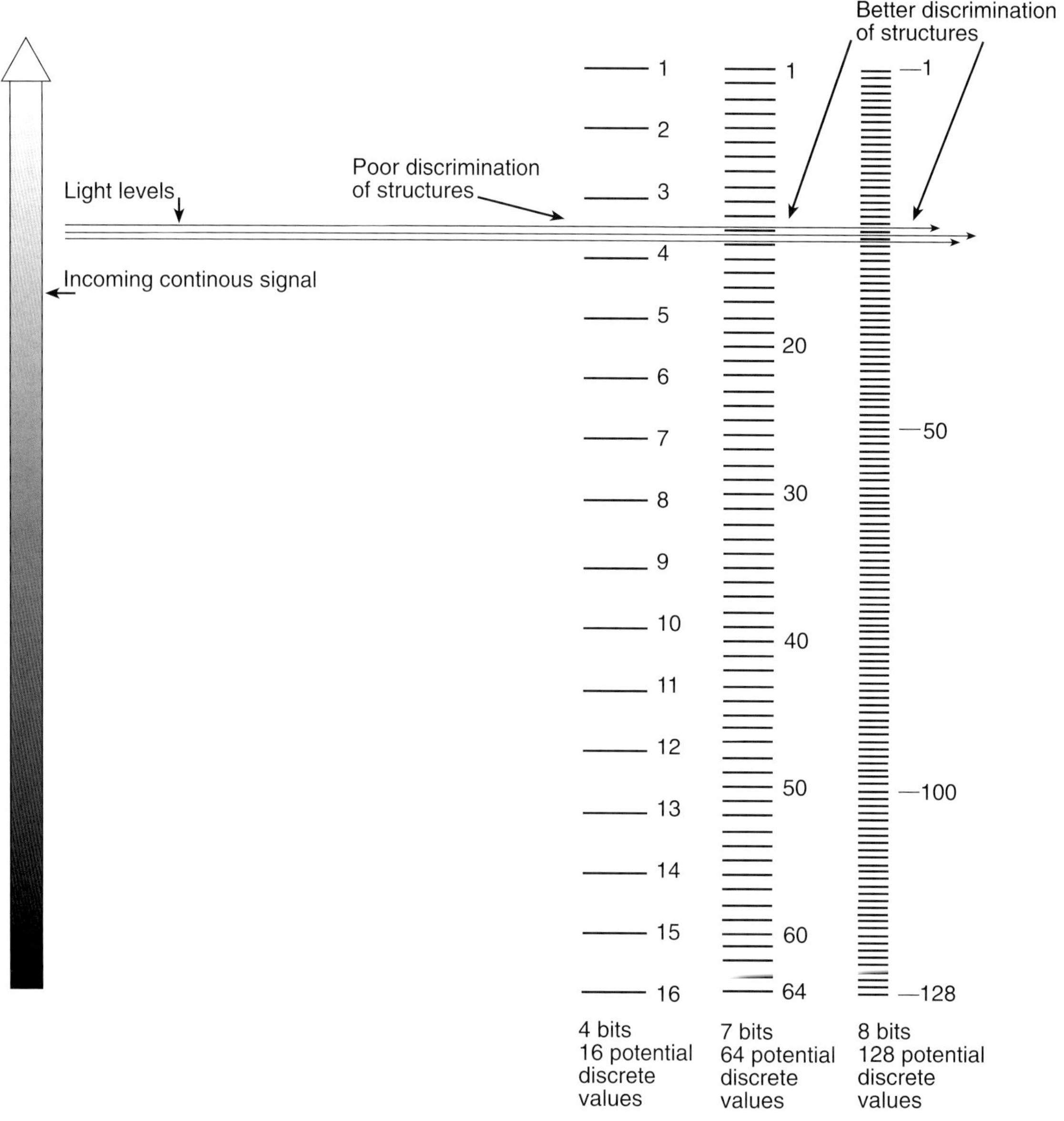

Figure 5.14. Analog-to-Digital Converter. The ADC converts the incoming continuous signal to a digital signal by giving light levels a numerical value. The bit depth of the ADC determines the contrast discrimination of the digital system. A greater bit depth results in the possibility of greater contrast discrimination. As illustrated here, the 4-bit depth system will not be able to discriminate these light levels; a 7-bit system separates the values better, and the 8-bit even more so.

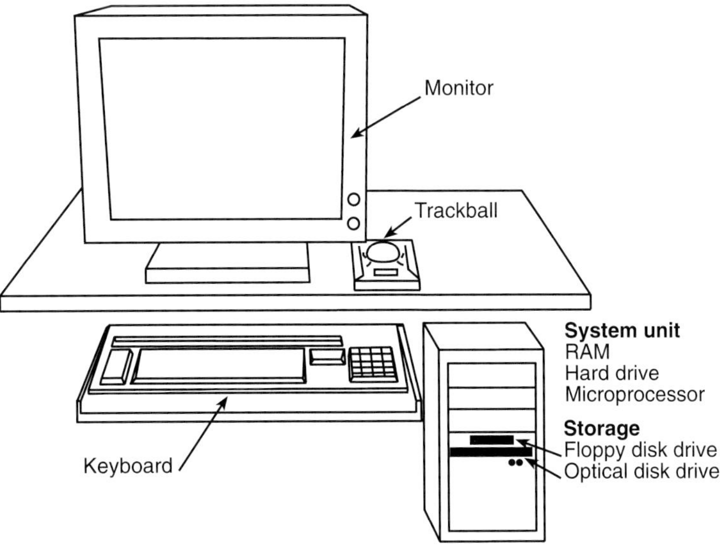

Figure 5.15. Digital Workstation.

pixel, and provides the environment for analysis of each individual value. Analysis of these values is the essence of digital imaging. Because each light intensity or level of gray is represented by a numerical value, it is possible to enhance or manipulate an image through image processing algorithms (see *Image Processing* section).

Bit depth—Bit depth sets an upper limit for the contrast resolution or the visibility of the image information available[13]. Although it sounds like a third dimension of the pixel, bit depth is not a physical dimension, but rather is related to the number of light levels the digital camera provides to describe the light levels coming into the CCD. As each pixel collects light, a voltage is produced in response to the light level. Through the analog-to-digital converter, this voltage is divided into a discrete set of light levels[13]. *The bit depth determines the number of light levels the system is capable of rendering* (Figure 5.14).

For example, if a certain level of signal is available for recording, a unit providing a bit depth of 8 bits allows the CCD output to be described in terms of 256 gray levels (determined by 2 to n power, where "n" represents the bit depth, in this case, 2 to the 8th power = 256). A unit with a depth of 12 bits would allow the same signal to be separated into about 4,000 levels. The greater bit depth will potentially yield greater discrimination of detail through better contrast resolution. SBB systems currently operate at a depth of 14 bits. This provides for a maximum of 16,000 levels per pixel. Since digital systems respond over a wide range of exposures, adequate bit depth is critical to the system. A system can have a large matrix with small pixel size and provide adequate signal-to-noise ratio, but without adequate bit depth, contrast resolution and visibility of detail are limited.

The Cooling System

The cooling system minimizes the amount of inherent electronic (dark) noise in the CCD. The CCD is cooled via an electronic cooling system to about -20° Centigrade. Reducing this source of noise increases the signal-to-noise ratio, particularly at low exposure levels, thereby improving image quality.

Workstation

The SBB workstation **(Figure 5.15)** provides the means for controlling the acquisition, processing, display, manipulation, and storage of digital images. It is also used to perform coordinate calculation for abnormality localization. The workstation houses the following components, allowing the digital unit to function and the user to interact with the system:

- Computer
  - Microprocessor
  - Random access memory
  - Storage disks
  - Monitor
  - Keyboard
  - Trackball
- Software

Microprocessor

The microprocessor is a complex integrated circuit in the computer that executes commands and performs calculations.

Currently, SBB systems use computers based on the Intel® 80486 microprocessor, with clock speeds of 50 megahertz or higher. The term "megahertz" describes the number of instructions (in millions) the processor will execute per second.

Memory and Storage Capacity

A computer stores information in "bits." A bit is the smallest possible unit of information. An SBB scout image typically consists of approximately 500,000 bytes (1 byte consists of 8 bits) of information. To avoid large numbers, the computer's memory and storage are described in megabytes. A megabyte is approximately 1,000,000 bytes. The computer must have adequate storage space and memory for the operating system and accompanying software, and should provide adequate space for acquiring new information, such as images and labels (or annotations).

A computer has temporary memory, referred to as random access memory (RAM) and online storage space, referred to as the hard drive or hard disk.

Random Access Memory—Random access memory provides the active working space in the computer. Anytime the user is acquiring, manipulating or targeting an image, he or she is using RAM. Having an adequate amount of random access memory is important to the efficiency and expediency with which the computer performs its functions. RAM provides the space to run the operating system (such as DOS) and the functional software. At the same time, RAM must be large enough to acquire images and related information and also run the software that allows image processing and manipulation. Large images, such as the one-half megabyte images for SBB, and the complexity of image processing algorithms, require large amounts of RAM.

Current stereotactic units operate with at least 16 megabytes of RAM. As image processing becomes more complex and images become larger (in terms of space requirements), the amount of random access memory will have to be increased to maintain efficiency.

Images or other information stored in RAM are not permanent. If power is interrupted or the computer is turned off, any information in RAM that has not been saved, that is, stored on the hard drive, will be lost. Therefore, all information in RAM must be saved onto the hard drive to become permanent.

Hard Drive—The hard drive provides permanent online storage of information for immediate recall. The information on the hard drive remains when the computer is turned off. The storage capacity of the hard drive is also described in megabytes, but is significantly greater than that of RAM. Hard drive storage space for SBB systems is currently 240 megabytes or more. However, with ongoing developments in computer technology, it would not be surprising to see this increase up to a gigabyte (1,000 megabytes) or more. Although the hard drive is for permanent storage, it is finite in size. For archival storage of the large numbers of images generated by SBB, a means to permanently *archive* images offline is needed.

Archiving—Because a typical image produced for SBB requires at least a one-half megabyte of storage capacity, it is not practical to store images indefinitely on the hard drive. *Optical disks* meet the need for large archival storage. Currently available optical disks provide two sides for storage for a total of 600 megabytes of space (usually 300 per side). Optical disks can be either permanent (write once, read many times [WORM]) or rewritable, which means the information can be erased and the disk reused. Transferring cases on a daily basis (or daily disk back-up) to an optical disk is recommended to free up hard drive space and reduce the chances of losing patient information. Some units provide an automatic optical disk back-up.

Hard copy—The digital systems for SBB can send images to a multiformat camera, or a remote laser imaging system, to produce hard copy images.

Monitor

The monitor is usually a high-resolution monochrome (black and white) cathode ray tube (CRT). The monitor typically displays a matrix with a bit depth of 8 bits (256 levels). Even though the CCD provides about 16,000 levels of gray per pixel, the monitor can only display 256 levels of gray. However, window and level adjustments allow viewing of any selected range of the entire 16,000 levels of gray, as necessary.

Matrix size, the range of brightness, the sharpness, and the noise in the displayed image vary with the quality of the monitor. Factors that influence monitor performance, such as spot size, spot shape, and matrix size (which contribute to detail/blur), as well as amplifier noise, phosphor grain noise, and photon noise are beyond the scope of this text, but are worth noting to emphasize the complexity of the monitor.

Other factors affecting the contrast of the image that can be directly affected by the user are as follows:

Luminance Levels—Luminance levels of a CRT are about 10 times less that of mammographic viewboxes[15,16]. Therefore, when viewing monitors, ambient light levels should be kept to a minimum to maintain contrast resolution, especially when looking for low-density abnormalities or fine microcalcifications.

Contrast and Brightness Control—Contrast and brightness settings are critical to perceiving the detail available to the monitor. The literature suggests the use of a test pattern to establish optimum settings[15,16,17]. A Society of Motion Picture and Television Engineers (SMPTE) pattern is one such device. While test patterns are unavailable on SBB digital systems, their use and other options are currently being evaluated. The use of screen savers that help maintain the integrity of the screen also are available on some SBB systems.

Window and Level Adjustments—The window and level capabilities of the system allow the user to scan or "map" through the 16,000 levels of gray without permanent image degradation. Window and level are discussed in greater detail in the next section.

Software

The most fundamentally important software program is the *operating system* , a program of basic commands that allows the machine to function. It enables the computer to perform the most fundamental tasks, such as booting up and running applications programs. The most common operating system today is DOS (disk operating system), which can be found on most SBB digital equipment. Other software programs are specific to the needs of the system's application. In general, SBB software programs provide a complete environment for image acquisition, processing, display, storage, and hard copy.

Image Processing

Image processing is one of the most distinguishing characteristics of the digital system. The principle objective of enhancement techniques is to process a given image so that the result is more suitable than the original image for a specific application[12]. Without image processing, digitizing the image would offer little added value. The purpose of image processing is to enhance image information for interpretation by the human eye. Since digital images are displayed as a discrete set of brightness points, the ability of the eye to discriminate between brightness levels is an important consideration in presenting image processing results[12].

Image processing allows the subjective adjustment of the displayed image to accommodate the user's eye. It is important to realize image processing or enhancement is not necessarily performed so that the image will become more esthetically pleasing, but rather to better visualize the clinically important information[18].

Initial image processing occurs before the image appears on the monitor. However, the operator can utilize postacquisition image manipulation processes to alter the image during display. The following section briefly describes the processes that occur both prior to and during display.

Prior to Display

Flat Fielding (White Fielding)

The x-ray beam and the subsequent visible image is nonuniform as a result of the heel effect. More important, the sensitivity of the intensifying screen to x rays and the sensitivity of the CCD's light detection may vary from pixel to pixel. Flat fielding, or white fielding, allows the computer to compensate for these nonuniformities so they are not included as part of the image.

Dark Fielding

Electronic current noise (inherent in the CCD) can also be compensated for by the image processor. In this way, digitization does not include the CCD signal associated with the dark current. Therefore, digitization levels are only used for CCD levels expected to be signal.

Histogram Formation

The image processor can produce a graphic representation of pixel values, referred to as a histogram. The histogram is not alterable; however, the user can utilize the histogram to determine sufficient exposure and thereby adequate signal-to-noise ratio, and to adjust window and level for optimal display of the region of interest **(Figure 5.16)**. The manufacturer usually recommends the histogram levels that offer adequate signal-to-noise ratio.

Postdisplay Image Manipulation

Image manipulation requires the user to learn to view the resultant image differently from how images are viewed using conventional methods. Since the image viewed on the monitor is a computer's representation of the image based on pixel values, it may be inaccurate to conclude that an image is unusable based on the initial computer reconstruction. In addition, changes in technique values *will not* have the same affect on the initially displayed digital image as they would in a screen-film image. The digital image that initially appears may not demonstrate the area of interest. In fact, in some cases, the image may not look usable.

The user cannot evaluate the digital image based on the conventional terms of density and contrast, at least not in a permanent sense. The term density is not permanently associated with the pixel value of a digital image, and contrast can only be discussed as a function of what appears initially. Instead, the operator can *evaluate and alter* brightness levels to properly demonstrate the area of interest (**Figure 5.17**). Other image processes allow the operator to enhance the image to bring out the subtle qualities of an abnormality for identification. When image manipulation fails to demonstrate the area of interest, the operator may decide that the image is unusable, reconsider signal-to-noise ratios, and alter technique accordingly. The following section discusses the various postacquisition image processes available for SBB.

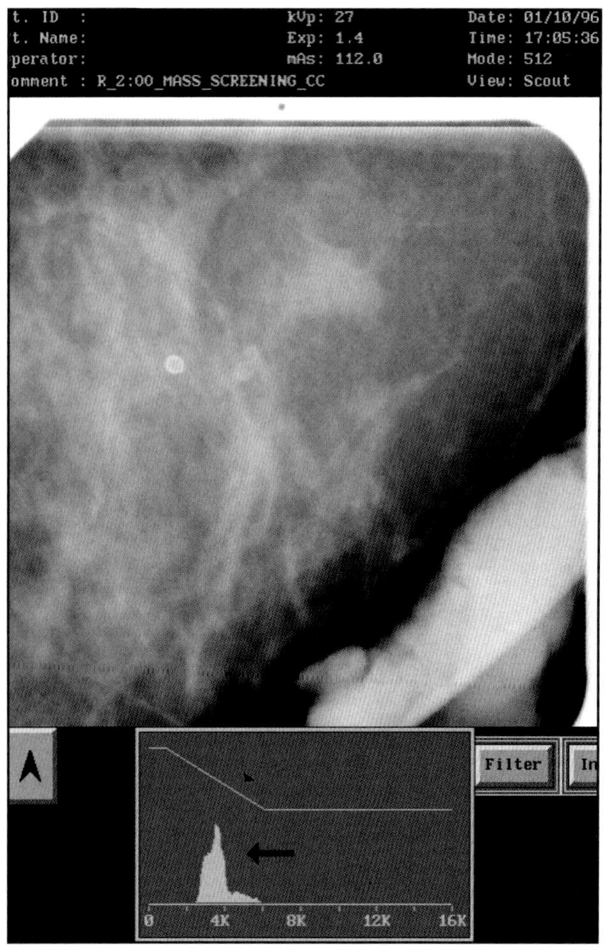

Figure 5.16. Histogram. The histogram **(arrow)** shows the number of pixels at each code value, where code value is proportional to x-ray signal. The histogram can be useful when adjusting technical factors. This figure shows a window and level **(arrowhead)**.

Window and Level

While each pixel of the captured image may be described by 14 bits (a number in the range 0 to 16,384 that reflects the exposure level), the display only allows 8 bits to specify one of the 256 shades of gray to be displayed on the monitor. This poses the problem of how to match the 16,384 possible input values to 256 available output values. One way to address this problem would be to map 64 levels of the captured image into each of the 256 shades of gray. For example, levels 0 through 63 of the input would be mapped to level 0 of the output; levels 64 though 127 would be mapped to level 1, etc. This would allow us to view all the possible levels of the captured image, but it would not allow us to reliably distinguish levels that were close together.

Fortunately, the exposure range of interest rarely includes all the possible levels of the captured image. It is possible, therefore, to have a subrange of the input pixel values mapped into the range of display values. Input values below this range are mapped into an output value of zero, and input values above this range are mapped into an output value of 256. *The size of the range of input values that are mapped into the entire range of the output values is called the* ***window width*** *or simply the* ***window*** (**Figure 5.18**). *The input value at the center of the input range, mapped into the center of the output range (pixel value 128), is called the* ***level*** (**Figure 5.18**).

Workstations normally perform two functions relating to window and level. First, the workstation automatically examines the range of pixel values in the image to be viewed, then it selects a window and level for initial presentation of the image. This normally gives a reasonable display of the entire image, although it may not optimally display the region of greatest interest. (In some cases, it may fail entirely when the image includes areas of very high exposure that might better have been collimated). However, workstations also allow manual manipulation of window and level.

With this capability, any desired window and level can be selected to optimally display any region of interest. *The ability to adjust window and level completely disassociates technique factors from the displayed density and contrast. This allows the use of technique factors to obtain the signal-to-noise needed for each particular SBB procedure.*

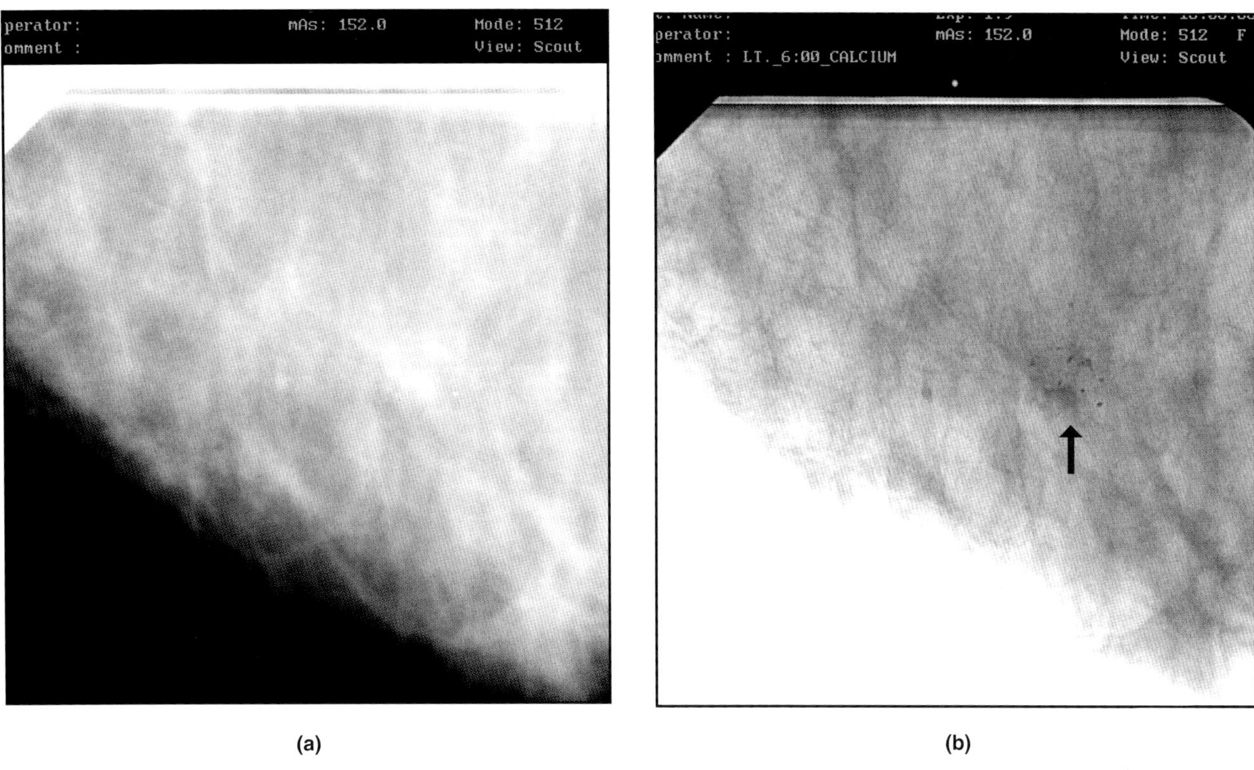

Figure 5.17 a and b. Image Processing. The beauty of digital imaging is its image processing capabilities, which enable the user to alter an image subjectively to bring out the area of interest. **Figure 5.17a** illustrates what appears to be a useless image. **Figure 5.17b** is the same image after image processing; note the minute calcifications that appear **(arrow)**.

Inverting

When a window and level adjustment has been selected either automatically or manually, the image will normally be displayed with the areas of lowest exposure bright (as with film, low density) and the areas of highest exposure dark (as with film, high density). The workstation provides the capability to reverse the polarity of the displayed image such that low exposures are rendered dark and high exposures bright. This is sometimes referred to as *black bone rendition* because of the appearance of bones in such images. Microcalcifications also appear black in inverted images. Inverting the image can sometimes be helpful for visualizing faint objects, particularly if the normally displayed image has large bright areas. Bright areas tend to lower the

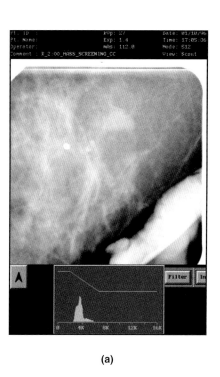

(a)

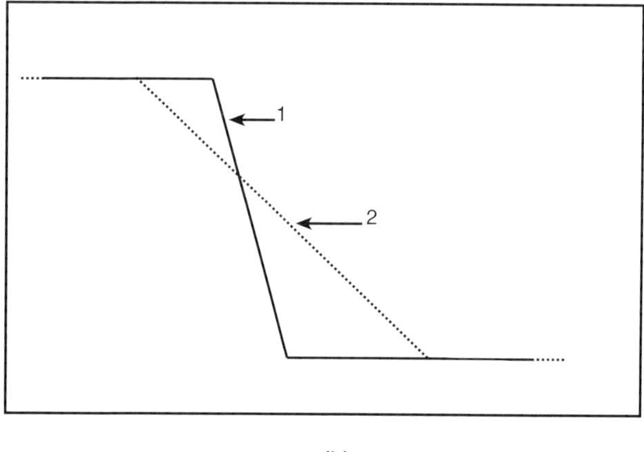

(b)

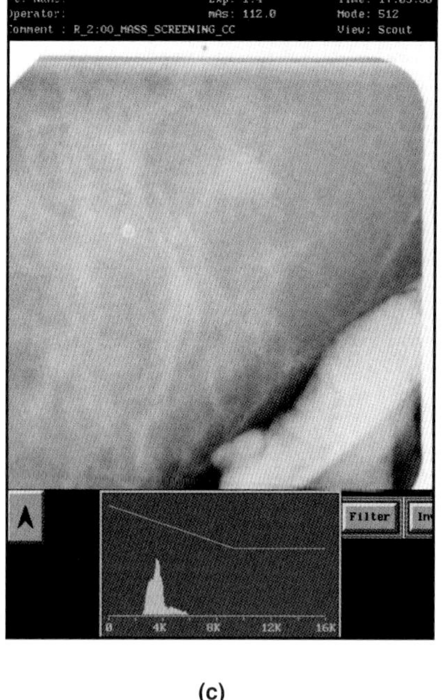

(c)

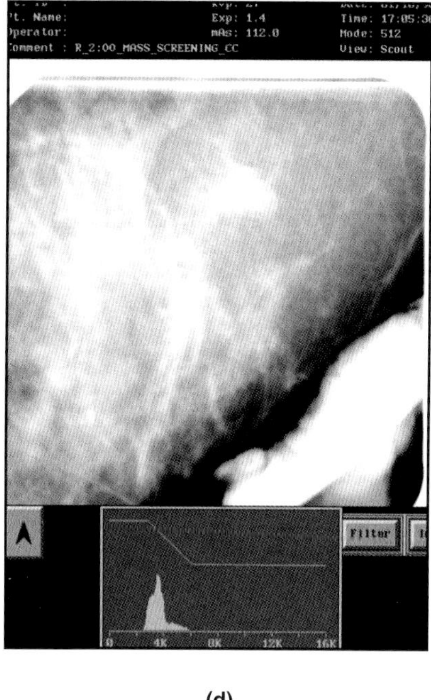

(d)

Figure 5.18 a-h. Window and Level**.** Window and level are perhaps the most useful image processes available to the user, allowing the alteration of brightness levels. **Figure 5.18a** illustrates an *unaltered image* with histogram and window and level curve. **Figure 5.18b** illustrates the *window function;* note the two curves in 1 and the flattening of the slope in 2. *Window is similar to adjusting contrast,* as illustrated in **Figure 5.18 c and d,** which show two extremes of the window function. **Figure 5.18e** illustrates the *level function;* note that the slope of the curve does not change, but that the whole curve shifts from right to left. *Level is similar to adjusting the brightness* of the image as shown in **Figure 5.18 f and g**, which illustrate the two extremes of the level function. In reality, the window and level functions are used together to render a usable image for the viewer, as illustrated in **Figure 5.18h**.

Figure 5.18 continued.

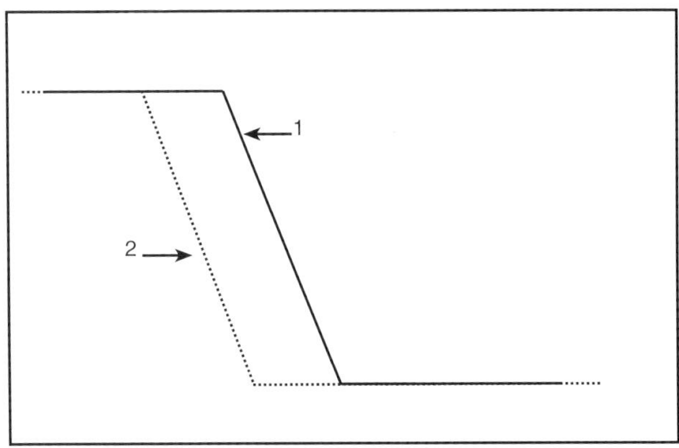

(e)

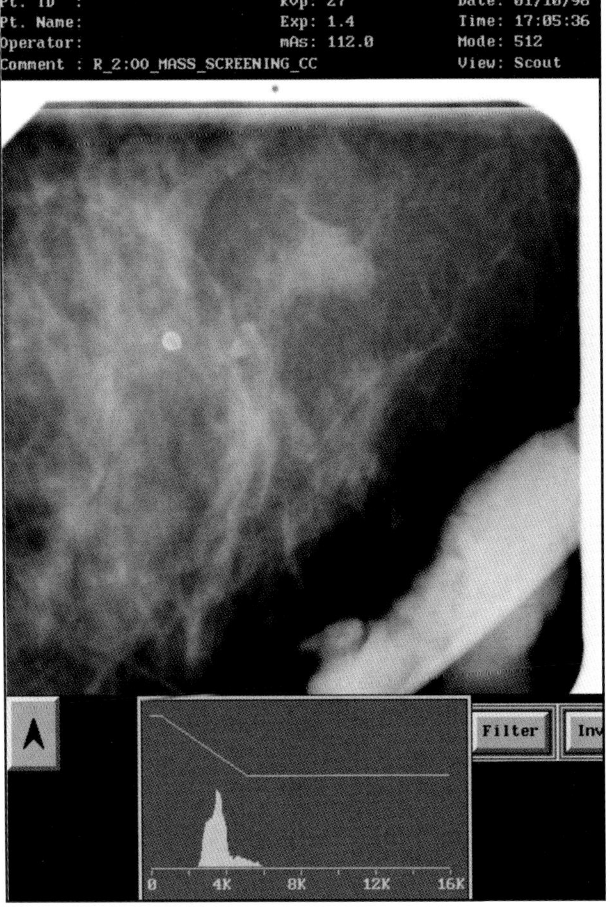

(f)

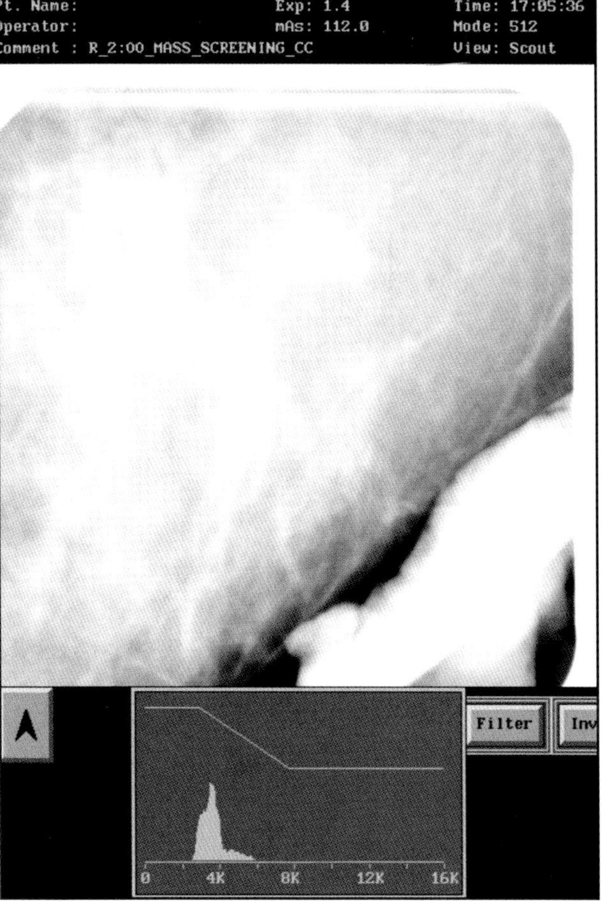

(g)

Figure 5.18 continued.

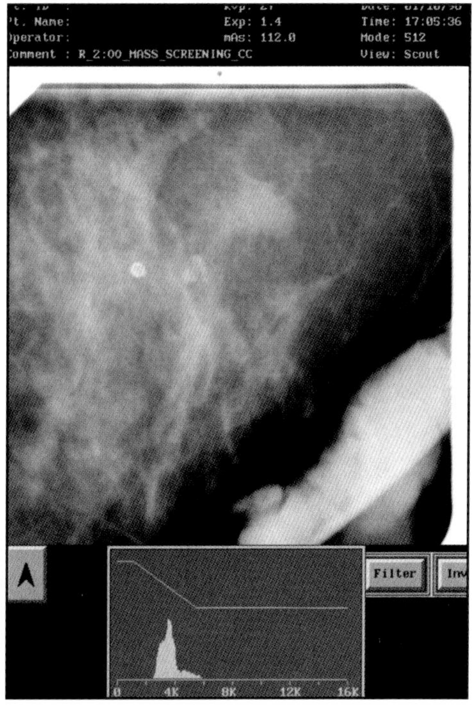

(h)

viewer's ability to see low-contrast objects in darker areas because the eye is flooded with light **(Figure 5.19 a and b)**.

Filtering

Filtering changes the degree to which different spatial frequencies are enhanced or suppressed before being displayed. A modest amount of high-pass filtering (sharpening) can help compensate for the loss of high-frequency signal caused by blurring in the detector and display. Sharpening does not, however, generally improve the signal-to-noise ratio, as both signal and noise at high frequencies are enhanced. Low-pass filtering (blurring or smoothing) is also available on the workstation to create a more tolerant image for the user. Workstations also provide a way of redisplaying the original unenhanced image. When this is done, the structures revealed by filtering are usually visible, although they may be less conspicuous **(Figure 5.19 c and d)**.

Technical Application

Image quality depends upon system design. However, technical application is equally important in achieving the best a system has to offer. The use of the digital modality is sufficiently different from a conventional screen-film system to warrant a discussion of technical application.

The imaging goal for SBB to identify rather than characterize an abnormality for targeting (on both the scout and stereo images) allows some flexibility in image acceptance, both in its appearance *and* information content. Image processing and enhancement provide a wide exposure range, creating a more technique-tolerant environment. Therefore, the imaging goal should be to provide as minimal a dose as possible, while maintaining abnormality identification.

The following factors affect the successful imaging of an abnormality:

- Signal-to-noise ratio
- Matrix
- Image in space

Signal-to-Noise Ratio

Aside from the inherent resolution of the system (that is, pixel and matrix size), signal-to-noise ratio will be the determining factor in visualization of an abnormality. A digital

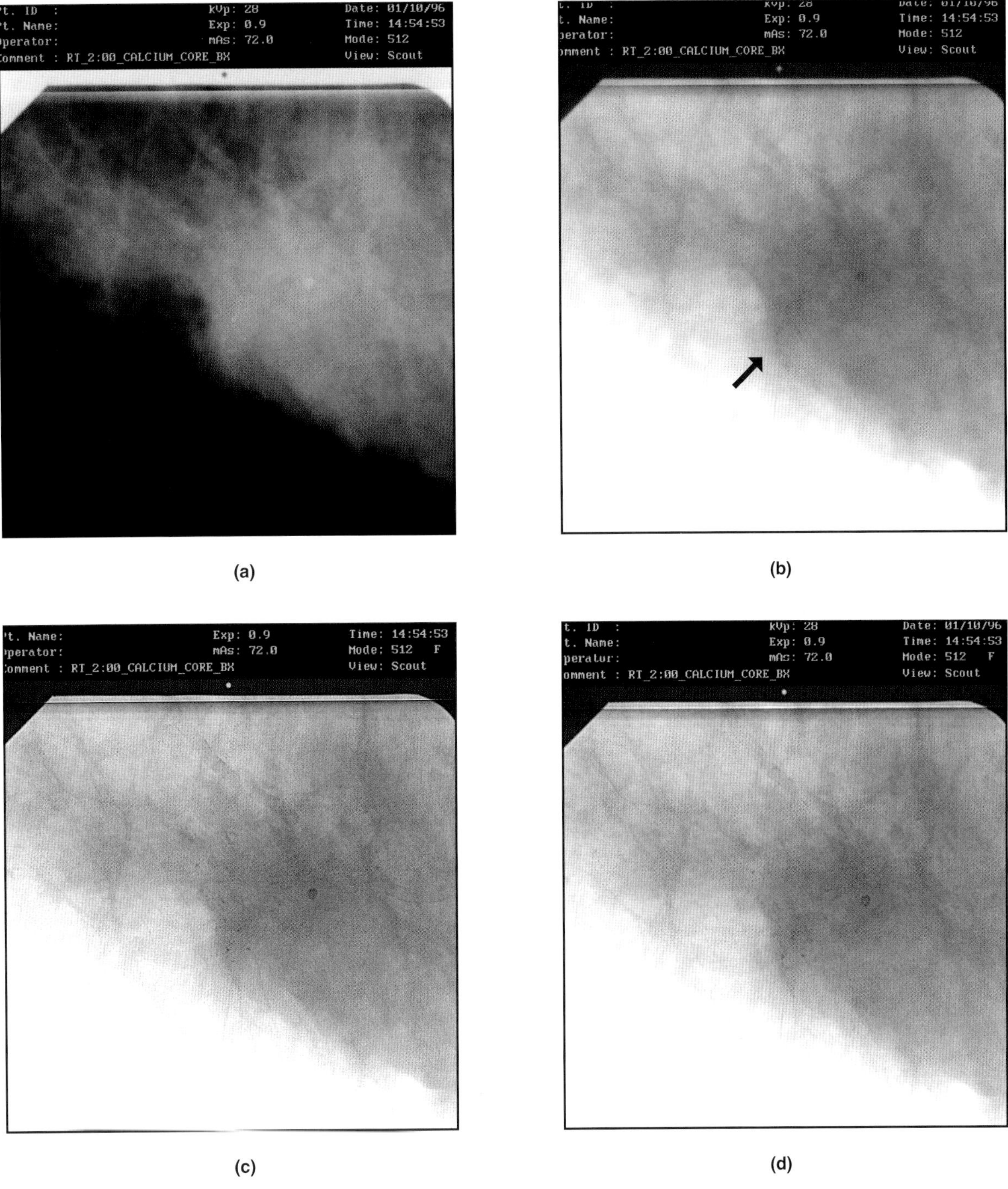

Figure 5.19 a-d. Inverting and Filtering. Inverting and filtering are two other image processing functions available to the user to alter the image for viewing. **Figure 5.19a** illustrates an unaltered image. **Figure 5.19b** shows the same image inverted; in some cases, this function will help the user to perceive calcifications **(arrow)**. **Figures 5.19 c and d** illustrate this inverted image in conjunction with the filtering function, which has an edge enhancement effect. **Figure 5.19c** illustrates the sharpening function of the filter process; note that even though the calcium becomes more visible, the visibility of noise also increases. The smoothing function of filtering "quiets" the noise to make the image more pleasing to the eye, as shown in **Figure 5.19d**. These two functions are usually used together.

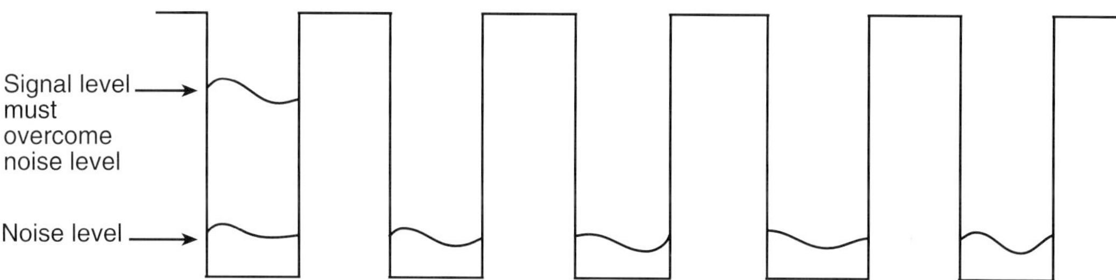

Figure 5.20. Noise Levels. The noise levels in each pixel of the CCD must be overcome with signal to enable faint signals to be seen.

receptor will almost always render what looks like a usable image, however, the image may not provide the necessary information because of a low signal-to-noise ratio.

As stated earlier, some noise is added by every level of the digital imaging chain (Figure 5.8). The noise associated with quantum mottle can be reduced by an increase in exposure. However, signal levels must be high enough to overcome the noise inherent in the CCD (**Figure 5.20**); this is the challenge of producing a usable image. The *goal of the user is to attain adequate signal-to-noise ratio based on the imaging needs of the pathology of interest, while minimizing dose.*

This is quite different from a screen-film system, where exposure is thought of in terms of achieving an optimal density range, based on breast thickness and composition. For example, with a conventional imaging system, a breast measuring 6 cm with a 2 cm mass would require just as much exposure as microcalcifications in the same breast. However, with a digital system, a breast measuring 6 cm with a 2 cm mass will require a lower exposure or signal-to-noise ratio to visualize the abnormality than microcalcifications in the same breast. While image processing and enhancement will provide an adequate image of the mass at a lower exposure, noise may interfere with the visualization of the calcifications. An increase in signal to noise ratio would be necessary to image the calcifications due to its smaller size and low contrast. With fairly obvious abnormalities, a reduction in dose may be realized, compared with a screen-film system. However, for *microcalcifications, low- density masses with poorly defined borders (no matter the size), and fine-lined architectural distortions, dose may need to be increased for adequate visualization.*

Exposure also depends on the tissue surrounding the pathology in question. Visualizing abnormalities against a background of fat generally requires less exposure than when in a background of glandular structures. Generally speaking, *greater contrast sensitivity requires a higher signal-to-noise ratio* (**Figure 5.21**).

Technical Factors

Technical factors are chosen based on obtaining an adequate signal-to-noise ratio.

Kilovoltage (kVp)

The contrast of the displayed image is relatively insensitive to kVp selection (see *Image in Space*). Higher kVp values can be chosen to reduce dose. The new role of kVp is to provide maximum signal-to-noise ratio for each specific imaging situation. Generally, a fixed kVp is recommended based on milliroentgens (mR) per mAs to provide the highest signal. KVp would only be increased for an extremely thick breast of very dense tissue composition, where a lower kVp would be inadequate to penetrate the breast and reduce signal-to-noise ratio.

Milliamperage and Time

A specific choice of milliamperage and time are no longer necessary to achieve density, but serve to provide adequate signal-to-noise ratio. Size and contrast requirements of the pathology in question may require an increase in mAs for successful abnormality visualization. Although reciprocity law failure is not an issue with CCD technology, exposure times should be at a level that minimizes patient motion.

Determining Appropriate Technique

Manual Technique with Histogram—Proper technique is determined based on abnormality identification. Histogram levels issued by the equipment manufacturer provide the basis to alter exposure. However, the user should use these levels as a guideline rather than as an absolute **(Figure 5.22)**. If the abnormality is well-seen for the purposes of targeting, then technique may be reduced for subsequent images (based on histogram levels) to reduce dose. If the abnormality eludes visualization, the histogram level is used to determine proper signal-to-noise ratios based on the manufacturer's instructions for each matrix. The user must remember to utilize image processing, that is, manipulate the display before determining nonvisualization.

Automatic Exposure Control (AEC)—Digital equipment utilizing AEC bases optimal exposure on preset pixel values. This may limit the user's judgment in selecting the exposure needed to visualize a particular abnormality at the lowest dose possible, unless a histogram is also available. Without the histogram, there is no parameter for determining under- or overexposure based on visualization of the abnormality.

Matrix Selection

Some units have a choice of matrix size (512 x 512 or 1024 x 1024) available for imaging. Generally, the 512 matrix provides higher contrast resolution than the 1024 matrix. As mentioned earlier, the 512 matrix has fewer pixels (about 250,000 pixels compared with over 1,000,000 pixels for 1024). A reduced number of pixels means lower noise levels, and lower noise levels require *less* exposure to maintain adequate signal-to-noise ratios. Greater signal-to-noise ratios are possible at the same exposure with the 512 matrix, compared with the 1024 matrix **(Figure 5.23)**, providing for increased contrast resolution.

For these reasons, the 512 matrix should be chosen whenever possible, as it reduces patient dose. The 512 matrix should also be used when high contrast is desirable, such as with low-density masses. Again, this depends somewhat on the spatial requirements of the abnormality. In our experience, the 512 matrix seems to be adequate for the

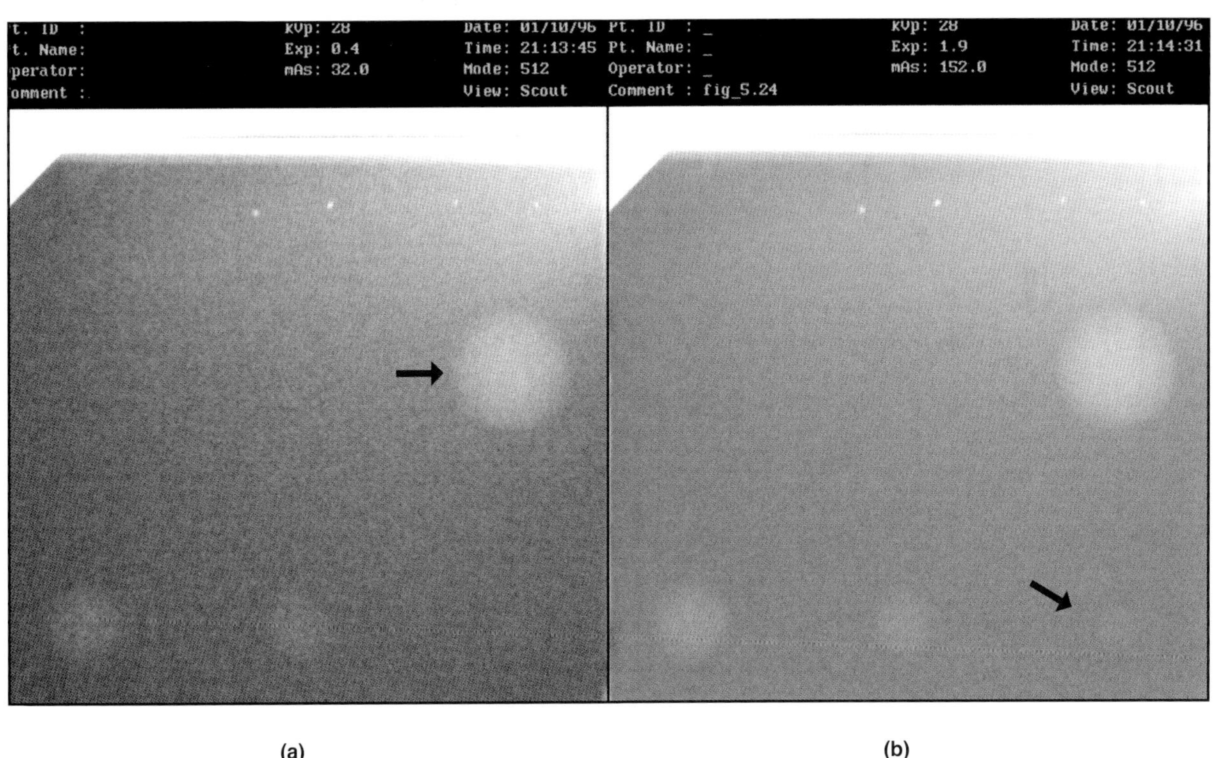

Figure 5.21 a and b. Contrast and Signal-to-Noise Ratio. A portion of the familiar ACR phantom is used to illustrate greater signal requirements for greater contrast needs. **Figure 5.21a** illustrates the large mass well **(arrow)** at a technique of 28 kVp and 32 mAs. However, the smaller masses are less well-seen or invisible. Increasing technique to 128 mAs [kVp remains constant] provides the greater signal-to-noise ratio required of the smaller masses **(Figure 5.21b)**. Note: the last mass is seen well enough for targeting **(arrow)**. This example illustrates the dose reduction possible with high-contrast abnormalities.

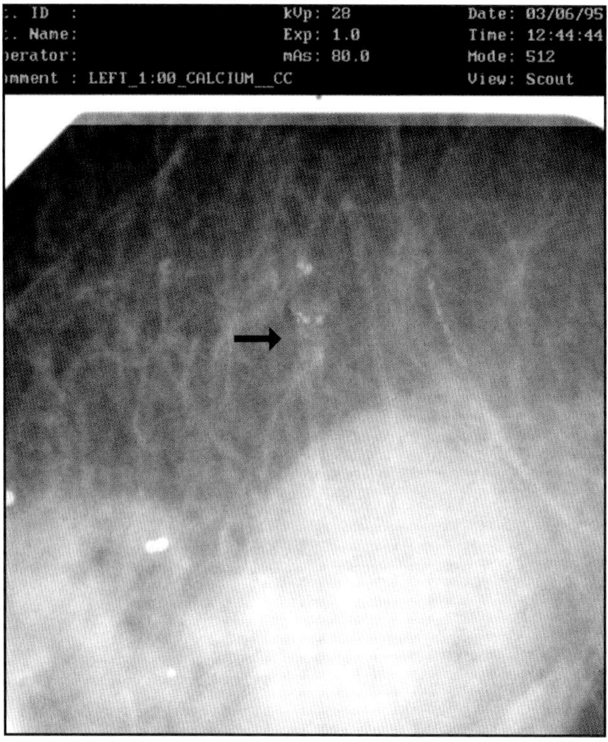

Figure 5.22. Technical Application. For SBB, technique should be determined based on identification of the abnormality, dose considerations, and histogram levels. Even though the manufacturer's recommended histogram level for this 512 matrix is 2-4K, the calcium in this 5 cm breast **(arrow)** is well-demonstrated at lower levels; always consider abnormality visualization as the goal of technique. If the abnormality of interest had not been visualized, then the histogram in this case would indicate a necessary increase in technique (see histogram in Figure 5.16).

purposes of SBB for the majority of abnormalities, mass or calcium **(Figure 5.24)**.

The decision to use the 1024 matrix requires the user to carefully balance the imaging requirements of the pathology and the composition of the surrounding breast tissue. *Determining whether high contrast or high resolution is necessary for visualization is the basis for choosing the appropriate matrix.* Pathologies of smaller size or lower contrast may require a 1024 matrix, if the resolution requirements are beyond that of the 512 matrix. However, there are those cases, specifically groups of microcalcifications, that appear to require the higher resolution matrix (1024). In practice, however, these calcifications escape visualization due to inadequate signal-to-noise ratio, which results from the increased noise levels at the 1024 matrix. This scenario is entirely possible because some abnormalities are beyond both the spatial and contrast resolution capabilities of the imaging system. However, because the entire abnormality does not have to be visible for SBB, if a few of the larger calcifications are within the spatial capabilities of the 512 matrix, then a greater signal-to-noise ratio is attainable, allowing identification of the abnormality.

Image in Space

The geometric principles of mammography are still the determining factors of visibility. Although a digital system provides greater contrast resolution over a wide range of exposures, visualization of an abnormality still depends on the quality of the image in space. Image manipulation and enhancement can improve the visibility of detail, but it *cannot* produce information that does not exist initially. Abnormalities of higher spatial frequencies are especially susceptible to nonvisualization because the image in space does not always provide the necessary information.

Because the digital unit is a separate piece of equipment, it functions within the design constraints of the mammography unit and/or the SBB system. In this sense, the capabilities or design of the host system may limit the digital system. Using a digital receptor with an upright unit can reduce procedure time. However, the limits of the host mammography unit combined with the SBB equipment may still limit abnormality visualization (see chapter 2).

Scatter Control

Although a digital system can reduce the effects of scatter on

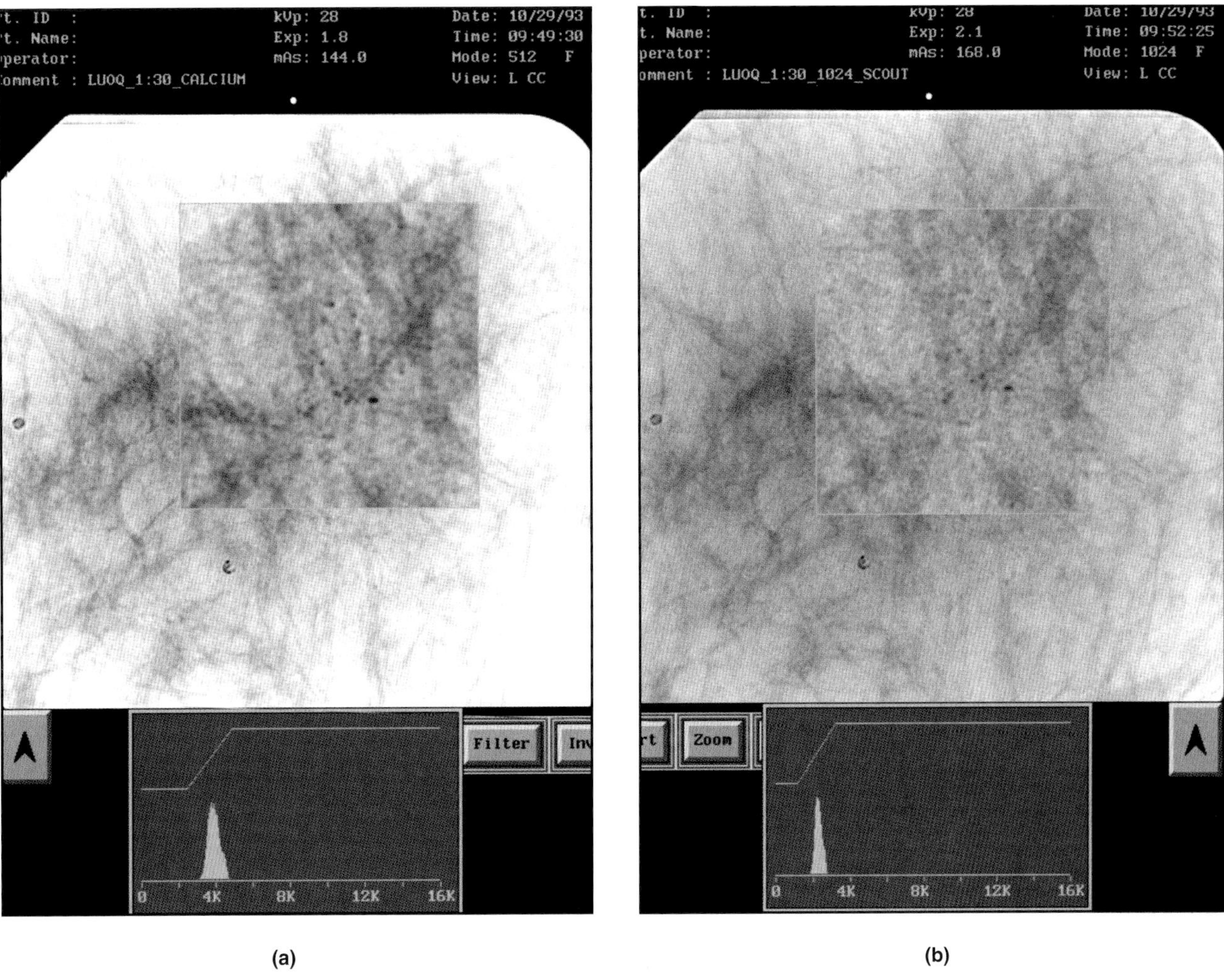

(a) (b)

Figure 5.23 a and b. Choosing a Matrix. Comparable levels of exposure illustrate the decreased signal-to-noise ratio of the 1024 vs. 512 matrix (histograms). More calcifications are visualized at reduced technique in the 512 matrix **(a)**, compared with the 1024 matrix **(b)**, because of greater signal-to-noise ratio. To get comparable levels of SNR in the 1024 matrix, mAs would have to be doubled, thereby increasing dose.

the viewed image, it is not free from the effects of scatter on contrast resolution. Moiré (cross-hatching) patterns caused by grids prohibit their use in SBB digital systems. The best a digital system can do is to provide an air gap to prevent some of the scatter from reaching the image receptor. Appropriate apertures to narrow the beam or imaging field will help reduce scatter. Scatter can also be decreased somewhat by compression. However, the open biopsy window and the length of the procedure disallow the compression levels of routine mammography. Furthermore, once the biopsy instrument is placed on the stage, a portion of the instrument will be visualized in the biopsy window. Scattered radiation, produced by the biopsy instrument, may reduce signal-to-noise ratio. This can be partially avoided by using a longer needle (16 cm rather than 10 cm), which will minimize the effect of the biopsy instrument on the field of view.

Positioning Aspects

Obtaining adequate visualization of an abnormality and maintaining visualization with stereo angles is discussed in detail in chapter 6 (*Positioning*). However, a few critical points are mentioned below.

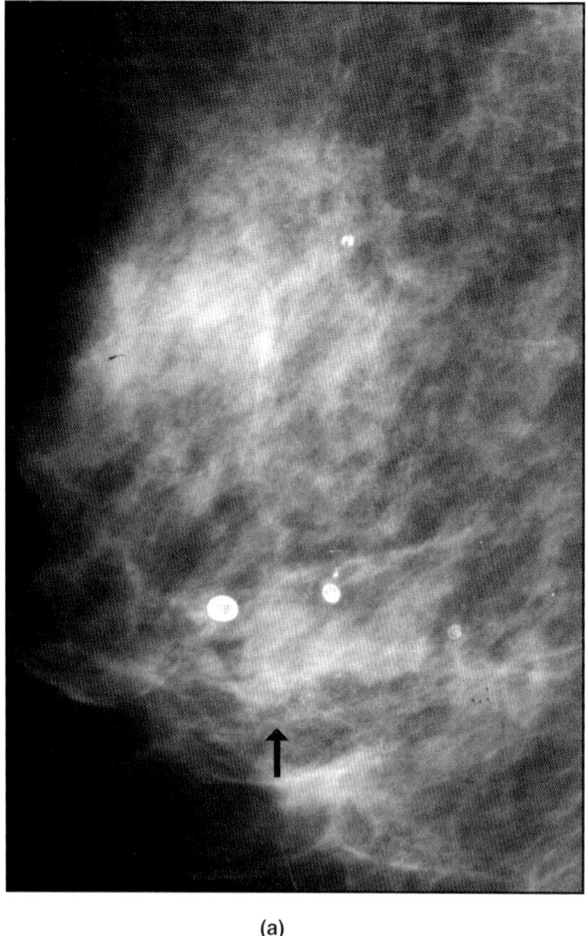

(a)

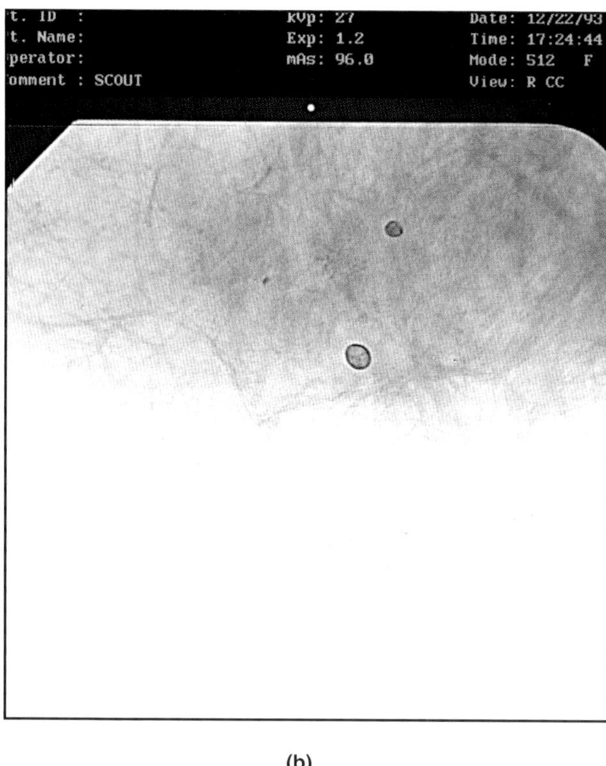

(b)

Figure 5.24 a and b. 512 Matrix vs. 1024 Matrix. The 512 matrix is adequate for most abnormalities for SBB. **Figure 5.24a** shows a 1.8x magnification view of calcifications. **Figure 5.24b** shows a digital image in the 512 matrix that demonstrates these calcifications for targeting. The 1024 matrix was not necessary, despite the minute size of these calcifications.

Demonstrating the Abnormality in Fat

Demonstrating the abnormality in fat, whenever possible, will provide the best contrast differentiation. This is especially important of abnormalities at higher spatial frequencies, where there will be a fine line between choosing one matrix over the other.

Coverage of the Biopsy Window

Maintaining compression on all sides of the biopsy window reduces motion and prevents "tenting" of the skin at needle insertion. In digital imaging, the need to "fill" the biopsy window is even greater. As outlined earlier in the image processing section, the image processor will produce an image based on pixel values. If a large portion of the biopsy window is *not* covered, the pixel values corresponding to that portion of the biopsy window will be very high. The balance of the biopsy window that demonstrates breast tissue will have normal pixel values. The image processor will detect the two ranges of pixel values and base the initial image processing on accommodating both ranges, thereby reducing the range of gray levels available for viewing visibility and detail in the region of interest. Chapter 6 discusses positioning methods to achieve maximum biopsy window coverage. When this is not possible, putty, clay, or lead can be placed in the x-ray field to equalize x-ray absorption.

References

1. Honeyman, J.C., Dwyer, III, S.J. 1993. Historical Perspectives on Computer Development and Glossary of Terms. *RadioGraphics* 13:145-152.

2. Schmidt, R. and Nishikawa, R.M. 1995. Clinical Use of Digital Mammography: The Present and the Prospects. *Journal of Digital Imaging* 8 (February) (1) (1): 74-79.

3. Shtern, F. 1992. Digital Mammography and Related Technologies: A Perspective from the National Cancer Institute. *Radiology* 183:629-630.

4. Kimme-Smith, C. 1992. New and Future Developments in Screen-Film Mammography Equipment and Techniques. *Radiologic Clinics of North America* 30 (January) (1).

5. Lucier, B. J., Kallergi, M., Qian, W., DeVore, R., Clark, R.A., Saff, E.B., Clarke, L.P. 1994. Wavelet Compression and Segmentation of Digital Mammograms. *Journal of Digital Imaging* 7 (February) (1): 27-38.

6. Karellas, A., Liu, H., Harris, L., D'Orsi, C.J. 1994. Digital Mammo Delivers Quick, Reliable Image. *Diagnostic Imaging* (February).

7. Karellas, A., Harris, L.J., Liu, H., Davis, M.A., D'Orsi, C.J. 1992. Charge Coupled Device Detector: Performance Considerations and Potential for Small-Field Mammographic Imaging Applications. *Medical Physics* 19 (July/August) (4).

8. Roehrig, H., Fajardo, L., Yu, T. 1993. Digital X-Ray Cameras for Real Time Stereotactic Breast Needle Biopsy. SPIE Vol. 1896. *Physics of Medical Imaging.*

9. Haus, Arthur G. 1994. Screen-Film Image Receptors and Film Processing, In Syllabus: A Categorical Course in Physics. Radiological Society of North America Publications.

10. Yaffe, Martin J. 1994. Digital Mammography, In Syllabus: A Categorical Course in Physics. Radiological Society of North America Publications.

11. Sprawls, Perry 1993. *Physical Principles of Medical Imaging* 2nd edition. Aspen Publishers, Inc.

12. Gonzalez, R.C., Wintz, P. 1987. *Digital Image Processing.* Addison-Wesley Publishing Co.

13. Balter, S., 1993. Fundamental Properties of Digital Images. *RadioGraphics* 13:129-141.

14. Hendrick, R.E. and Parker, S.H. 1994. Stereotaxic Imaging, In Syllabus: A Categorical Course in Physics. Radiological Society of North America Publications.

15. Blume, H., Roehrig, H., Browne, M., Ji, T.L. 1990. Comparison of the Physical Performance of High Resolution CRT Displays and Films Recorded by the Laser Image Printers and Displayed on Light-Boxes and the Need for Display Standard. SPIE Vol. 1232. Medical Imaging IV: Image Capture and Display.

16. Muka, E., Blume, H., Daly, S. 1995. Display of Medical Images on CRT Soft-Copy Displays: A Tutorial. SPIE 2431.

17. Parsons, D.M., Kim, Y., Haynor, D.R. 1995. Quality Control of Cathode-Ray Tube Monitors for Medical Imaging Using a Simple Photometer. *Journal of Digital Imaging* 8 (February) (1) 10-20.

Positioning in Stereotactic Procedures

Kathleen M. Willison
Debra S. Saunders

6

Introduction

The goal of positioning for stereotactic breast biopsy is to appropriately center and visualize an abnormality to allow adequate needle sampling. The technologist is primarily responsible for positioning, however, the clinician should be aware of the complex issues and challenges. Positioning is multifaceted, ranging from the relatively simple task of positioning the abnormality in the projection it was best seen to more challenging issues.

The complex conditions of positioning that exist for mammography also exist for stereotactic biopsy. Even though the focus is imaging a specific area of the breast rather than the entire breast, the same factors apply, that is, body habitus, placement of the breast on the body, and breast composition. In addition to these sometimes troublesome elements, other more critical and demanding factors influence the ultimate approach to positioning for SBB, the most notable being positive stroke margin (see chapter 2). Access to an abnormality's location may also be difficult. The technologist must identify the abnormality on the scout image, as well as maintain clarity on the stereo projections. Other important factors include overlying blood vessels and patient comfort.

This arduous set of tasks can be overcome with a positive attitude, an open mind, and a willingness to master new techniques. The technologist achieves proficiency with experience in a variety of circumstances. Canceled procedures should be limited to restrictions imposed by the patient or the stereotactic unit, rather than the technologist's reluctance to investigate new positioning options. The technologist can facilitate the positioning process and narrow the learning curve by adhering to the following guidelines:

- Be knowledgeable about the stereotactic unit by learning both its advantages and limitations.
- Understand the rudiments of stereotactic biopsy, grasping the concepts of stroke and the calculation of stroke margin.
- Become adept at approximating abnormality location in the breast, based on the two-view mammogram.

Understanding these elements and the positioning basics discussed below will provide a strong foundation to develop and build positioning skills.

The use of a live model to practice positioning will provide the technologist with valuable insight into positioning issues. Practicing with a phantom (homemade or commercial) will further enhance technical experience.

Positioning Basics

Patient Motion

The technologist should fully understand the negative effects of patient motion. The results of motion can increase dose, add an excessive amount of time to the procedure, and may complicate the biopsy process. If the patient moves her breast, thereby moving the abnormality, any time after acquisition of the stereo images, the coordinates may no longer be useful. Motion may result in the need to reposition the breast in the biopsy window, retake the stereo images, retarget the abnormality, and in some cases may require a second skin incision. Additional prefire stereo images will be necessary to again check for correct needle placement. With the use of a Cartesian coordinate system, reacquiring *stereos* may not be necessary; a simple measurement and adjustment is possible. However, *prefire* stereo images are necessary to verify accurate needle placement. It is vital, therefore, that the technologist does everything she can to assure the patient does not move during the procedure. To aid in the observation of patient motion the technologist should mark the breast **(Figure 6.1)**. The guidelines described below will help diminish the causes of motion and ensure a smoother biopsy procedure.

Applying Antiseptic

Apply antiseptic sparingly to cleanse the skin. An excessive amount can seep between the breast and the biopsy compression plate, allowing the breast to slip from compression.

Patient Cooperation

As with any clinical procedure, patient cooperation is vital to success. Achieving patient cooperation involves creating an atmosphere of trust and understanding. Sensitivity to the patient's genuine concerns about the results is critical. Her fear of carcinoma is justifiable, even if there is a low probability of cancer.

Most patients are relieved and pleased to learn that a less invasive option to open biopsy exists. However, the patient may still be uneasy about the biopsy procedure. Anxiety levels are often high, but a confident, compassionate technologist can help alleviate some of the patient's ambivalence. While the technologist can never offer reassurance as to the outcome of the biopsy, she can let the patient know her fears are understandable and acceptable. Inform the patient that the team is here to help her through the procedure with as little discomfort as possible. During the procedure, it is imperative to communicate with the patient to inform her of the progress and also to help pass the time for her. Some biopsy suites have piped in music or headsets for the patient, with choices of music or sounds of nature to create a more soothing atmosphere. *The patient should never be left alone in the biopsy room,* regardless of whether a prone or upright unit is being used.

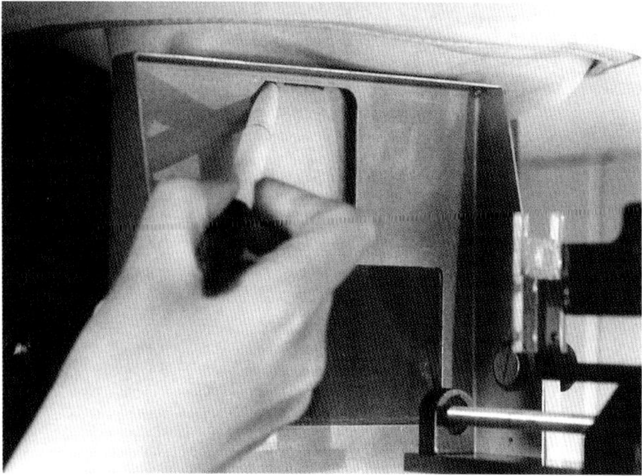

Figure 6.1. Marking the Breast for Motion. The technologist can mark the breast for observation of patient motion.

Explanation of the Procedure

A description of the biopsy procedure from beginning to end allows the patient to prepare for the process. Begin with a brief explanation of positioning. Achieving the appropriate biopsy projection can require a considerable amount of time; in fact, it may require more time than the actual biopsy. The patient should be made aware that this is normal. Gently stress the need to remain immobile for the length of the procedure, outlining the consequences of motion.

Inform the patient that during the procedure, there will be some conversation among team members to facilitate the smooth performance of the biopsy procedure. Then explain the sampling procedure step-by-step. Always use sensitivity in explaining the procedure. Avoid words such as gun, fire, and needle. Allow time for questions, directing diagnostic inquiries to the radiologist or supervising clinician.

Prior patient response confirms that pain is usually confined to needle insertion for local anesthesia. Once this numbing occurs, the patient will feel a minimal amount in her breast. After anesthesia, a small skin incision will be made that will barely be visible when it heals.

It is very important to explain the tissue sampling or "firing" of the biopsy instrument. Explain or demonstrate the noise of the biopsy instrument, never bringing the loaded instrument into her view. Without giving a definite number, inform the patient that multiple samples are necessary to adequately sample an area. If the abnormality involves calcifications, it is best to briefly explain the time period associated with specimen radiography, and the possibility of subsequent samples.

Tell the patient that most women do not experience pain at the firing of the biopsy instrument but feel a "thumping" sensation. However, request that if she does feel pain, let the team know. If possible, the clinician can administer additional anesthesia.

The combination of sound and sensation may startle the patient at the firing of the biopsy instrument. To avoid motion at this point, let the patient know that prior to sampling, she will be verbally reminded about the "thump," and that the technologist will place a firm but gentle hand on her shoulder to prevent a startled response.

During postbiopsy compression, the technologist can

explain follow-up contact and care. These instructions should also be given to the patient in written form before she leaves.

Patient Comfort

For most patients, the most uncomfortable part of the biopsy procedure may be remaining in one position for an extended period of time. Explain this to the patient in advance and make every effort to make her as comfortable as possible. Recommend that the patient use the lavatory prior to the beginning of the procedure. Also have her remove earrings or any other apparel that might interfere with the x-ray beam or her comfort. Prior to final positioning of the breast, allow the patient to remain in position for a few minutes so she can identify awkward positions or points of pressure. Offer a blanket to keep the patient warm.

Prone Tables

For prone tables, the patient is *normally* in a slight right anterior oblique (RAO), or left anterior oblique (LAO) position, depending on the breast and the location of the abnormality (see later discussion on positioning). Points of pressure often include the ipsilateral shoulder and inferior ribs. When addressing comfort issues, be careful not to excessively raise the shoulder or ribs from the table. This can raise the breast out of the table aperture, limiting posterior access. Placing a soft but thin sponge or other material between the shoulder, ribs, and table will help alleviate discomfort. A nonsterile surgical glove minimally filled with water, or a thin silicone-filled pad, creates a nice cushion between pressure points and the table without excessively raising the breast out of the table aperture.

The neck is another area that may be uncomfortable during prone biopsy. A thin, warm water bottle, supportive sponges, or a rolled towel placed beneath the hollow formed by the neck and table can offer support and comfort. *It is important not to place anything beneath the head* **(Figure 6.2).** This causes additional stress and strain on the neck and shoulder (and possible carotid compression). However, if access to the posterior breast is not necessary, offer a small, thin pillow to give both head and neck support in the same plane. Be sure that the contralateral breast is also comfortably placed. If it is necessary to have the contralateral breast over the table opening, a sling can be made from the patient's gown to hold the breast up and out of the way. During the procedure, if the patient complains of stiffness or loss of sensation in the neck or arm, the technologist can massage the area to alleviate discomfort.

The lower back may also need support to prevent an uncomfortable lordotic curve. Place a small pillow beneath the abdomen to prevent discomfort, or provide a pillow for support beneath the bent leg.

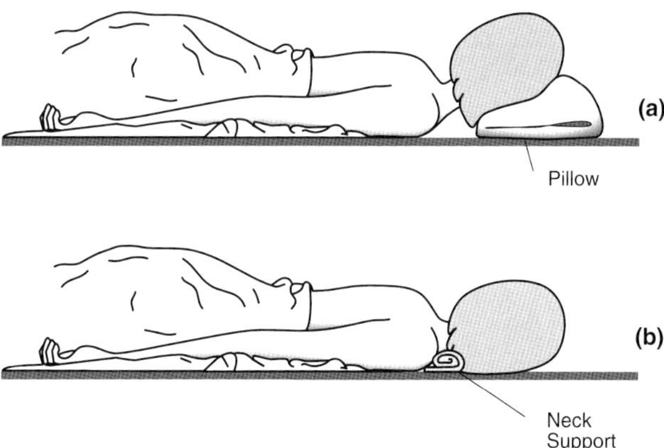

Figure 6.2. Neck Support. Placing a pillow under the head when the patient is prone may result in discomfort to neck and shoulder **(a)**. Placing a pillow for neck support is more appropriate **(b)**.

Add-on Units

Speed is of the essence for upright procedures. Reduction of procedure time is possible with standard processing (versus extended) and/or a digital receptor. The biopsy team must become comfortable with their roles and adept with equipment to achieve proficiency with a procedure. In the beginning of a biopsy program, procedures may be sparse, so it is crucial for the technologist to practice with a phantom to maintain skill with the stereotactic equipment.

Adapting a dedicated mammography unit for biopsy with add-on stereotactic equipment presents many challenges for the technologist. The biopsy team should first attempt a complete analysis of the positioning situation prior to patient arrival. This will shorten procedural time, and reduce complications. Awareness of the following issues will help provide the best possible environment for the patient while maintaining the requirements of stereotactic biopsy.

Support—For the patient to remain motionless in an upright position during the entire biopsy procedure, the technologist must ensure patient comfort. Very little effort should be expected of the patient to maintain the biopsy position. Back support is particularly important. Pillows or other similar props can provide the necessary support. Sufficient back support will hold the patient in position, diminish fatigue, and reduce the opportunity for motion. Support for the feet and legs also provides stability. Without foot support, the legs suspend freely, which counters the patient's ability to lean forward for breast positioning. This also places unnecessary stress on the lower back, making it increasingly uncomfortable and difficult for the patient to remain motionless during the extended period of time of the biopsy procedure. The floor can provide foot support if the chair is low enough, or use a footstool if a footrest is not provided on the biopsy chair. Although it might be advantageous for the biopsy chair to be on wheels, this may be a hindrance if the wheels do not lock for final positioning.

Bleeding—Extensive bleeding at the biopsy site is not a routine occurrence, however, always drape the lower half of the patient's body to prevent staining clothes or skin.

Vaso-vagal Response—Vaso-vagal response should always be a concern in any procedure where the patient is upright[1]. Diminishing vaso-vagal response with upright procedures depends on a number of factors. Every effort should be made to position the patient in a way that shields her view from the biopsy procedure and sterile tray. The technologist has to assure that she is comfortable and well-supported. The clinician and technologist should communicate with her at all times during the exam, especially when waiting for film processing.

Vaso-vagal response may also increase with limitations on food intake. There is no need to limit food intake for core biopsy or FNAC, assuming the patient will not be proceeding to surgical postbiopsy.

Technical Considerations for SBB Positioning

X-ray Field Size

Biopsy Field—Each stereo unit has a specified x-ray field size. The technologist should be aware of the actual dimensions of the field, as this may differ from the size of the biopsy window available on the compression plate. The imaging field for digital systems, typically 50 mm x 50 mm, may be smaller than the imaging field of screen-film systems.

Scout Field—A wider aperture may be available with a matching compression paddle. This wider field is useful for scouting purposes, providing a larger portion of the breast for imaging. It helps if the scout paddle is fenestrated (has openings), so the technologist can mark the location of the abnormality on the skin.

Centering and Abnormality Shift

Projectional shift of the abnormality occurs in the horizontal plane with stereo acquisition (see chapter 2). Centering of the abnormality in the horizontal plane (X or H-axis) of the biopsy window is critical to maintain visualization at stereo acquisition. However, nonvisualization of the abnormality can occur on one or both stereo images despite proper centering. The abnormality may not be within the confines of the image receptor or x-ray field. The probability of nonvisualization also increases as compression thickness increases. Nonvisualization becomes more critical when the image-receptor field size is limited, such as with digital imaging systems. The abnormality could also elude visualization as a result of system design. This can occur on systems that do not allow for increased compression thickness, usually above 6 cm (see discussion below).

Centering in the vertical plane (Y-axis) is not necessary, as the stereo projections do not affect vertical placement. However, a certain vertical placement within the biopsy window may facilitate the exam by creating easier access for the biopsy team.

Compression Thickness and the Breast Support

An adjustable breast support is most helpful with the use of a digital receptor. As described above and detailed in chapter 4, nonvisualization of the abnormality can occur with stereo acquisition when the abnormality is outside the field of view. This effect increases with compression thickness. A movable breast support **(Figure 6.3)** prevents this phenomenon from occurring, so that there is never a failure to image an abnormality as a result of compression thickness.

The technologist adjusts the breast support on the basis of compression thickness. However, some units do not have an adjustable breast support. In this instance, the technologist must reposition the breast to decrease compression thickness. If, after repositioning, the abnormality still eludes visualization on one or both stereo images, targeting is not possible. Never reduce the angle of stereo acquisition to maintain visualization, *unless* recommended by the manufacturer.

Tissue Coverage within the Biopsy Window

When positioning, always strive to completely cover the biopsy window with breast tissue **(Figure 6.4)**. Compression of the breast from all sides of the biopsy window reduces the possibility of motion. Coverage of the biopsy window increases stability of the breast for needle insertion and better tissue sampling. Window coverage also ensures coverage of the entire x-ray field, thereby diminishing scatter. In addi-

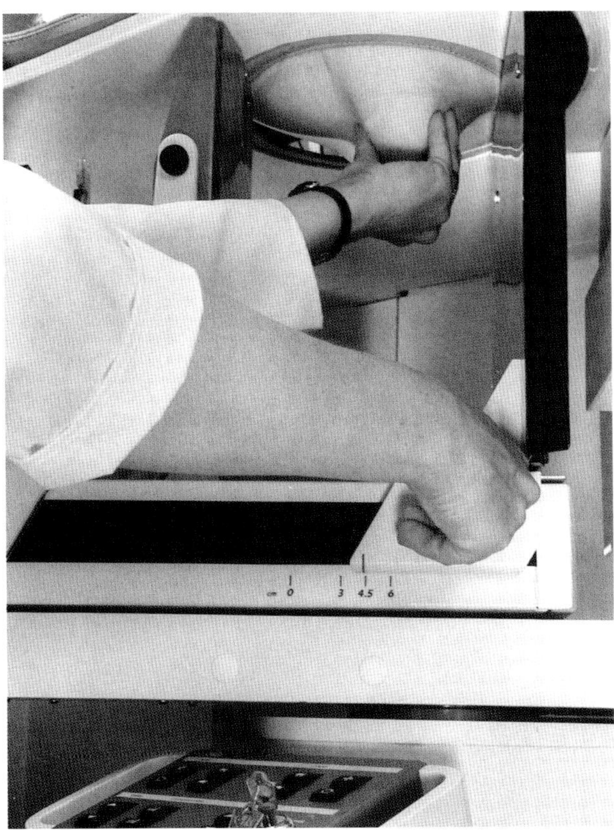

Figure 6.3. Movable Breast Support. Adjustment of a movable breast support allows visualization of the abnormality with stereo shift with all breast thicknesses.

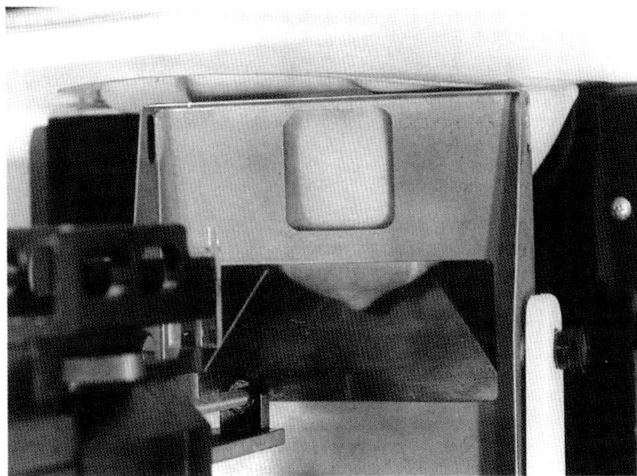

Figure 6.4. Coverage of the Biopsy Window. Coverage of the biopsy window with breast tissue prohibits breast movement and provides stability for needle insertion.

tion, when employing a digital receptor, the computer will reconstruct the image, interpreting any uncovered portion of the x-ray field as a structural part of the breast. This may result in an extremely small latitude for subsequent image processing (window and level functions), thereby inhibiting visualization of the abnormality. Images of retroareolar abnormalities are especially susceptible to incomplete filling of the biopsy window. If possible, it is best to rotate the breast upward or downward to fill the biopsy window rather than profiling the nipple. When this is not possible, place a small amount of single-use putty or modeling clay in the uncovered portion of the imaging field to act as a wedge filter, which will decrease pixel overexposure (see chapter 5) **(Figure 6.5)**.

Compression

Compression has a two-fold purpose in stereotactic biopsy. It holds the breast immobile to prevent motion and tightens the skin surface to facilitate the passage of the needle through the skin surface. The vigorous compression associated with routine mammography is not necessary for stereotactic biopsy. Compression should be applied until there is a "spring" to the skin when touched. Since compression over the biopsy area is prohibited by the open window, the technologist should spread the skin over the area, using her thumbs to make the skin tight **(Figure 6.6)**. This creates tension on the skin surface and minimizes inward "tenting" with needle insertion. Inward tenting may result in breast or abnormality movement, and may prohibit the cutting edge of the biopsy needle from passing through the skin.

Visualizing the Abnormality

Although optimal image technique is responsible for detecting the abnormality on the original mammogram, the circumstances of stereotactic biopsy are sometimes in direct conflict with the technical factors that apply to efficient

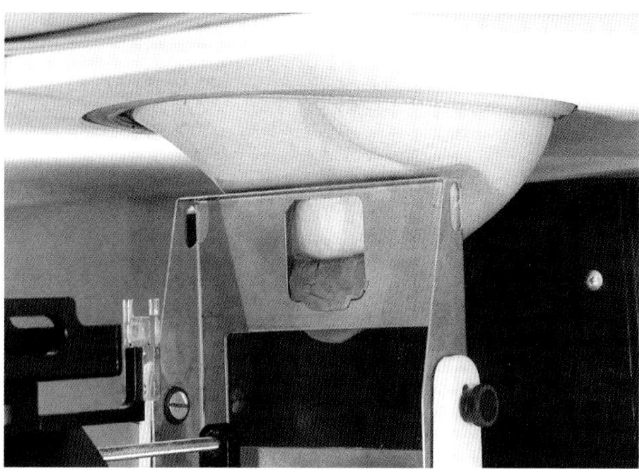

Figure 6.5. Noncoverage of the Biopsy Window. The technologist can place clay or putty in the uncovered portion of the biopsy window to provide better image quality.

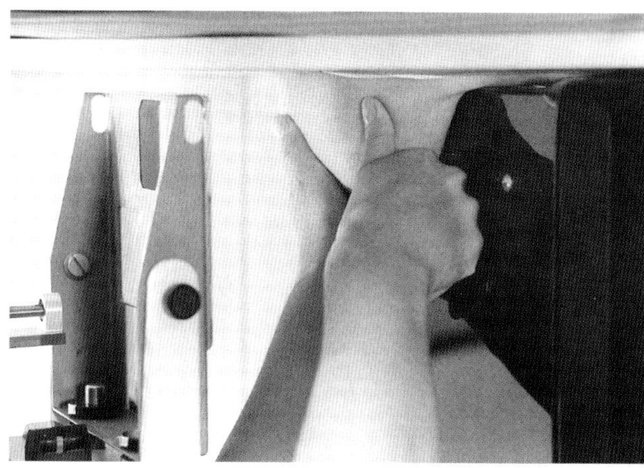

Figure 6.6. Tightening the Skin. The technologist spreads the skin with both thumbs while compressing to tighten the skin surface. This minimizes "tenting" and facilitates needle insertion.

imaging. For example, fine microcalcifications and low-density masses may be susceptible to nonvisualization as a result of 1) the loss of subject contrast due to decreased compression and increased breast thickness over the area of interest, and 2) increased geometric unsharpness due to the increased object-to-image receptor distance.

These undesirable effects become even greater with units using a substandard stationary grid, or no grid, as is the case with most add-on units. Units that allow the x-ray beam to *angle* against the image receptor upon stereo acquisition also introduce distortion.

The technologist must be aware of these compromises to apply the necessary technical skills to image the abnormality. The best the technologist can do in positioning is to select the projection that allows the thinnest compression, which also provides for positive stroke margin. A thinner breast compression will also decrease geometric unsharpness and scatter.

Greater subject contrast can also improve abnormality visualization. Positioning the abnormality against a background of fat will improve subject contrast **(Figure 6.7)**. The glandular parenchyma is distributed with the majority of breast tissue in the subareolar and upper-outer quadrants. This characteristic pattern allows the technologist to take advantage of the fatty areas of the breast. If the technologist and clinician consider the distribution of a patient's glandular parenchyma, they can choose a projection (see *Projections for SBB* later in this chapter) that allows an abnormality to be imaged against a background of fat **(Figures 6.8 and 6.9).**

Logistics for Add-on Units

C-arm Rotation—When choosing a position for biopsy, the technologist must be aware of the logistics of the c-arm swing for stereo images. The patient must be unencumbered by the x-ray tube head and the image-receptor mount of the mammography unit during stereo rotations. The technologist will learn to avoid projections that inhibit c-arm movement. For example, when the technologist positions the patient for a cranio-caudal projection, she may have to move the patient's head to accommodate tube rotation for stereo acquisition. This will increase the chances of breast and abnormality movement. Even if the SID of the unit allows stereo rotation without interference with the patient's head, her head may still interfere with the path of the x-ray beam. The inferior aspect of the c-arm has to clear the patient's lower body with stereo rotation. The technologist should consider another projection if the patient has to move to accommodate tube shift. For example, in the above case, a 20° oblique in the medio-lateral or latero-medial projection would replace the cranio-caudal projection **(Figure 6.10).** This projection should be sufficient to allow clearance for tube shift.

The technologist must also consider efficiency and ease of access from the clinician's perspective. For example, any reverse oblique projection, where the clinician is working from the inferior aspect of the breast, may introduce difficulty into the biopsy procedure.

Cassette Retrieval—The technologist should make sure that she has access to retrieve and replace the film cassette, without having to move or pinch the patient's body.

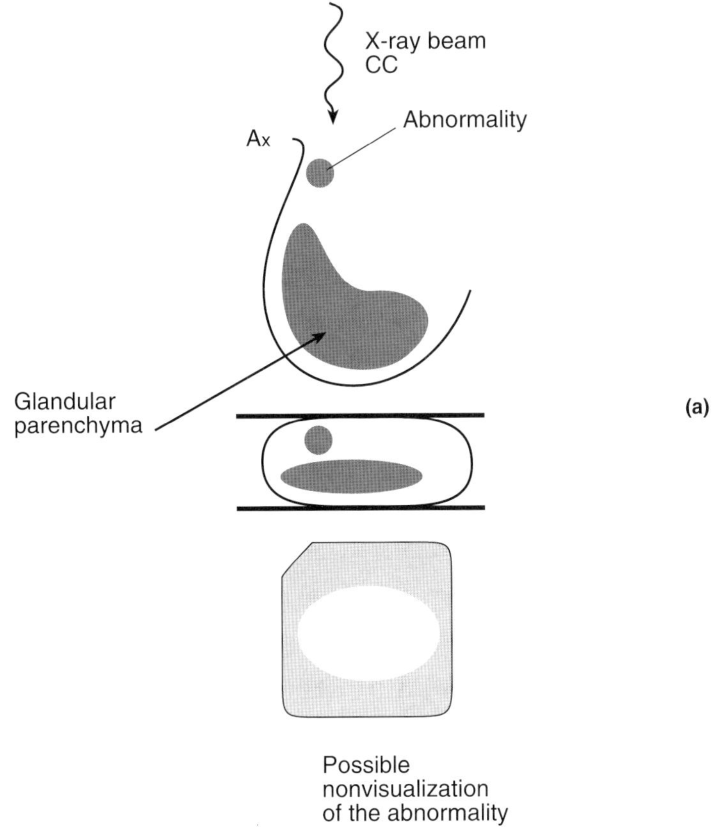

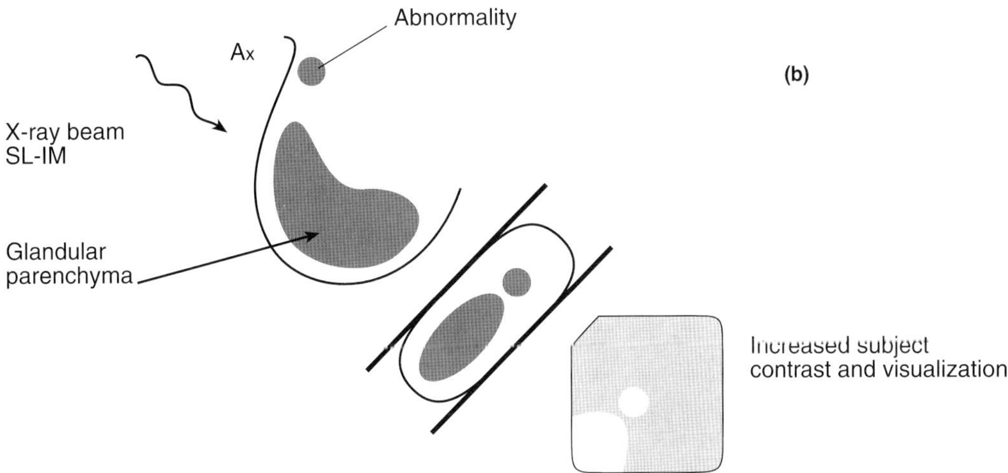

Figure 6.7. Increasing Subject Contrast. Demonstrating an abnormality against a fatty background increases subject contrast. The CC projection will superimpose the abnormality over glandular structures, resulting in possible nonvisualization **(a)**. A Supero-Lateral to Infero-Medial (SL-IM) projection would project the abnormality over the fatty area of the medial breast, increasing subject contrast and visualization **(b)**.

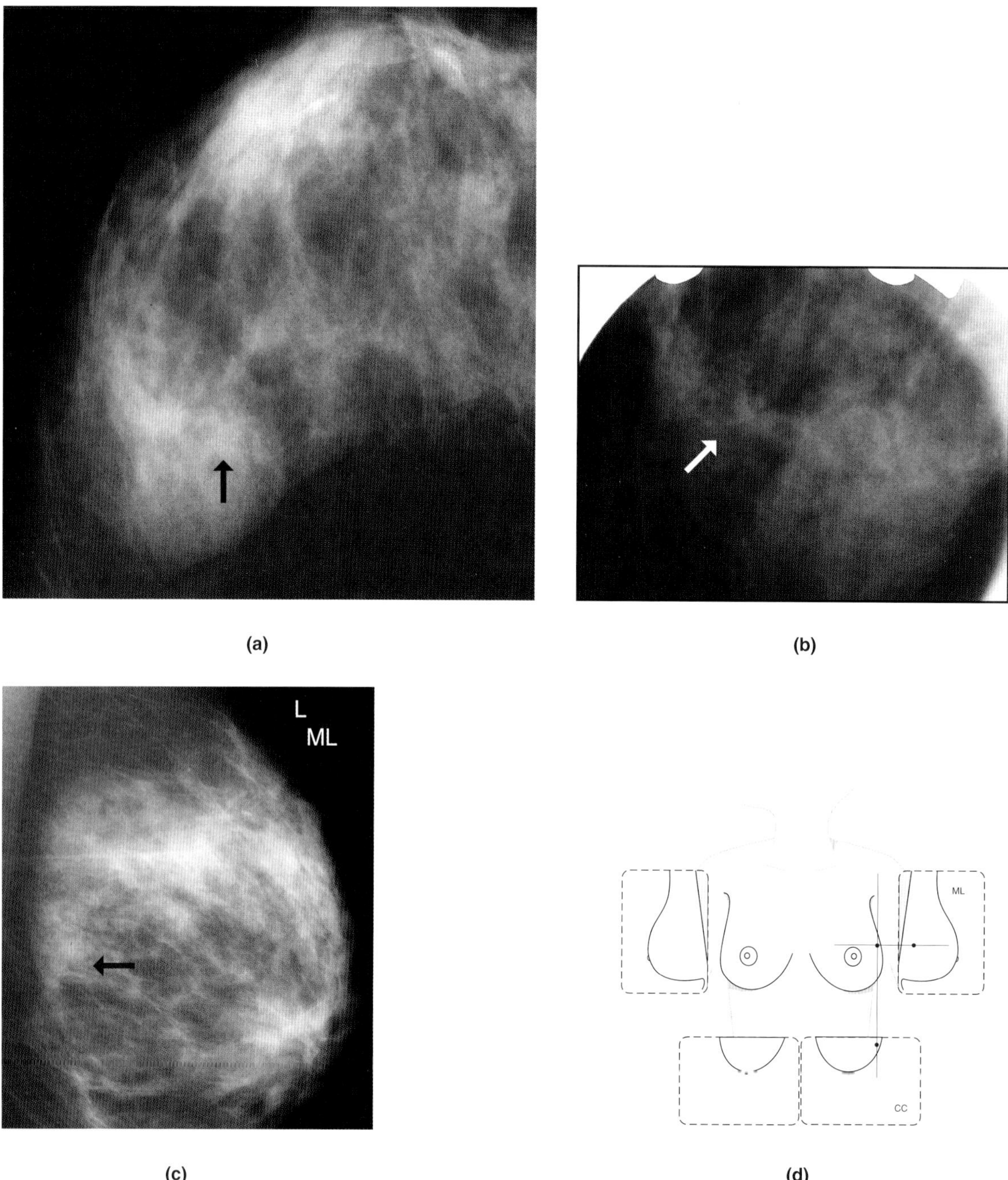

Figure 6.8 a-g. Subject Contrast. The cranio-caudal mammogram **(a)** demonstrates an area of architectural distortion **(arrow)** in the lateral aspect of the left breast. A coned-down magnified view **(b)** acquired in a 30° supero-lateral to infero-medial (SL-IM ACR-SIO) projection demonstrates this abnormality **(arrow)** in fat, increasing the subject contrast and substantiating a real abnormality rather than a pseudo mass. A medio-lateral projection **(c)** localizes the abnormality **(arrow)** at approximately 2:00 in the left breast **(d)**. For biopsy, the team did not attempt a CC or CC-FB due to abnormality depth from the skin surface in these projections. A latero-medial scout projection **(e)** demonstrates the abnormality **(arrow)**. However, visualization is not maintained on the stereo images, preventing localization. Reproduction of the 30° SL-IM projection, where the abnormality is imaged against a background of fat, demonstrates the abnormality **(f) (arrow)** on the scout projection. Visualization of the abnormality is maintained on both stereo images **(g) (cursors)** (Carcinoma).

Figure 6.8 continued.

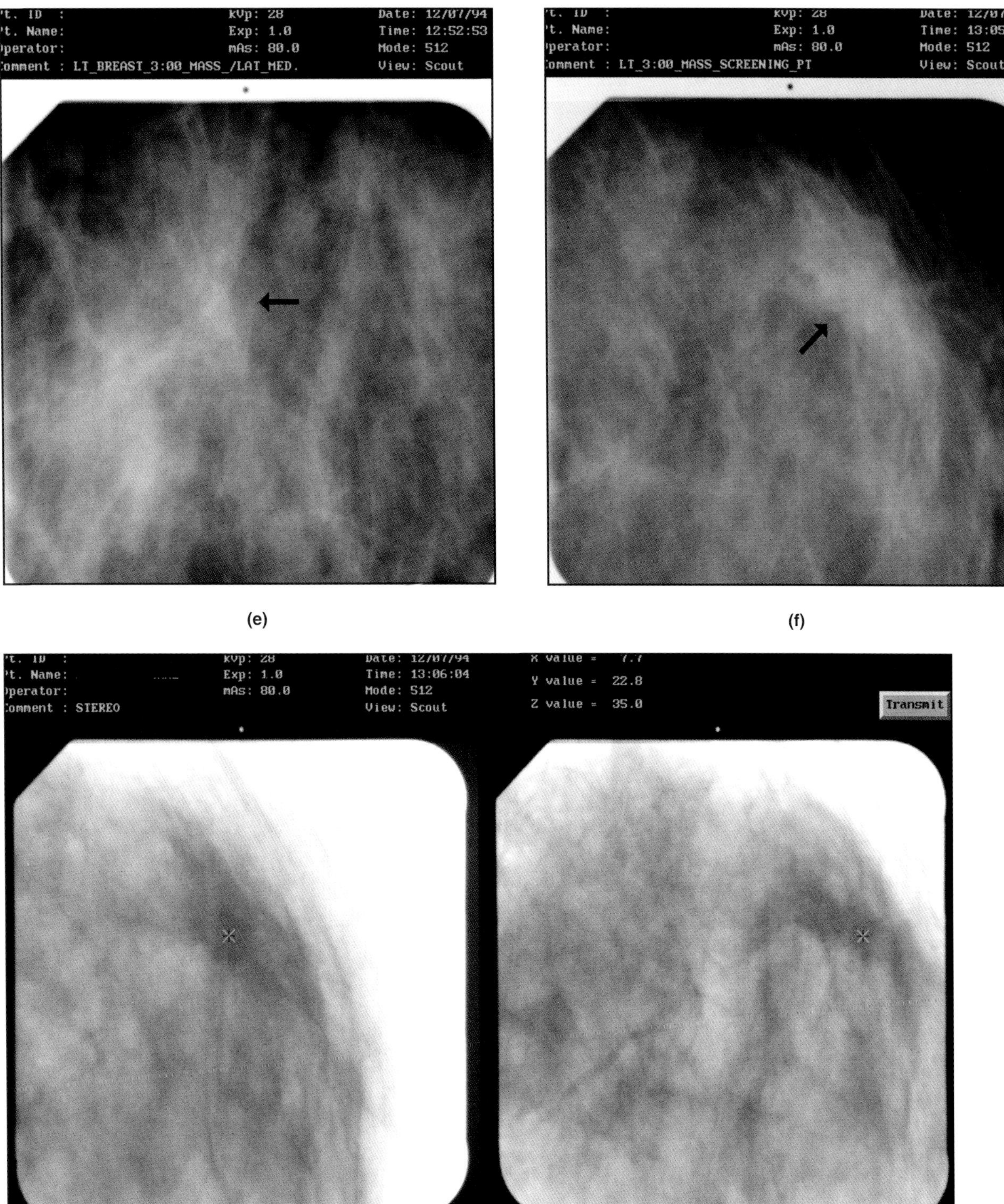

(e) (f)

(g)

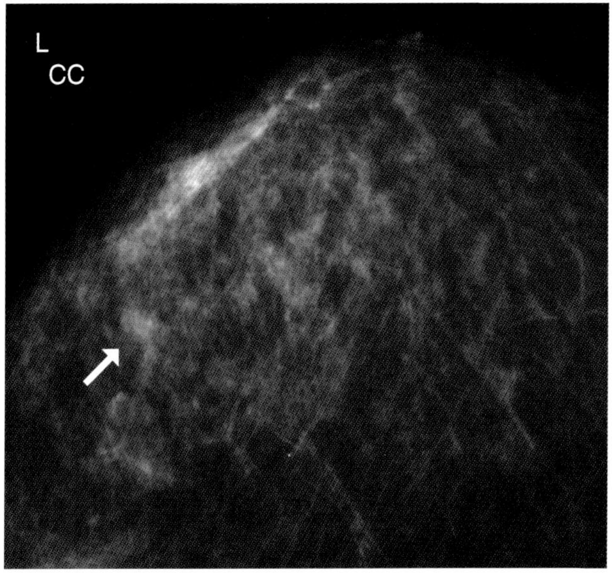

(a)

Figure 6.9 a-g. Subject Contrast. This routine screening mammogram **(a,b)** reveals a new area of asymmetry **(arrows)** in the lower outer quadrant of the left breast at approximately 4:00 **(c)**. A coned-down magnified 20° SL-IM projection **(d)** demonstrates this abnormality **(arrow)** to be suspicious. This same projection is not useful for biopsy because of negative stroke margin. A scout image in the latero-medial projection fails to adequately demonstrate the abnormality **(e)**. Reversing the SL-IM approach will give the same view of the abnormality from the opposite direction; a scout image **(f)** in an IL-SM projection demonstrates the abnormality **(arrow)**. Visualization is maintained on the stereo images **(g)** **(arrows)** (Carcinoma).

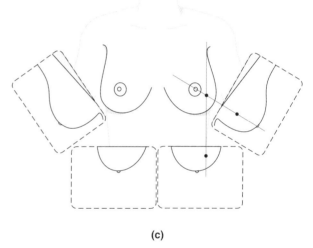

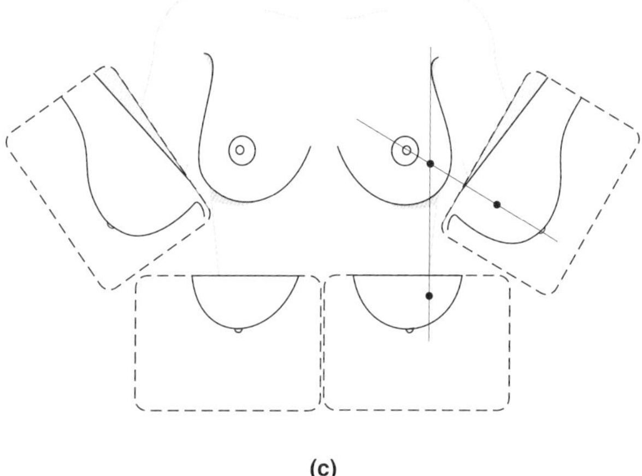

(c)

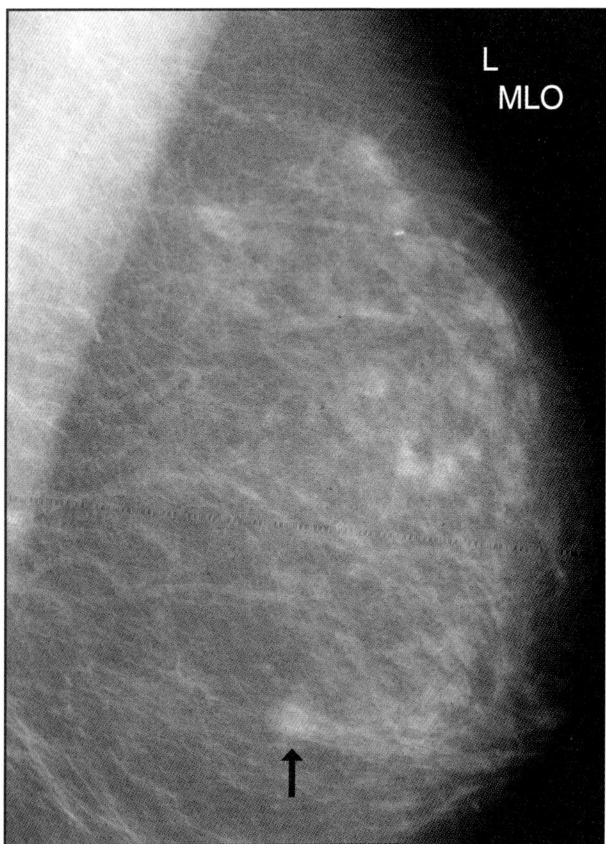

(b)

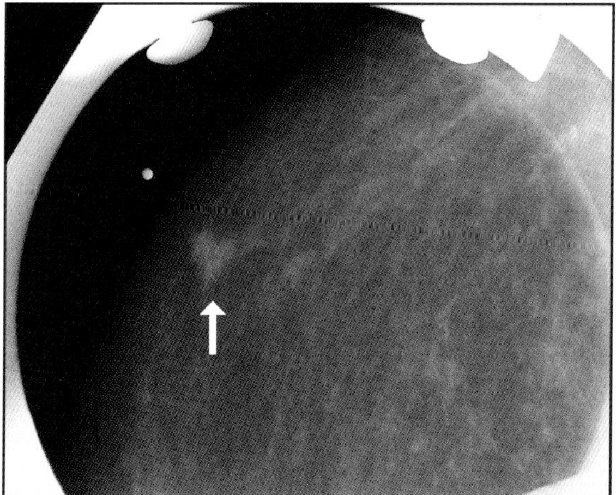

(d)

Figure 6.9 continued.

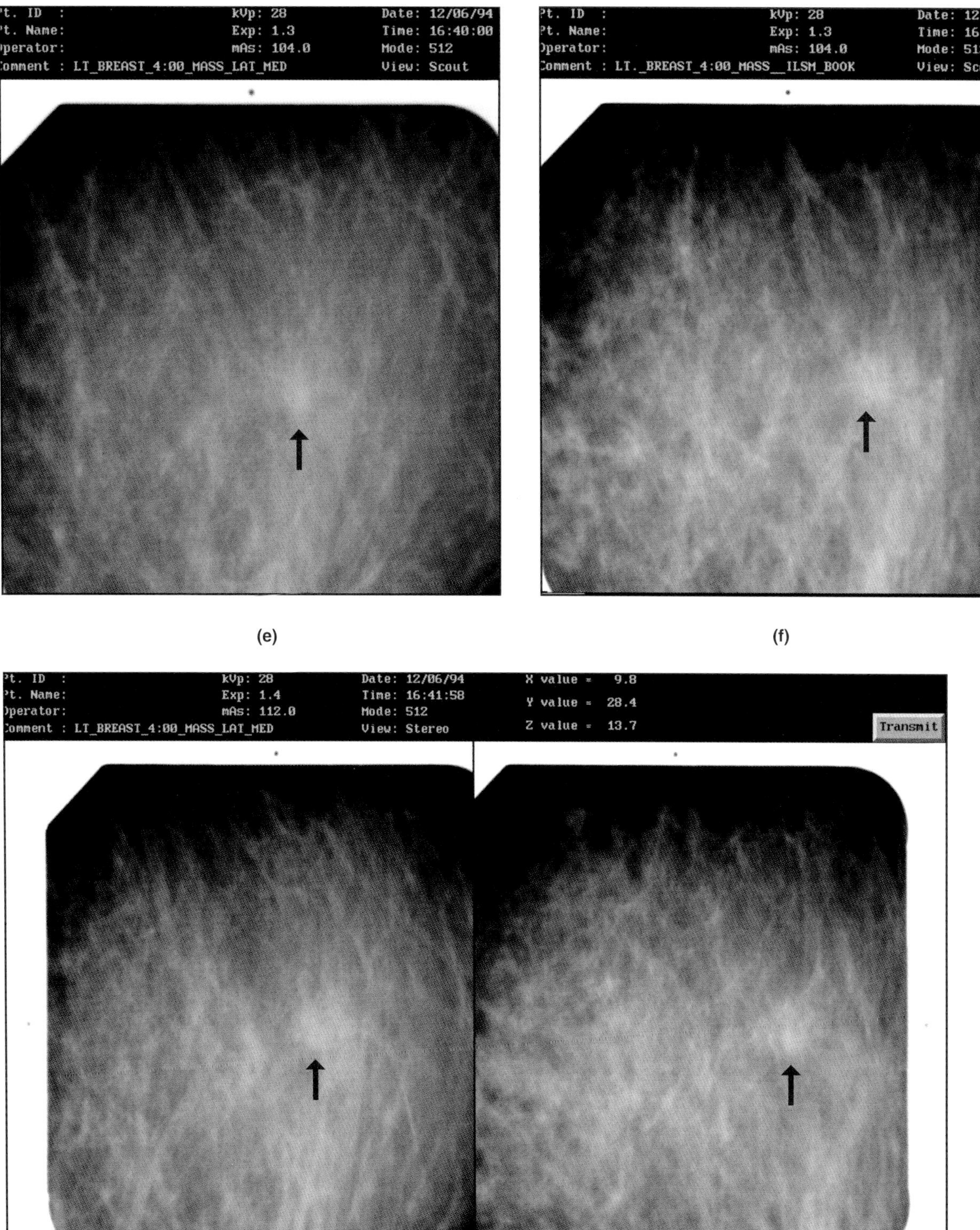

(e)

(f)

(g)

Positioning the Breast

Once the patient is comfortable, the technologist can focus on positioning the breast. This section discusses the various positioning factors for stereotactic biopsy, focusing primarily on prone positioning. However, many of these methods apply to upright positioning. As mentioned earlier, positioning can be straightforward, requiring minimal planning, or it can be complex. For example, if an abnormality is well-demonstrated in one of the routine mammographic projections and this projection allows for positive stroke margin for needle core biopsy (see chapter 2), then use that projection. There is no need to complicate a simple application or situation. Conversely, some situations will require flexibility and the application of technical skills. Use common sense and apply technical expertise.

The technologist's creativity will be critical in difficult cases where convention does not work. In general, a solution can be found for a difficult set of circumstances, but there will also be cases where needle core biopsy is not possible for any number of reasons. The following section provides a basis upon which to build positioning skills.

Purpose

The task of positioning for BNB is to visualize the abnormality on the scout image and to maintain visualization on both stereo images. If the abnormality is occult on either one or both of the stereo images, and subsequent repositioning fails to remedy the situation, biopsy should be canceled. Positioning must also allow positive stroke margin for needle core biopsy.

Team Approach

The clinician and technologist together as a team should decide on a starting projection for biopsy. But the technologist should have the freedom to alter the projection when

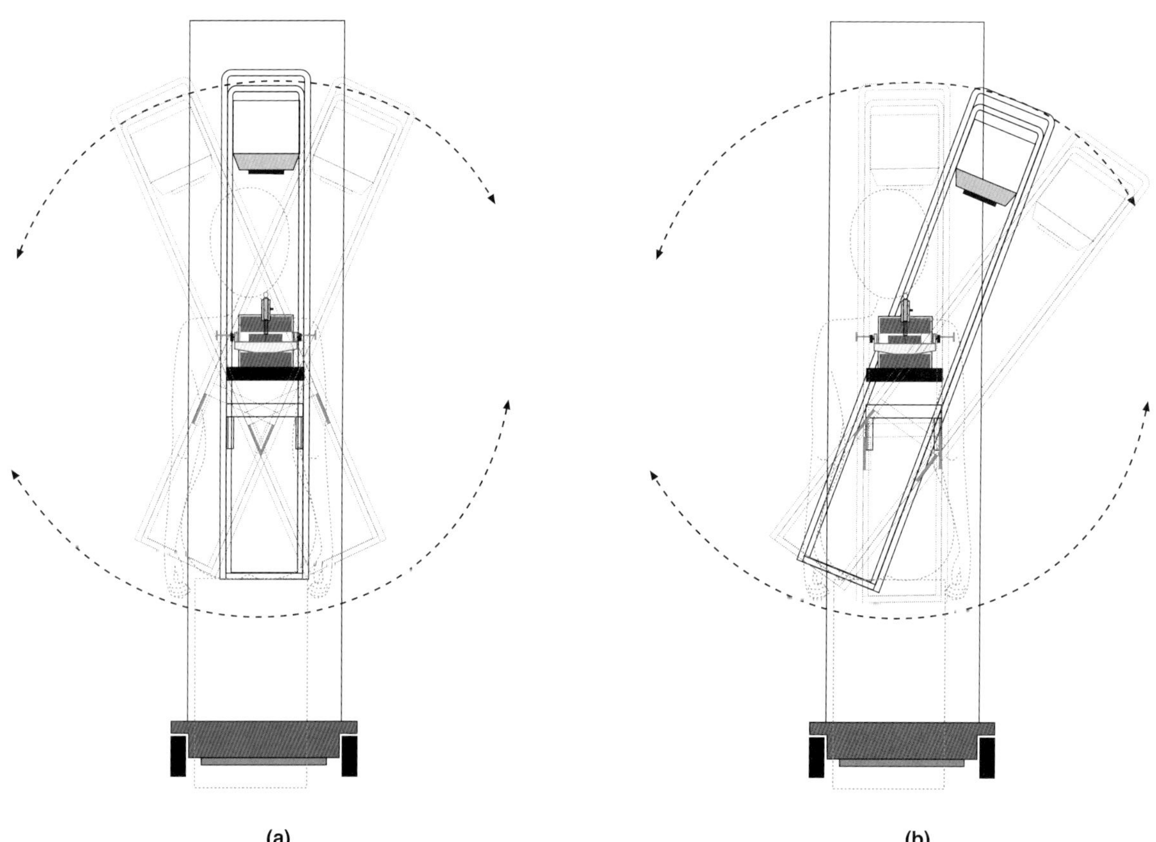

Figure 6.10. Logistics with Upright Add-on Equipment. The technologist should choose a projection that inhibits patient motion. This figure demonstrates positioning of the patient using a CC projection **(a)**. The patient's head will interfere with stereo angulation. A better approach would be to use a SL-IM oblique or a SM-IL oblique of some degree, eliminating interference of the patient's head **(b)**.

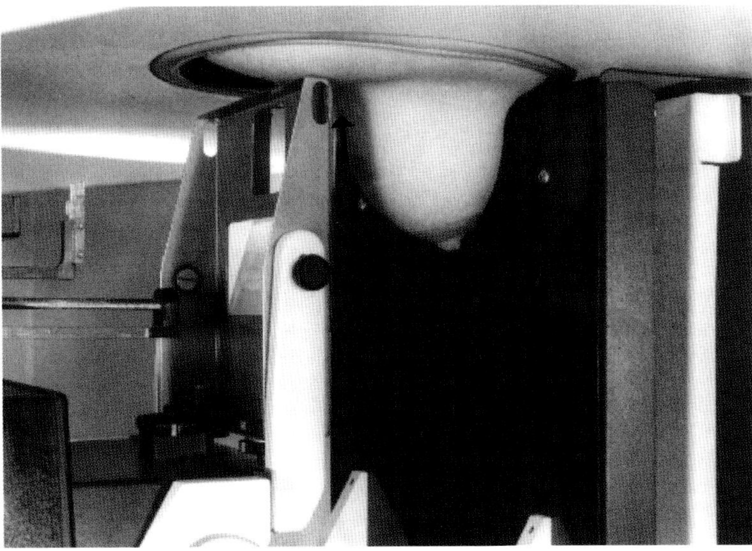

Figure 6.11. Altered Perspective with Prone Units. The technologist may experience disorientation with prone positioning. In this *oblique* projection, the arrow indicates 2:00 and not 12:00 as it seems to appear.

necessary. When in doubt, the technologist will need the clinician to confirm identification of the abnormality on the scout image. It is possible the scout image will demonstrate the abnormality, but escape identification on one or both stereo images. The technologist may want to consult with the clinician before abandoning the projection. The ultimate responsibility to properly position the breast remains with the technologist. An increase in work, frustration, and procedure time will occur if the technologist depends on the clinician to continually intercede in positioning decisions. The clinician who gives the technologist the freedom and responsibility to complete the positioning process helps create a more effective, efficient biopsy team.

Altered Perspective with Prone Units

When utilizing a prone unit, the technologist may at first find positioning disorienting because of the altered perspective of the breast and the disassociation of the breast from the body **(Figure 6.11)**. For example, the 12:00 area of the breast may shift more medial or lateral when the breast is dependent, or the breast will seem to pull or turn in one direction or the other. Positioning can be especially perplexing when using a projection other than a cranio-caudal or lateral projection. In addition, the abnormality location in reference to breast landmarks may change when the breast is dependent. For example, when the breast is dependent in a lateral or near-lateral projection, the abnormality will consistently appear more inferior than expected. Reorientation takes some adjustment. Placing a marker on the breast at the approximate location of the abnormality can help maintain perspective **(Figure 6.12)**. The technologist can also reorient the breast as it would be for the cranio-caudal projection, noting the 12:00 position and the approximate location of the abnormality from this point.

Choosing the Biopsy Approach

Projections for SBB

Once the clinician and technologist determine the approximate location of the abnormality (see discussion below), they can identify the appropriate c-arm approach. To maximize the use and effectiveness of the stereotactic unit, the team must be aware of the positioning choices available from the system, and the application of each projection. There are eight possible projections and many possible oblique angles that the team can use in stereotactic biopsy with a system that provides 360° access. **Figures 6.13-6.20** demonstrate each of these projections on a prone system. Although some of these terms may seem awkward

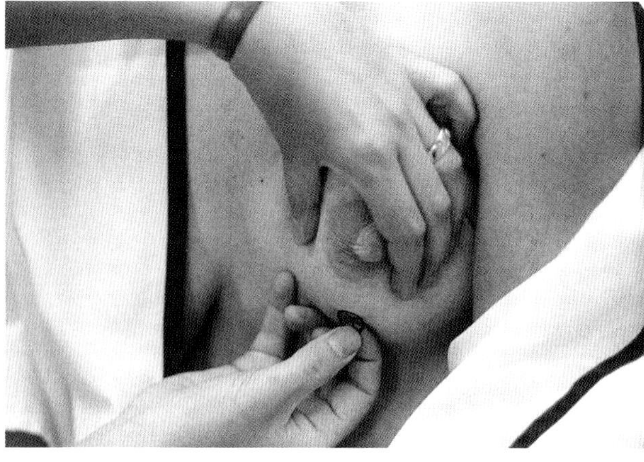

Figure 6.12. Placing a lead marker at the approximate location of the abnormality can aid the technologist in the positioning process.

initially, the following projections† will become commonplace with experience.

Cranio-Caudal - CC
Caudal-Cranial - CC-FB
Latero-Medial- LM
Medio-Lateral - ML
Supero-Medial to Infero-Lateral Oblique* - SM-IL (ACR - MLO)
Supero-Lateral to Infero-Medial Oblique* - SL-IM (ACR - SIO)
Infero-Medial to Supero-Lateral Oblique* - IM-SL
Infero-Lateral to Supero-Medial Oblique* - IL-SM (ACR - LMO or Reverse)

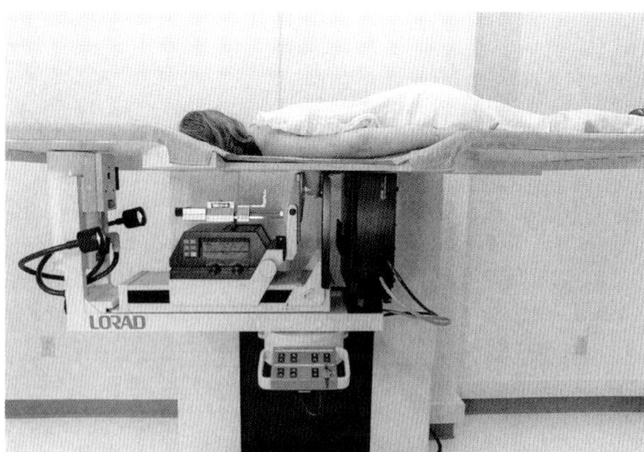

Figure 6.13. The Cranio-Caudal (CC) Projection.

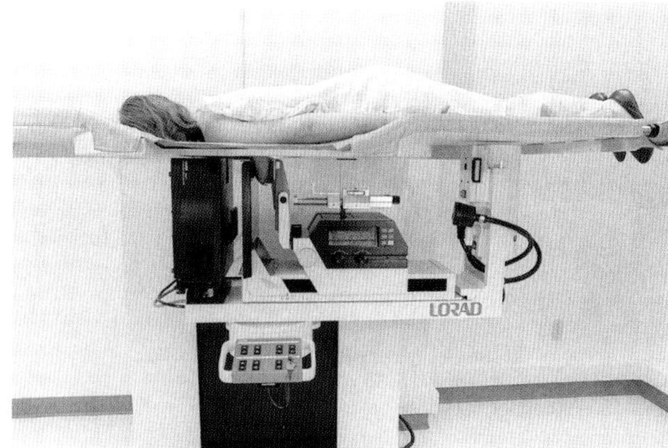

Figure 6.14. The Caudal-Cranial (CC-FB) Projection.

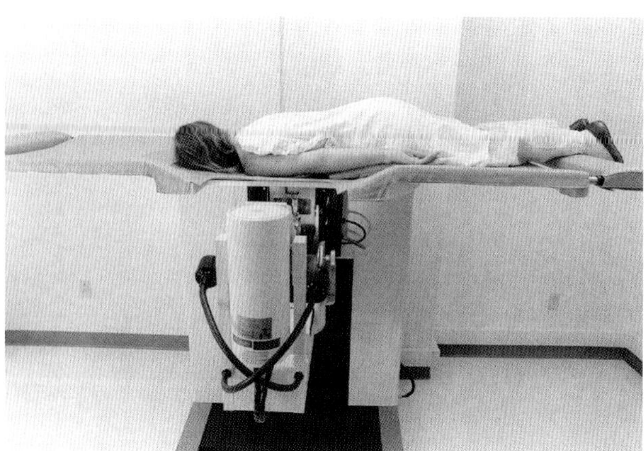

Figure 6.15. The Latero-Medial (LM) Projection as Demonstrated on the Left Breast.

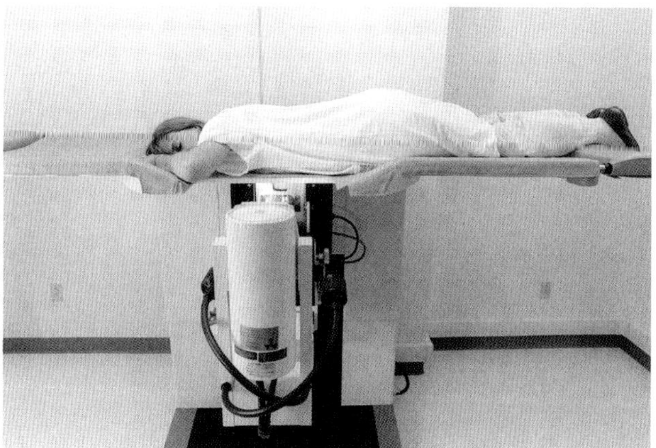

Figure 6.16. The Medio-Lateral (ML) Projection as Demonstrated on the Right Breast.

†The terminology is taken from the National Council on Radiation Protection report draft SC72 on mammography. The terminology set forth by the American College of Radiology is put in parenthesis when possible. The NCRP terminology is extremely specific and not open to interpretation.
*The degree of obliquity depends on the location of the abnormality.

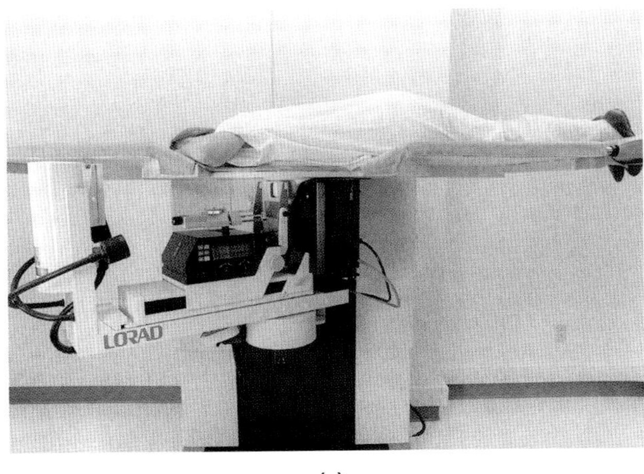

(a)

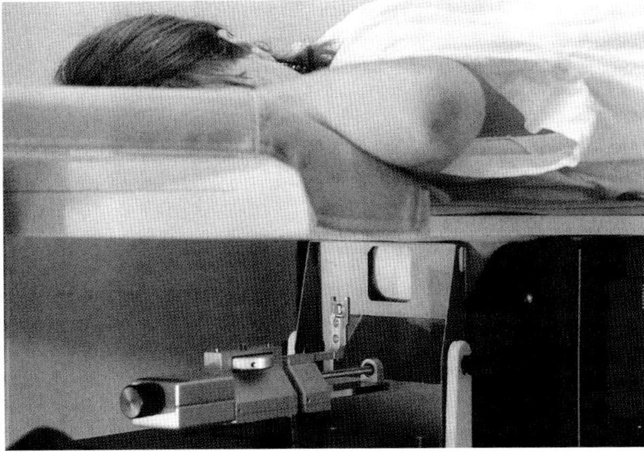

(b)

Figure 6.17 a and b. The Supero-Medial to Infero-Lateral Oblique (SM-IL, ACR-MLO) Projection. Demonstrated on the right breast **(a)** and close up **(b)**.

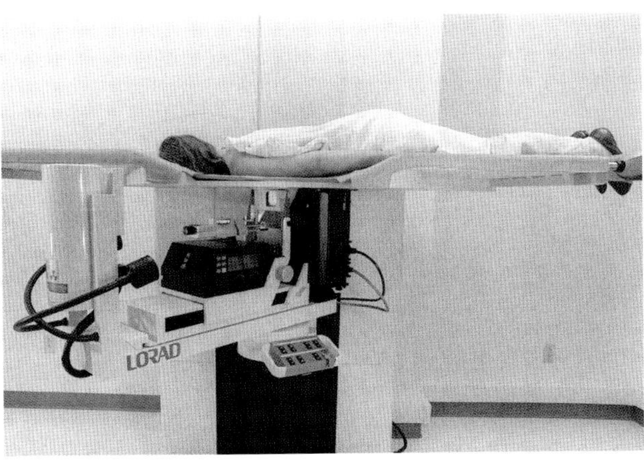

(a)

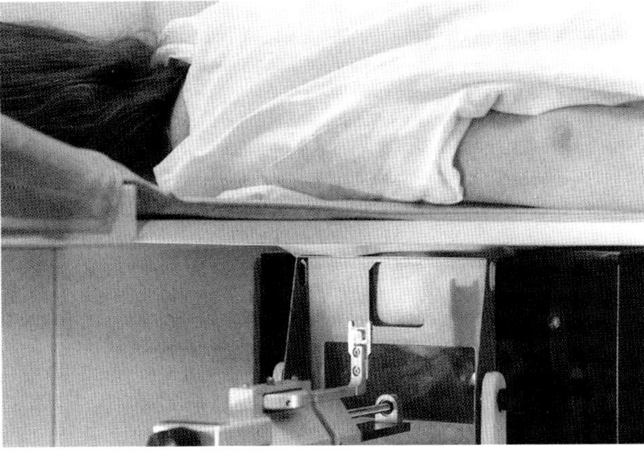

(b)

Figure 6.18 a and b. The Supero-Lateral to Infero-Medial Oblique (SL-IM, ACR-SIO) Projection. Demonstrated on the left breast **(a)** and close-up **(b)**.

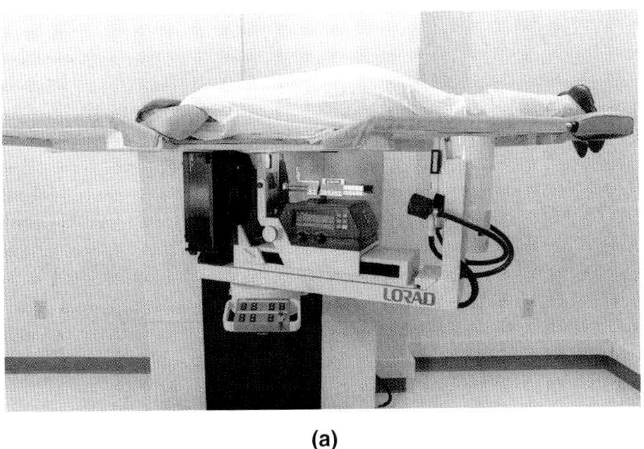

(a)

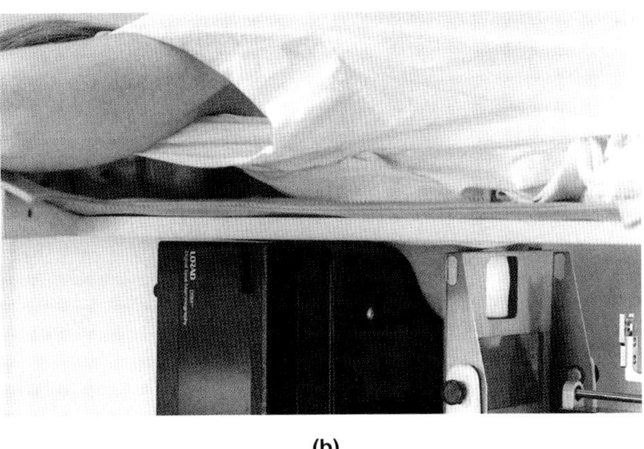

(b)

Figure 6.19 a and b. The Infero-Medial to Supero-Lateral Oblique (IM-SL) Projection. Demonstrated on the right breast **(a)** and close up **(b)**.

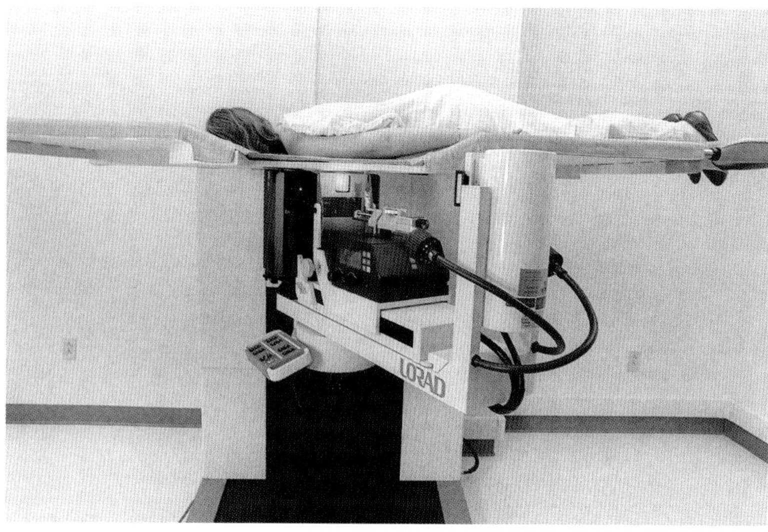

(a)

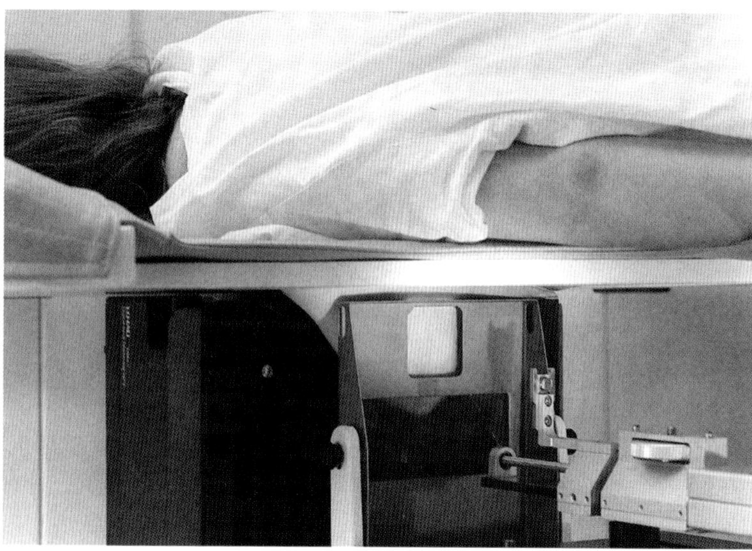

(b)

Figure 6.20 a and b. The Infero-Lateral to Supero-Medial Oblique (IL-SM, ACR-LMO or Reverse) Projection. Demonstrated on the left breast **(a)** and oloco up **(b)**.

Figure 6.21 illustrates the application of these projections in accessing the four quadrants of the breast. The technologist will have only the following five projections available for positioning, if the system offers only 180° access: CC, ML, LM, SM-IL and SL-IM.

The more versatile the unit, the easier it will be to achieve successful imaging and biopsy of the majority of abnormalities. Continual rotation around the breast that allows imaging at any point permits the most flexibility. Furthermore, 360° access will allow imaging and biopsy of abnormalities that would otherwise be eliminated from biopsy as a result of nonvisualization, accessibility, or negative stroke margin. For example, inferior abnormalities that cannot be approached in a medio-lateral or latero-medial projection can be approached with a caudal-cranial, IL-SM, or IM-SL oblique angle **(Figure 6.22)**, depending on location. Be aware that even though upright units may mechanically provide 360° access, other limitations may prohibit the use of the full 360° rotation. For example, while an upright unit may have the capability to provide a caudal-cranial

Stereotactic Projections								
	Cranio-Caudal	Caudal-Cranial	Medio-Lateral	Latero-Medial	(SM-IL) (ACR-MLO)* Supero-Medial to Infero-Lateral Oblique	IL-SM* (ACR-LMO or Reverse) Infero-Lateral to Supero-Medial Oblique	SL-IM(ACR-SIO)* Supero-Lateral to Infero-Medial Oblique	IM-SL* Infero-Medial to Supero-Lateral Oblique
Location of abnormality	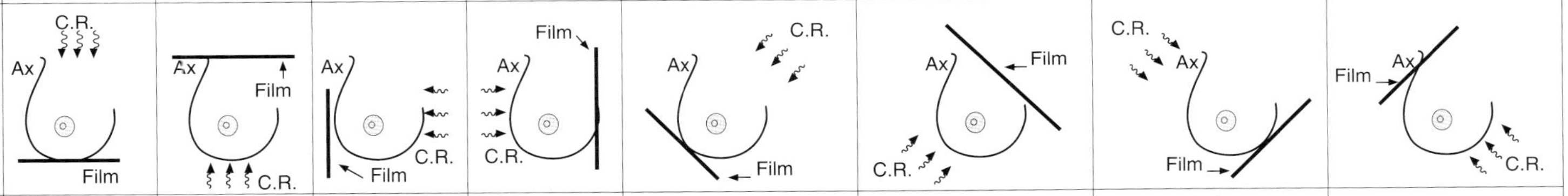 C.R. Ax Film	Ax Film C.R.	Ax Film C.R.	Film Ax C.R.	Ax C.R. Film	Ax Film C.R.	C.R. Ax Film	Film Ax C.R.
Upper Outer Quadrant	X			X	X slight oblique only	X	X	
Upper Inner Quadrant	X		X		X		X	X
Lower Inner Quadrant		X	X		X	X		X
Lower Outer Quadrant		X		X		X	X	X

*The degree of obliquity depends on the location of the abnormality.

Figure 6.21. This table correlates access to the four quadrants with the possible projections available.

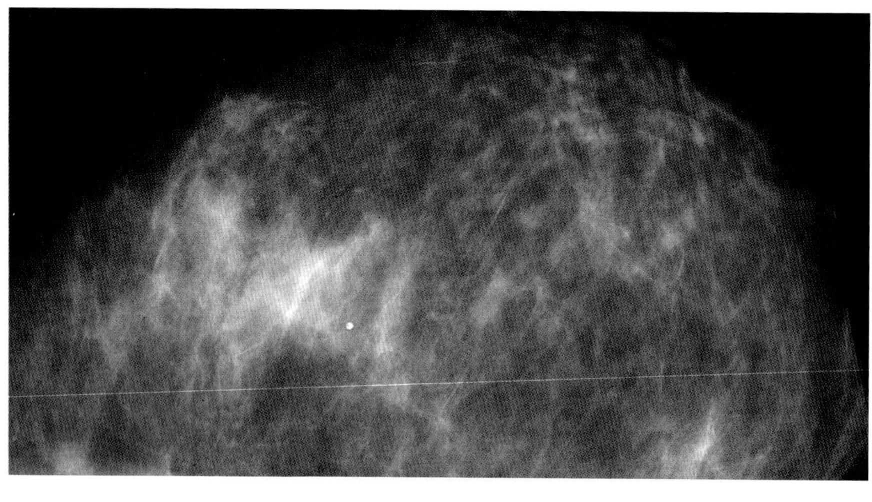

(a)

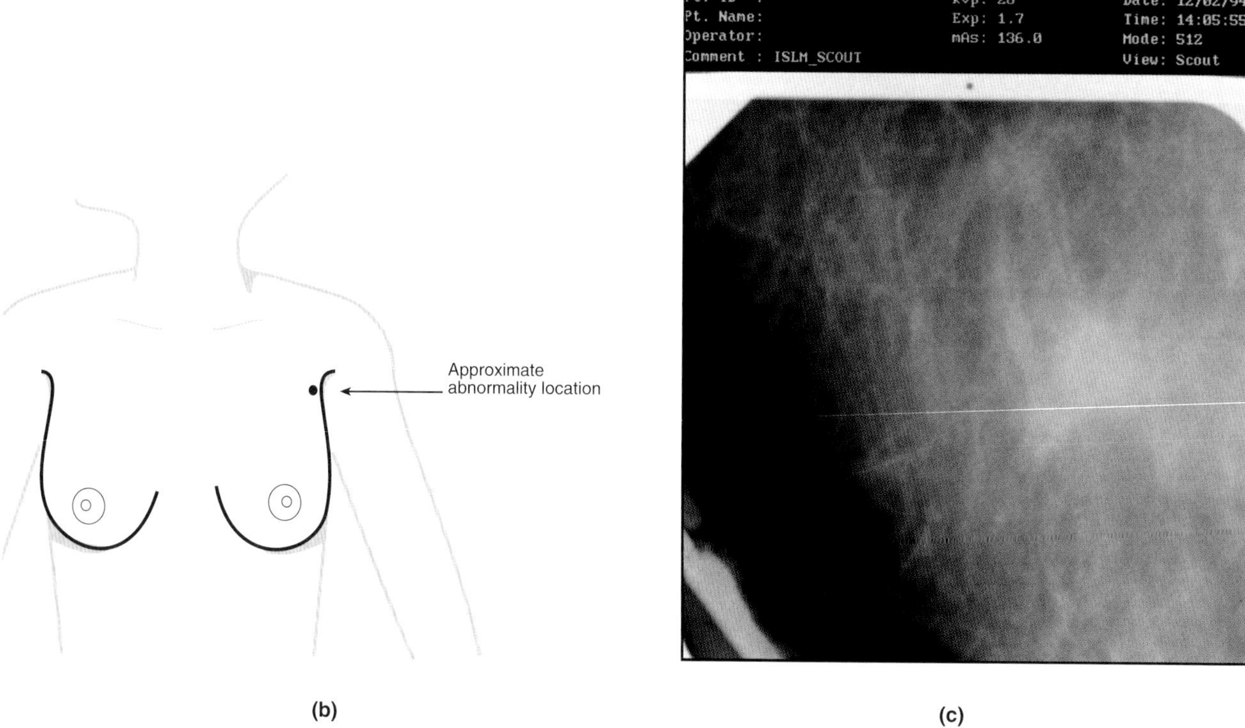

(b) (c)

Figure 6.22 a-c. Importance of 360° Approach. A patient presented for a second opinion with a mammogram, demonstrating an 8 mm irregular density on the left MLO (SM-IL) projection only (not shown). A 20° oblique **(a)** demonstrates this abnormality in the extreme posterior upper outer quadrant at 2:00 **(b)**. An attempt to reproduce this projection (SM-IL of 20°) on the prone table failed to visualize the abnormality. Reproducing the MLO (a SM-IL of 45°) resulted in negative stroke margin. Reversing the approach from a SM-IL projection to an IL-SM projection demonstrates this abnormality on the scout image **(c)**.Visualization of the abnormality is maintained on both stereo images (not shown). Targeting of the abnormality yielded positive stroke margin. (Carcinoma.)

approach, this would present an awkward approach for the biopsy team and would require the patient to straddle the tube head.

Blood Vessels

Blood vessels that project over the abnormality may be at risk for puncture, creating unnecessary complications during needle biopsy **(Figure 6.23).** The technologist must examine the scout image to check for vessels over the abnormality. The vessels over an abnormality may be out of needle range. An examination of the mammogram can help determine the proximity of blood vessels. Targeting of the abnormality and blood vessel can also reveal to the technologist where the blood vessel is in relation to the abnormality. If necessary, roll or reposition the breast. The technologist can simply rotate the breast or c-arm slightly, 5-10°, to modify the projection and to eliminate the risk of vessel puncture.

Full Breast Scout

A large fenestrated compression paddle with a matching aperture provides a larger field of view to locate an abnormality when visualization is elusive. The technologist can

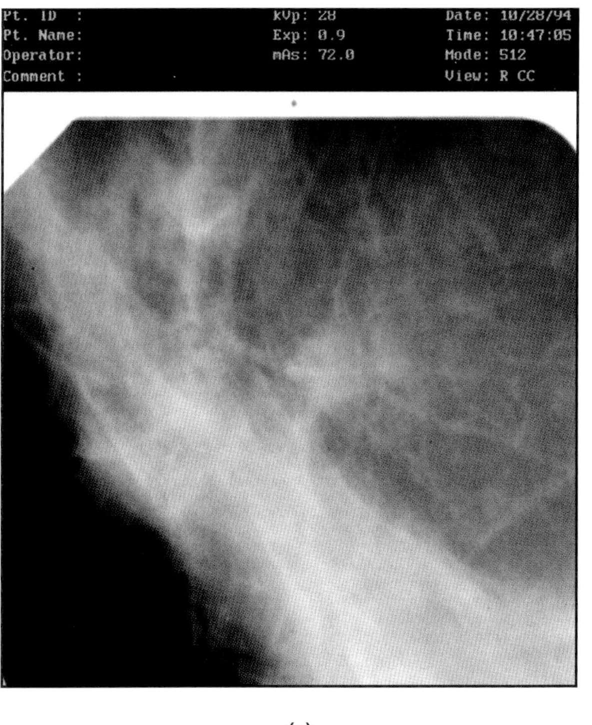

(a)

Figure 6.23 a and b. Checking for Blood Vessels. The technologist should check for overlapping blood vessels **(a)** that are subject to puncture, causing hematoma **(b)** and possibly complicating the procedure. (Benign.)

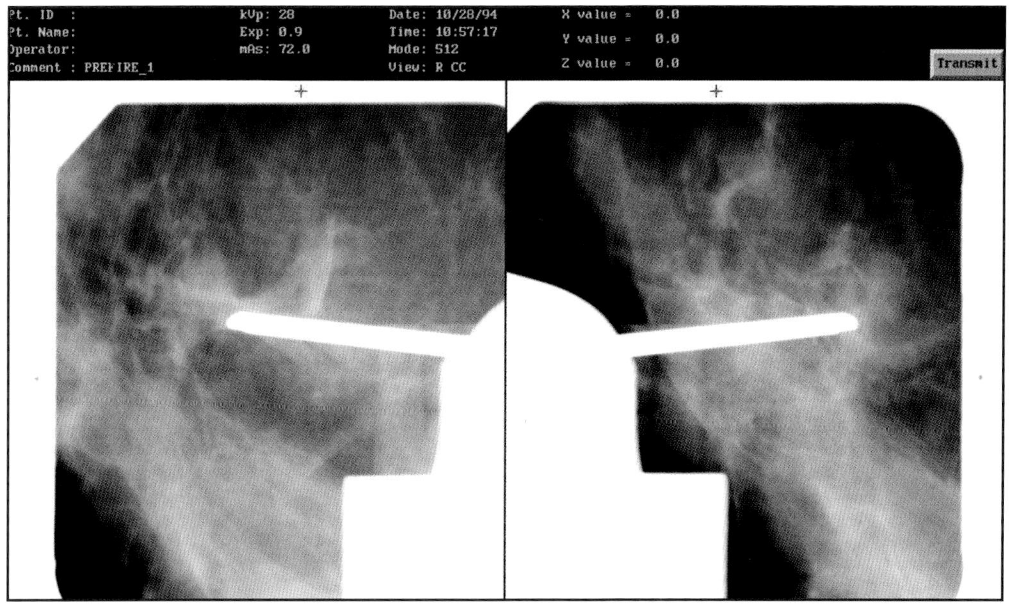

(b)

acquire a full breast scout image using a screen-film combination (digital receptors are limited in field size). The scout image reveals in advance the approach that best enables visualization. Such a scout view can reduce the number of small-field scout images, diminishing the technologist's frustration and the patient's discomfort. The ample-sized scout is especially helpful for extremely posterior abnormalities, fine microcalcifications, and low-density abnormalities that are difficult to define from the surrounding glandular structures.

Technologists who are new to stereotactic biopsy may want to use the scout routinely until they become adept at positioning. The scout image may also be useful in providing a comparison for the clinician who is new to digital imaging, where the increase in contrast of all breast structures engenders perception difficulties.

When the technologist discovers the proper approach and location through the larger scout image, marking the breast with ink or a lead marker provides a landmark for positioning in the smaller biopsy window **(Figure 6.24a)**. The technologist should always repeat the scout image using the smaller biopsy window and aperture **(Figure 6.24b)**. This will ensure adequate centering of the abnormality prior to stereo acquisition.

Locating the Abnormality for Positioning

One of the most effective skills the technologist can acquire is fully understanding the three-dimensional information available from the two-view mammogram. In doing so, she can determine the quadrant and approximate clock time of the abnormality. This skill will greatly assist the technologist in accomplishing a difficult set of positioning tasks. Understanding the abnormality's position will help the technologist to choose the appropriate projection for biopsy and to utilize the SBB equipment more effectively.

Abnormality Demonstrated on Two Views

If *any* two mammographic projections demonstrate an abnormality, the technologist can determine approximate location by using **triangulation**. **Figure 6.25** demonstrates a very simple method of triangulation, showing direct correlation with the mammogram. This method will render the quadrant and approximate clock time of the abnormality. The technologist can also estimate the approximate depth of the abnormality from the nipple by measuring from the nipple to the abnormality on either mammographic image. These localization techniques render approximate location and serve as a guideline only. Once the technologist determines location, it might be useful to place a mark using ink or a lead marker on the patient's skin, correlating to the approximate location of the abnormality. Note that when the breast is dependent in the prone position, location of the abnormality may change somewhat.

Abnormality Demonstrated on One View

If only one mammographic projection demonstrates the abnormality, triangulation is not possible. The stereotactic

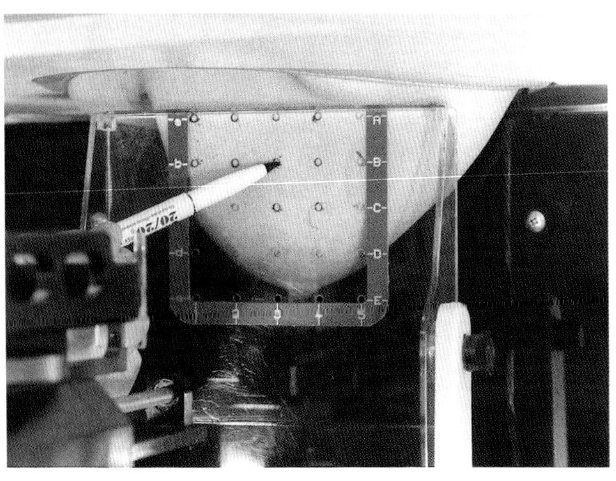

(a)

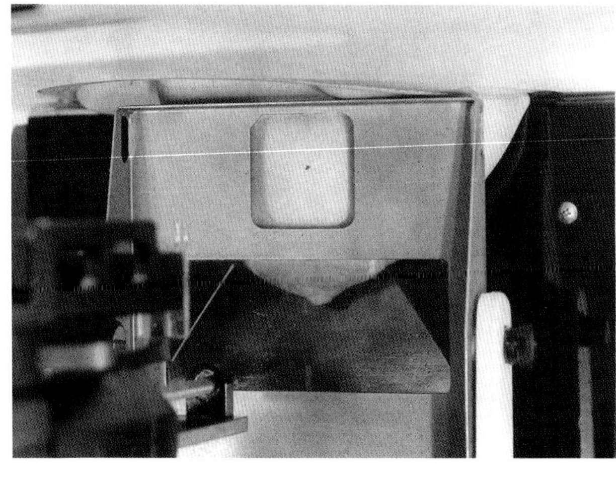

(b)

Figure 6.24 a and b. Full Breast Scout. A scout paddle with a larger field of view assists the technologist in finding a difficult to visualize abnormality. Once the image is acquired, the approximate abnormality location is marked **(a)**. The technologist reacquires the scout with the smaller aperture and biopsy/compression plate to assure proper centering **(b).**

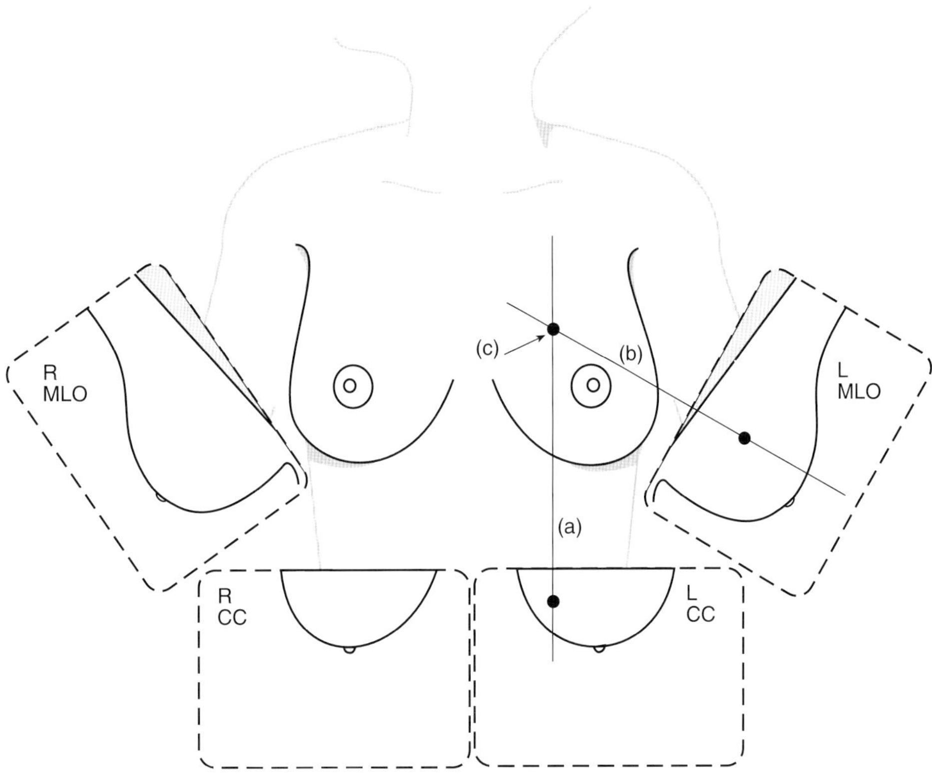

Figure 6.25. Triangulation. The technologist can use this simple method to approximate the location of an abnormality. Since the x-ray beam always remains perpendicular to the image receptor in routine mammography, follow a perpendicular line back through the breast from the abnormality on both the CC **(a)** and MLO **(b)** projections (or any two projections). The two lines will bisect at the approximate location of the abnormality **(c)**.

unit is especially useful in these cases because it accurately provides the location of the abnormality and, most important, the depth coordinate. Under these circumstances, it is best to "scout" in the projection that demonstrates the abnormality. After stereo acquisition, the team targets the abnormality and determines stroke margin. The team can complete biopsy with a positive stroke margin. However, if there is a negative stroke margin, repositioning in the reverse projection will best serve the team and patient for biopsy **(Figure 6.26)**.

For example, an MLO projection demonstrates an abnormality, not readily identifiable on the CC projection. For stereotactic biopsy, replicate the MLO projection (supero-medial to infero-lateral, SM-IL). If the depth coordinate will not allow positive stroke margin, then positioning in the reverse projection (infero-lateral to supero-medial IL-SM) will permit the shortest skin-to-abnormality distance and positive stroke margin.

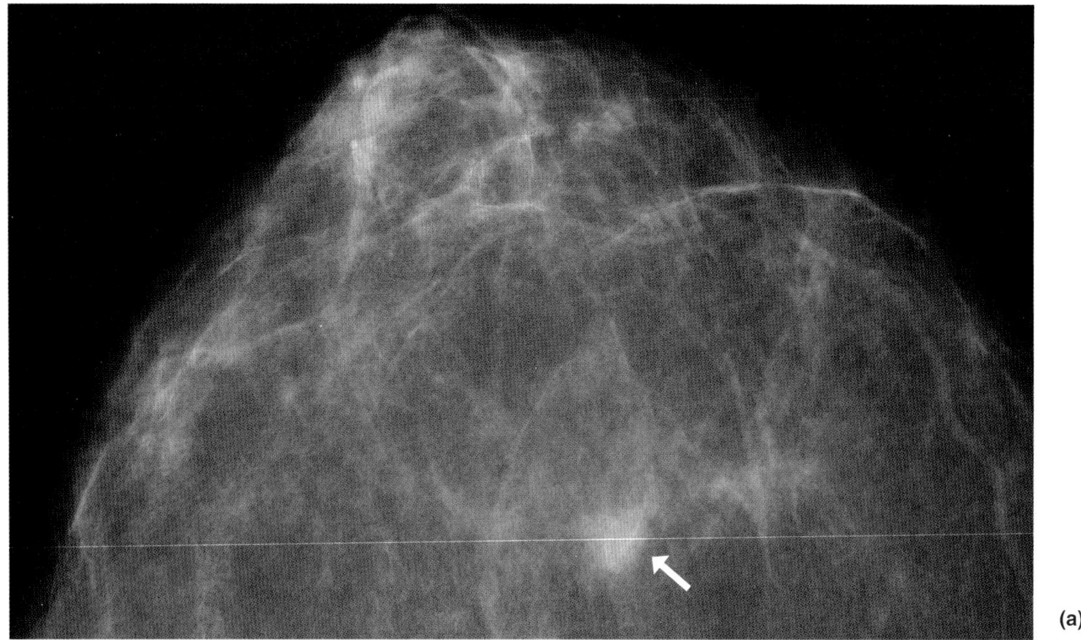

(a)

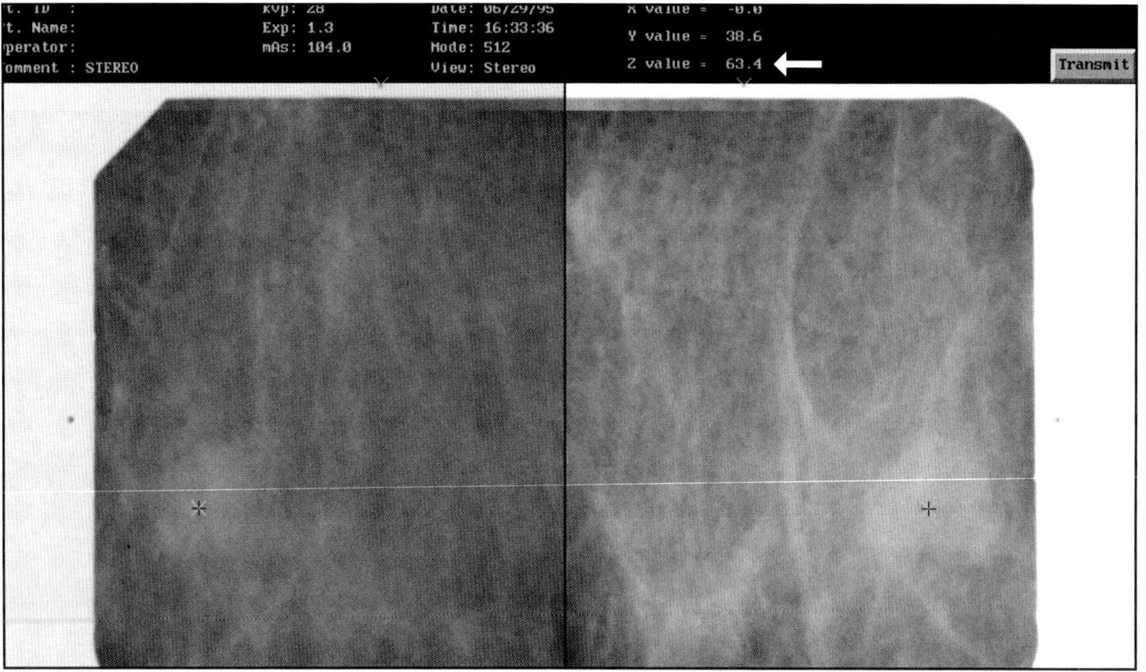

(b)

Figure 6.26 a-d. Abnormality on One View. The CC projection **(a)** demonstrates an ill-defined mass density **(arrow)**. The abnormality was not demonstrated on either the MLO or lateral projections. The scout cranio-caudal projection for stereotactic core biopsy demonstrated this abnormality, which maintains visualization on both stereo images (note the wide shift, typical of deep abnormalities on this unit) **(b) (cursors)**. Coordinate calculation **(arrow)** renders a depth coordinate of 63.4 mm with total breast compression measuring 72 mm, producing a negative stroke margin. Reversing the position of the c-arm for a caudal-cranial approach demonstrates the abnormality on the scout image **(c)**. The abnormality maintains visualization on both stereo images **(d)** (note reduced shift, indicating, for this unit, a more superficial location). Retargeting renders a depth coordinate **(arrow)** of 43.3 mm (with a total compression approximately the same as previously indicated), resulting in a positive stroke margin.

Figure 6.26 continued.

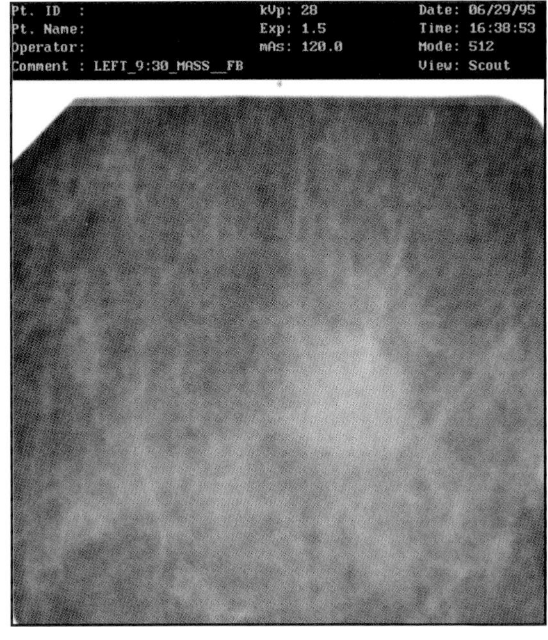

(c)

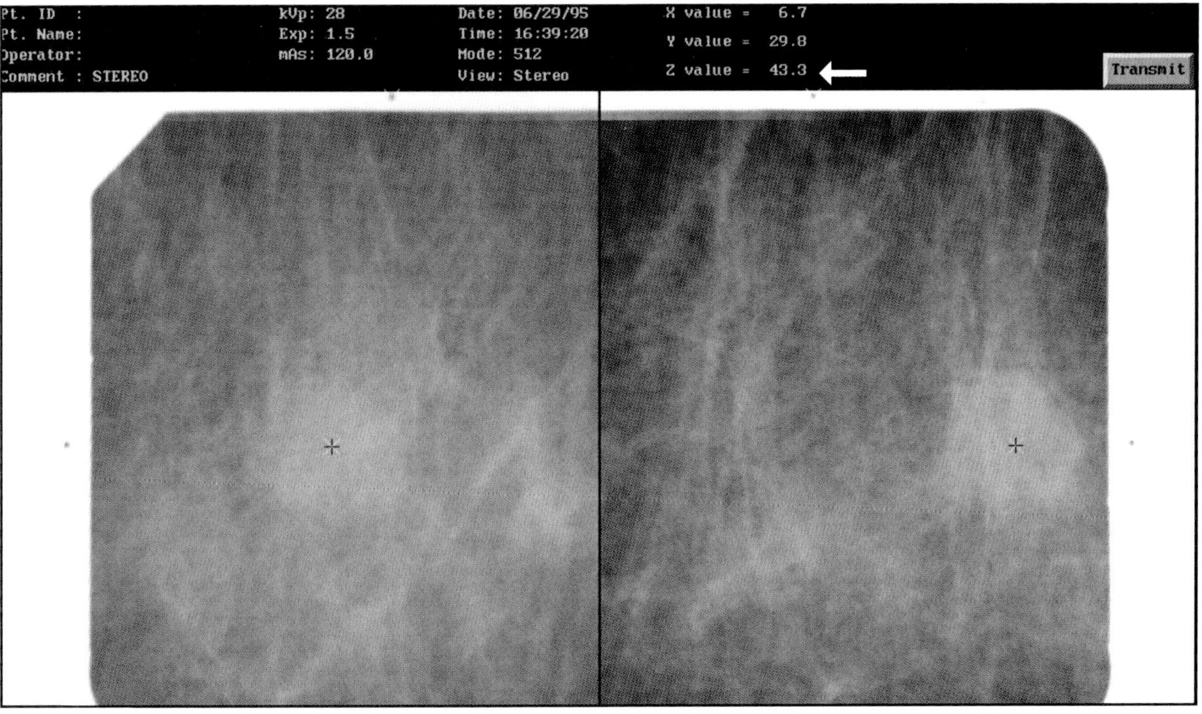

(d)

Shortest Skin-to-Abnormality Distance and Positive Stroke Margin

When possible, the team should confine positioning choices to those projections that provide the shortest skin-to-abnormality distance and also allow abnormality visualization on the scout and stereo images (**Figure 6.27**). This will minimize trauma to the breast and provide for positive stroke margin during needle core biopsy. The shorter skin-to-abnormality distance also ensures minimal excursion of the biopsy needle into the breast. The deeper the needle travels, the greater the length available for deflection (**Figure 6.28**). This is especially important with the smaller needle gauges in use for FNAC.

It is possible that the projection providing the shortest skin-to-abnormality distance will not demonstrate the abnormality. In this case, the team should choose the projection that allows visualization and positive stroke margin, regardless of the shortest skin-to-abnormality distance.

It is not always possible to determine positive stroke margin *prior* to final positioning. If the technologist is in doubt as to whether positive stroke margin exists, she can perform a cursory targeting of the abnormality to determine if repositioning is necessary.

Placing the Patient for Prone Positioning

The technologist can facilitate positioning by appropriately placing the patient on the table. In general, with a center table aperture, the technologist should position the patient so that the half of the breast containing the abnormality is availible for 180° rotation. This allows the maximum number of projections for accessing the breast. A notable exception to this rule applies when the technologist uses a slight SM-IL oblique projection (5-20°) for upper outer quadrant abnormalities. In this case, position the patient so that the half of the breast of interest would be near

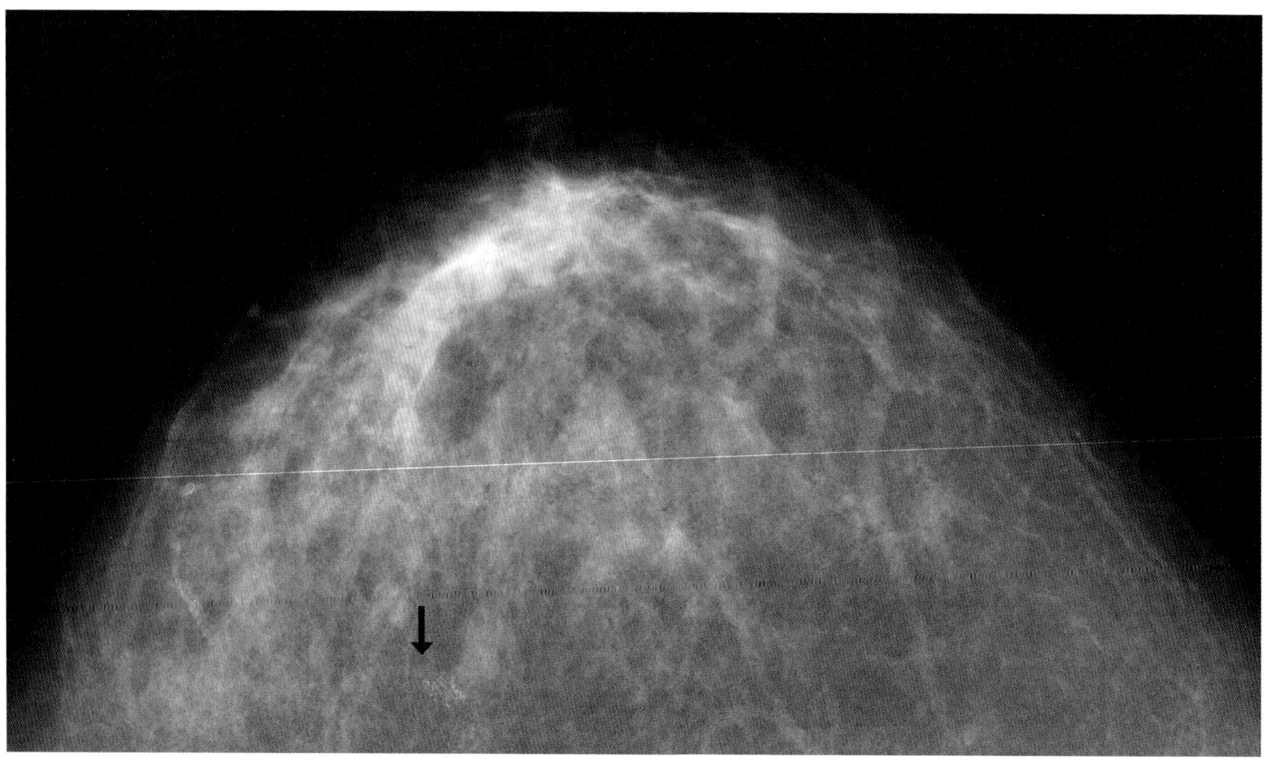

(a)

Figure 6.27 a-c. Shortest Skin-to-Abnormality Distance and Positive Stroke Margin. The cranio-caudal **(a)** and MLO **(b)** projections demonstrate this abnormality to be at about 1:00 in the left breast. Although the LM would be an appropriate projection, the breast compresses to only 3 cm in this position, producing a negative stroke margin. Using a SL-IM projection **(c)** provides the shortest skin-to-abnormality distance. The breast in this projection compresses to 4 cm, providing for positive stroke margin.

Figure 6.27 continued.

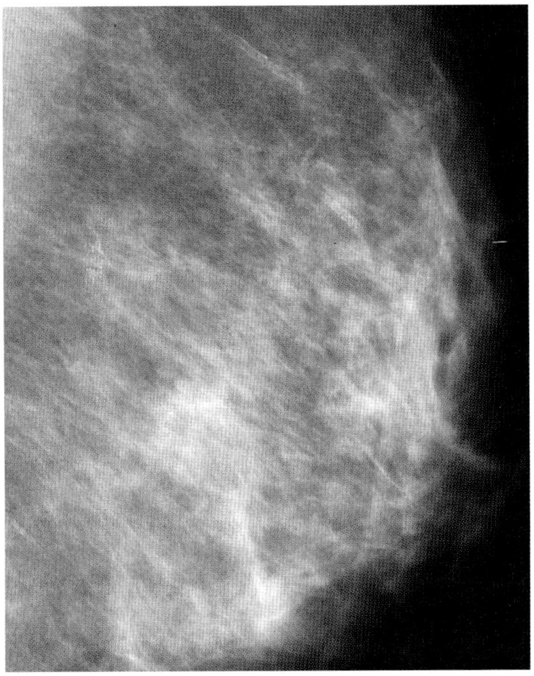

SL-IM projection

Breast support
SL-IM projection

(b)

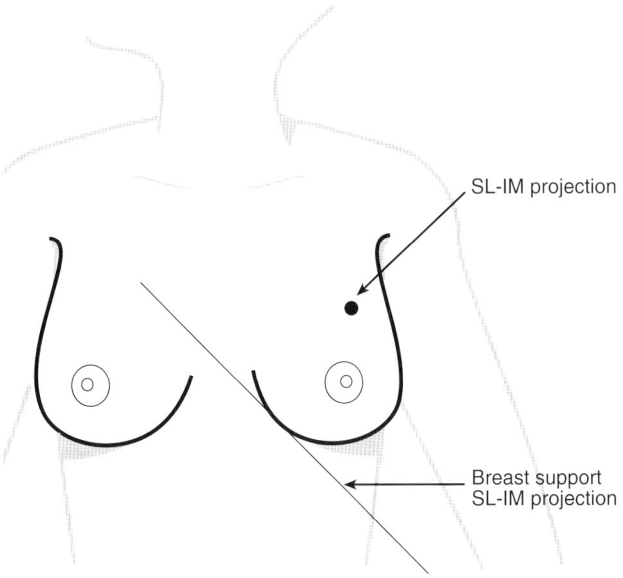

(c)

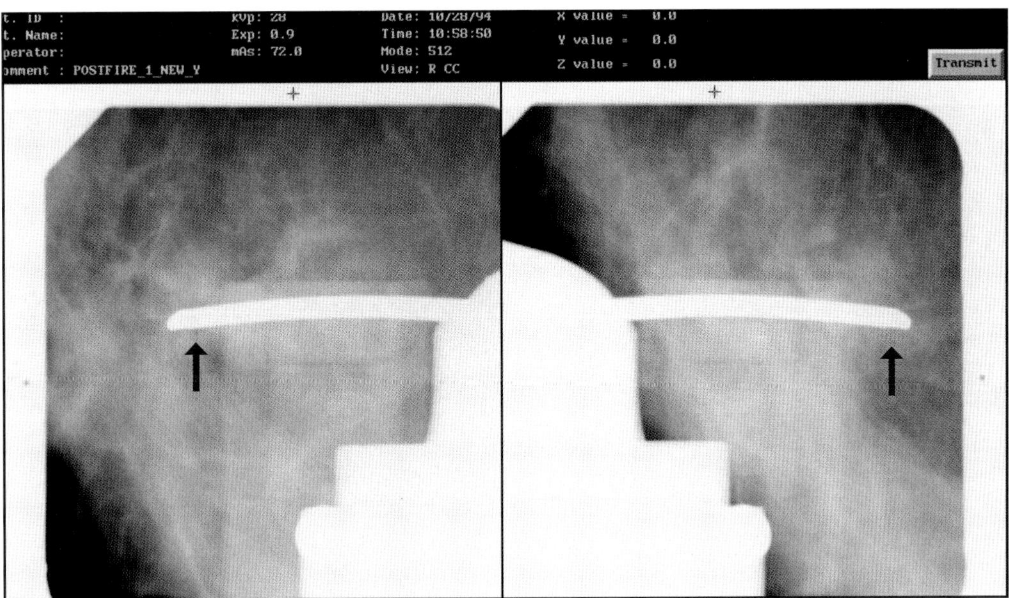

Figure 6.28. Needle Deflection. The CC approach to this abnormality, at approximately 9:00 in the right breast, allows a greater amount of needle to be available for deflection **(arrows)**. Other projections that might have provided visualization and a shorter skin-to-abnormality distance include an LM, SL-IM, or IL-SM.

Table with a Center Aperture

Right Anterior Oblique

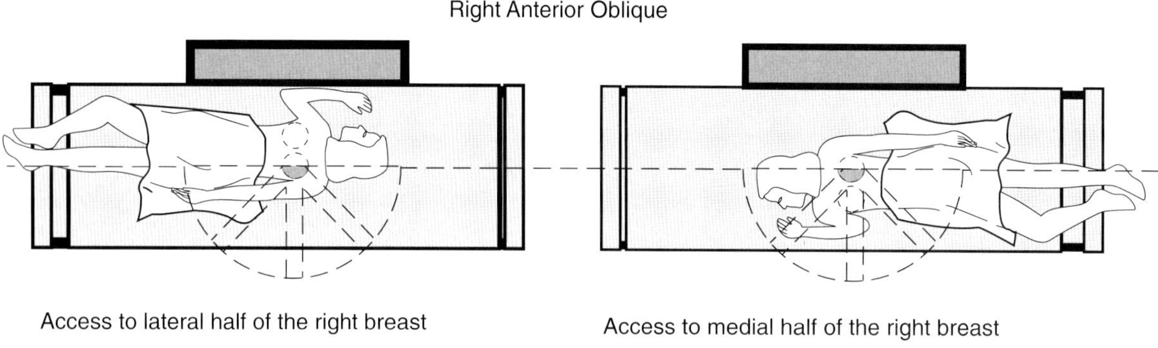

Access to lateral half of the right breast

Access to medial half of the right breast

Left Anterior Oblique

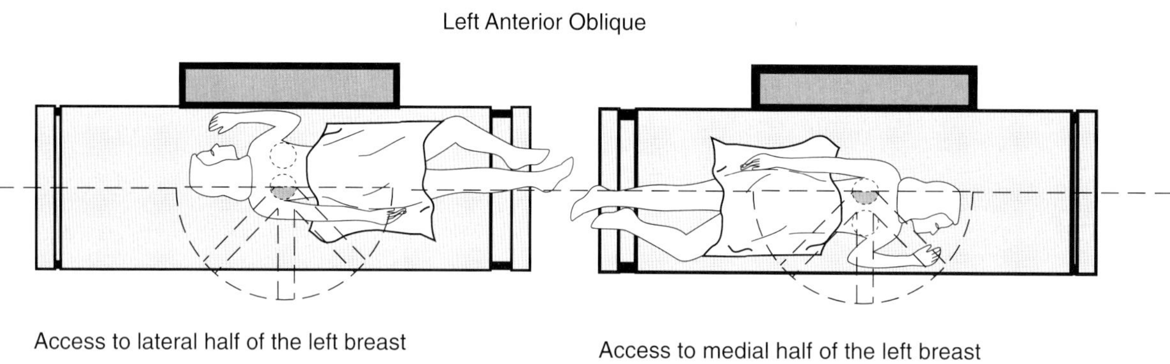

Access to lateral half of the left breast

Access to medial half of the left breast

Figure 6.29. Placing the Patient for Prone Positioning. In general, the patient is placed in an RAO projection for access to the right breast and an LAO projection for access to the left breast.

the support side of the table. In most cases, placing the patient in a right anterior oblique (RAO) will provide access to the right breast, whereas the left anterior oblique (LAO) will provide access to the left breast **(Figure 6.29)**. The ipsilateral arm is placed at the patient's side and the contralateral arm is flexed and up at the patient's head, allowing the breast to completely suspend through the table opening.

Generally, the technologist will gain greater access if she centers the breast in the table aperture. This permits the patient's chest wall to fully descend into the table aperture, allowing greater maneuverability of the breast. Accessing some abnormalities will require the patient to lie completely flat; others will require further adjustments, depending on the location of the abnormality and the selected c-arm approach.

Recommendations for SBB Positioning

The methods described below will aid the technologist in effectively positioning the breast for stereotactic biopsy. Not all methods will be successful with all patients, but having many methods available will help to achieve success. Some of these methods are specific to prone units, others have application for both prone and add-on units.

Maximizing Breast Support Placement

In general, the technologist can achieve greater access, especially for posterior abnormalities, by moving the breast support as close to the breast as possible. This maneuver is the same principle that Eklund[1] describes in elevating the inframammary fold for routine mammography, resulting in greater access. For stereotactic positioning, perform this maneuver in any projection by moving the breast support forward behind the breast, allowing visualization of more proximal tissue. The technologist can overemphasize this maneuver by sacrificing breast tissue nearer the breast support **(Figures 6.30-6.32)**, thereby increasing chest wall proximity.

Position Parallel with the Clock Time

To gain optimal maneuverability of the breast, choose the projection where the x-ray beam is parallel to the clock face location of the abnormality **(Figure 6.33)**. For example, if the abnormality is at 12:00, use a CC projection; whereas,

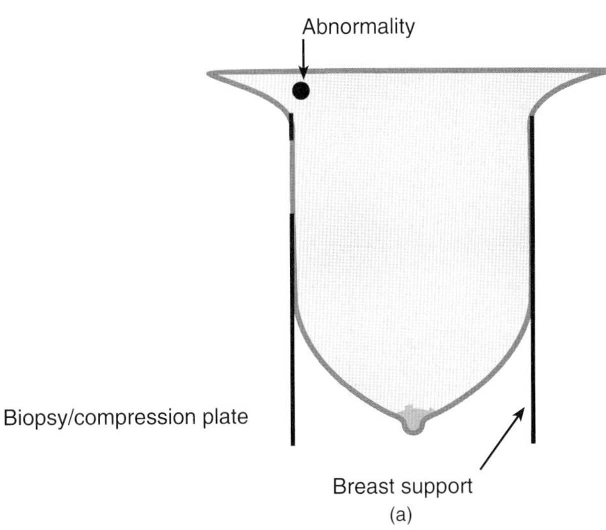

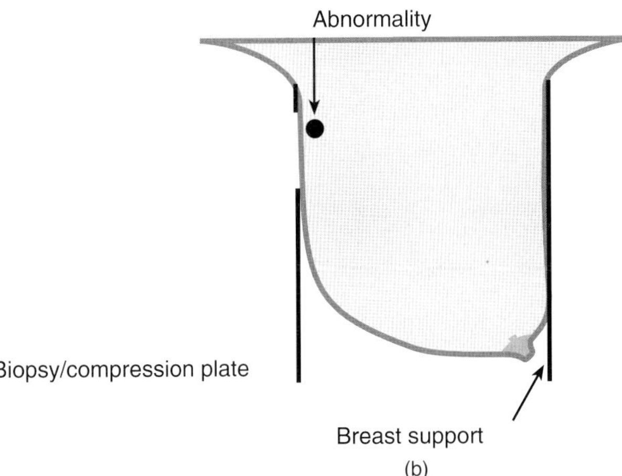

Figure 6.30. Maximizing Breast Support Placement. Greater access to posterior abnormalities is possible by moving the breast support forward behind the breast, sacrificing distal breast tissue.

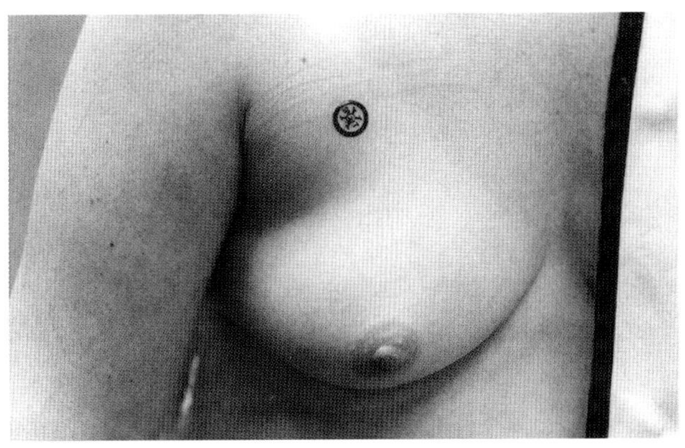

(a)

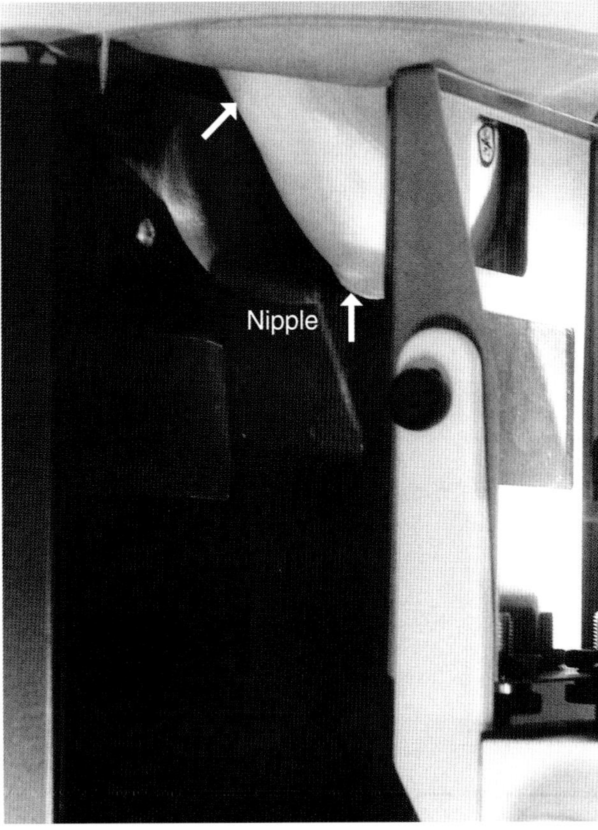

(b)

Figure 6.31 a and b. Breast Support Placement. Moving the breast support forward behind the breast allows greater access to chest wall abnormalities **(a)** nearer the biopsy/compression plate, usually causing the nipple to roll under. Figure **(b)** demonstrates completed positioning of this abnormality. Note how tissue near the breast support trails off **(arrow)**, allowing greater proximity to chest wall abnormalities.

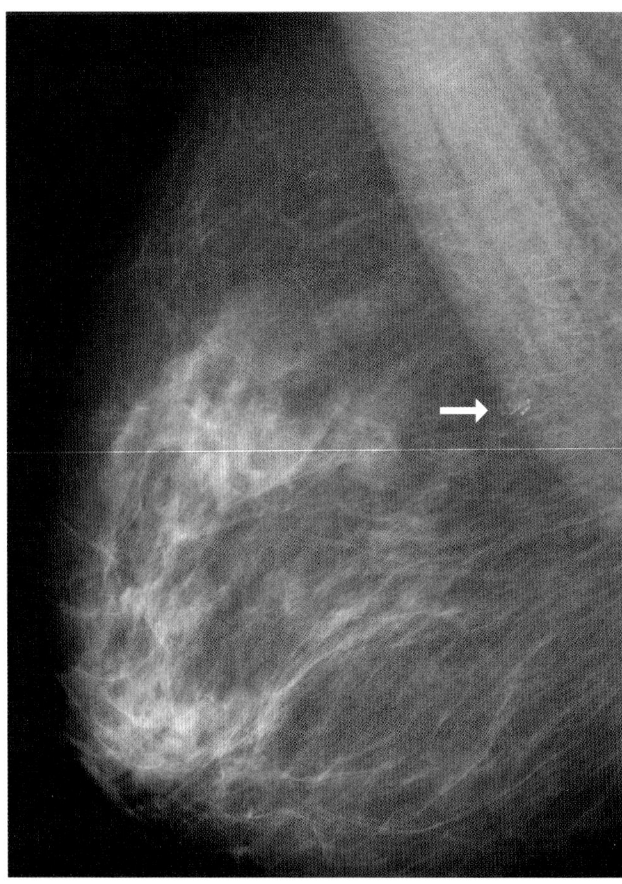

(a)

Figure 6.32 a-d. An Example of Accessing an Abnormality in the Upper Outer Quadrant of the Right Breast. The routine screening mammogram demonstrates an area of calcifications in the superior aspect of the MLO projection **(a) (arrow)**; the CC projection did not demonstrate the abnormality. An exaggerated CC (XCCL) **(b)** localizes these calcifications **(arrow)** in the upper outer quadrant of the right breast at about 10:00 **(c)**. A latero-medial projection allows access to this abnormality with extreme lateral movement of the breast support, sacrificing medial tissue. The scout image **(d)** demonstrates these calcifications **(arrow)** for biopsy.

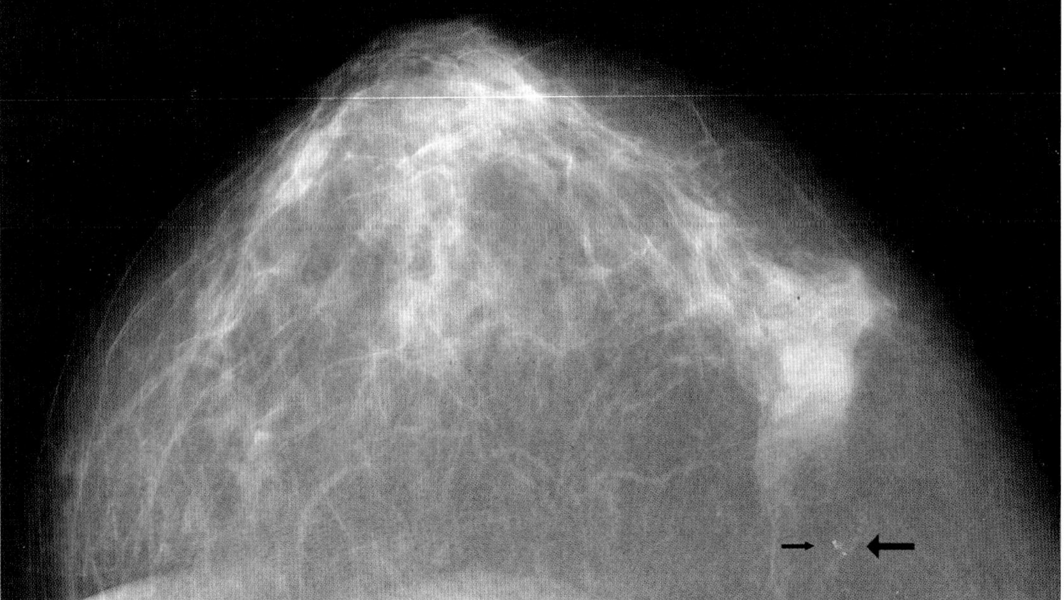

(b)

Figure 6.32 continued.

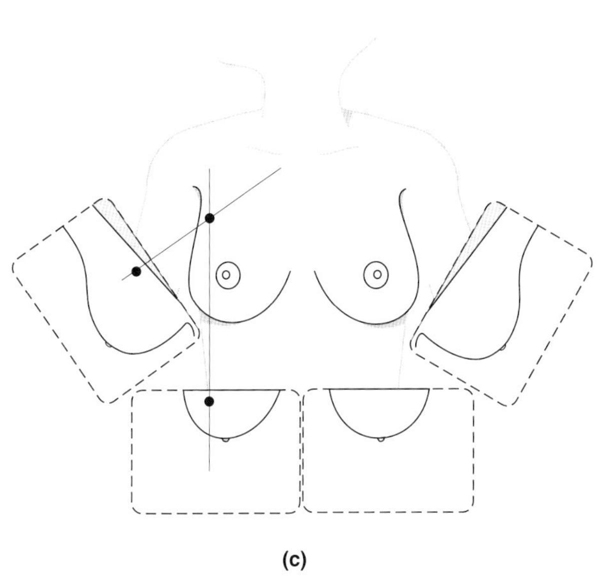

(c)

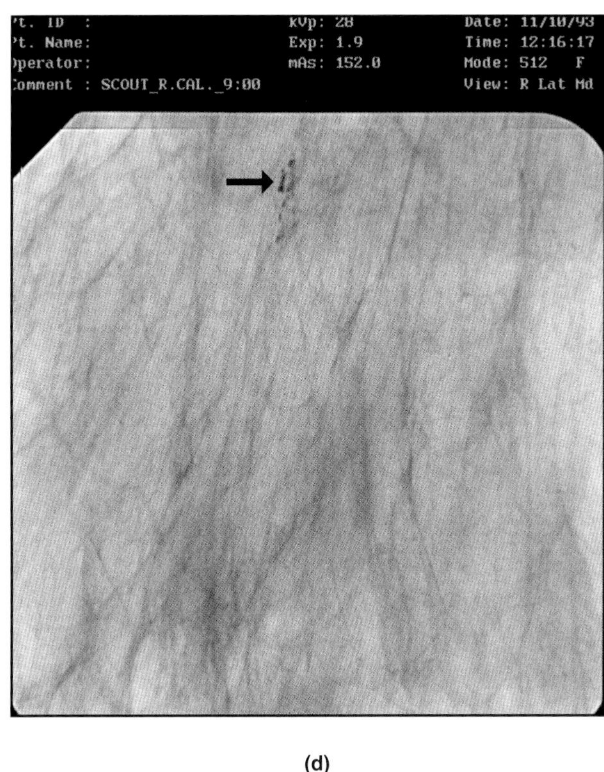

(d)

X- ray beam parallel with clock position (of abnormality)

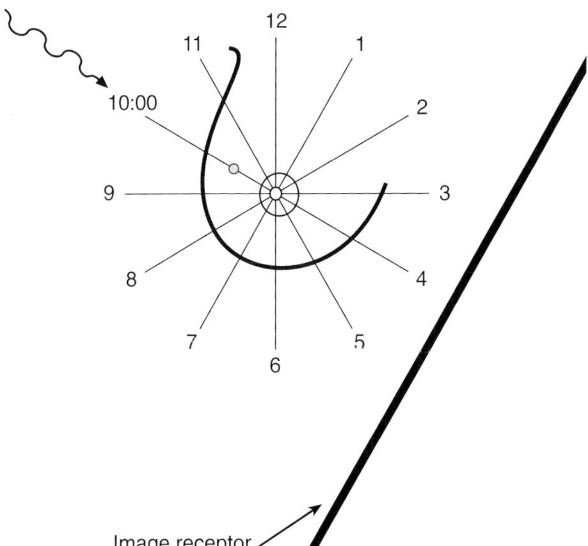

Figure 6.33. Positioning Parallel to Clock Time. The technologist can gain greater posterior access and breast mobility by choosing a projection that parallels the x-ray beam with the clock time of the abnormality.

if the abnormality is at 10:00 in the right breast, use a 45° SL-IM (**Figures 6.34**). This method allows greater mobility of the breast (**Figure 6.35**) and movement of the breast support closer to the compression plate.

Posterior Abnormalities

The technologist can successfully image what seem to be inaccessible posterior abnormalities that are near the chest wall. The team should never base their decision not to biopsy solely on the location of the abnormality on the mammogram. For example, a posterior location on the mammogram does not always indicate difficulty with stereotactic positioning. Always enlist the patient's cooperation; for example, request her to relax her rib cage into the table aperture. Gentle manipulation and downward pulling of the breast and adjacent tissue can also extend more posterior tissue through the opening. With large, heavy breasts, the weight of the breast in the pendulous position aids in lowering the posterior portions of the breast through the table aperture for greater access. The technologist will have greater success at imaging posterior abnormalities by making use of these suggestions and by varying the biopsy approach. The following methods may also work in some cases.

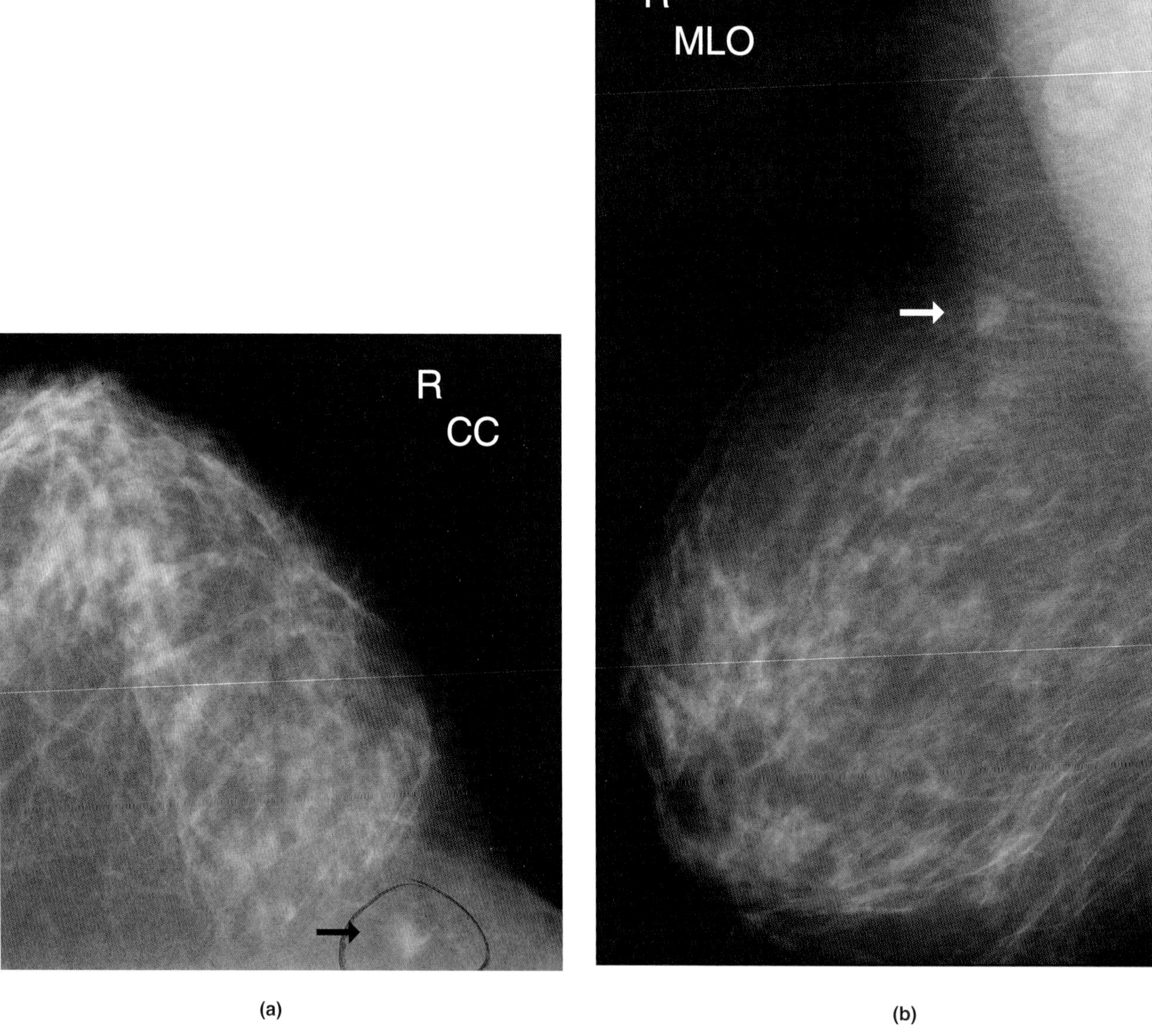

Figure 6.34 a-e. Positioning Parallel to Clock Time. This routine screening mammogram **(a,b)** demonstrates a mass density **(arrows)** in the extreme posterior aspect of the upper outer quadrant at about 10:00 **(c)** in the right breast. A lateral approach failed to access the abnormality for biopsy. Positioning the x-ray beam parallel to the clock time of the abnormality **(d)** results in a supero-lateral to infero-medial (SL-IM) projection, allowing greater mobility of the breast and access to this extremely posterior abnormality. The scout **(e)** image demonstrates the abnormality for biopsy. (Carcinoma.)

Figure 6.34 continued.

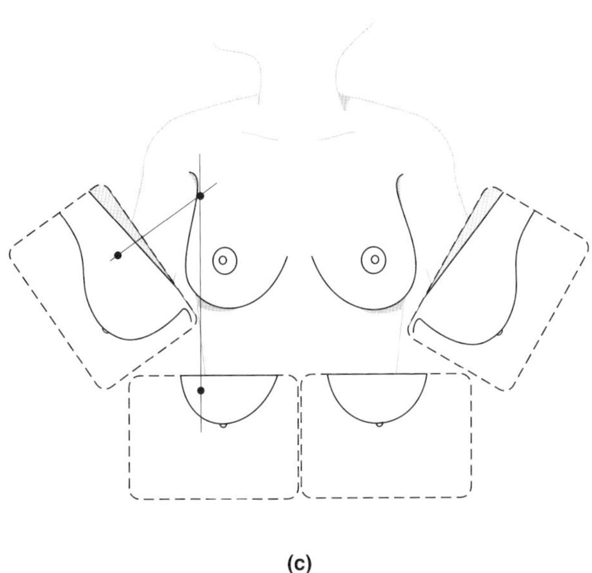

(c)

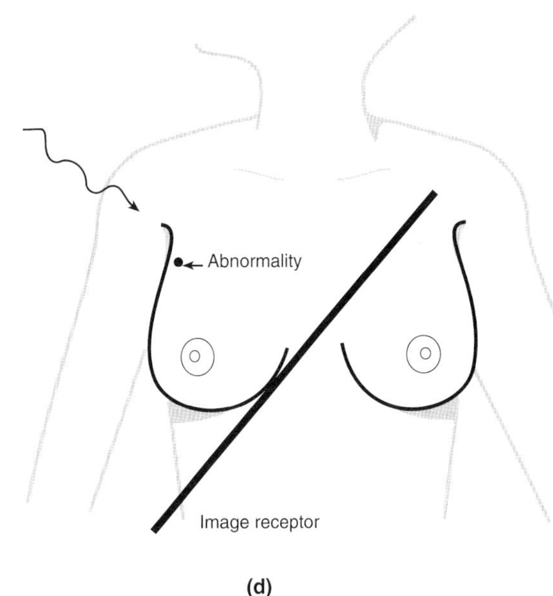

(d)

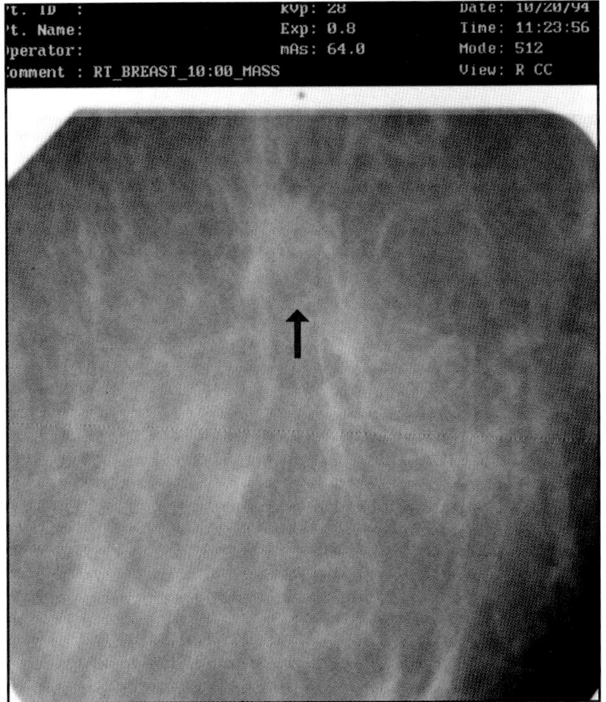

(e)

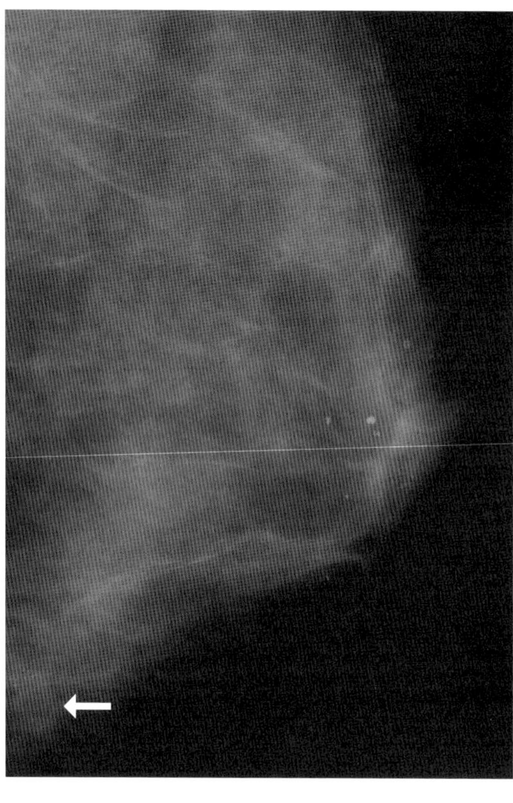

(a)

Figure 6.35 a-c. Positioning Parallel to Clock Time. This patient, referred for a second opinion, demonstrates an area of calcifications **(a) (arrow)** in the lower inner quadrant of the left breast at approximately 7:30. The patient was asthenic, with small breasts compressing to about 3 cm in both the caudal-cranial and lateral projections, disallowing these positions for biopsy because of negative stroke margin. The team selected an approach that placed the x-ray beam parallel to the clock time of the abnormality **(b)**; an infero-medial to supero-lateral (IM-SL) projection of approximately 45° provides 4.5 cm of compressed breast for positive stroke margin and the mobility to access this portion of the breast for abnormality visualization on both the scout **(c) (arrow)** and stereo images (not shown).

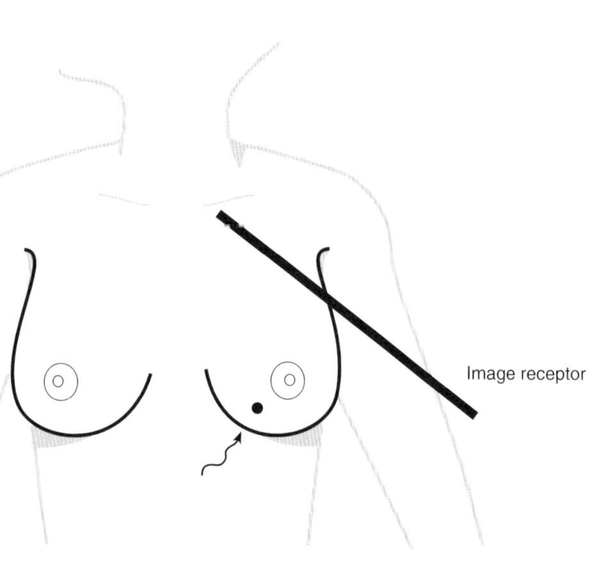

(b)

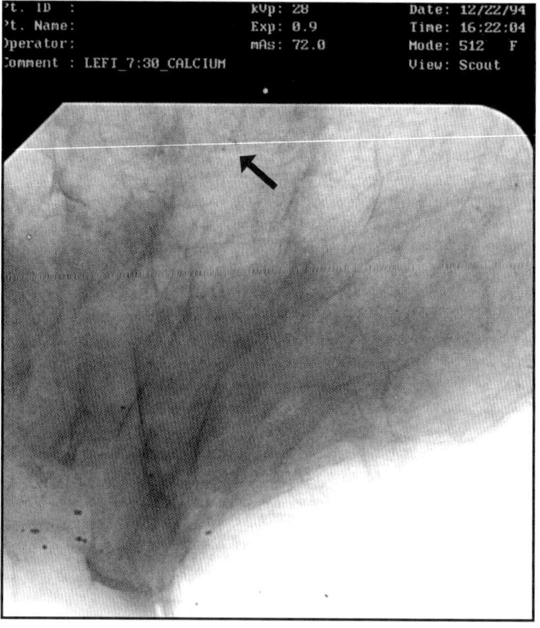

(c)

Shoulder Placement

When positioning the patient on the table, the technologist can place the ipsilateral shoulder at the very rim of the table opening, or allow the shoulder to drop through the opening **(Figure 6.36)**. This allows the patient's torso and breast to drop lower into the table aperture, providing greater access to posterior tissue.

Steeper Oblique

There are situations where placing the ipsilateral arm up near the head rather than at the side, and rolling the patient into a steeper oblique, nearly on her side, will be beneficial. Abnormalities that are extremely posterior and lateral in location may be easier to access with this maneuver. The amount of tissue that is accessible in this position depends on the total volume of lateral breast tissue **(Figure 6.37).**

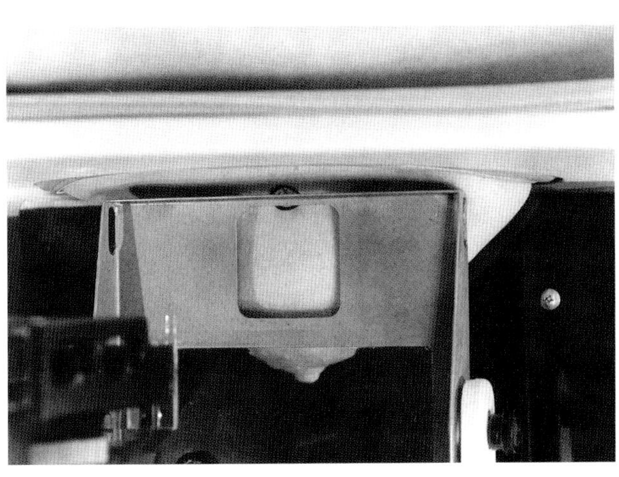

(a)

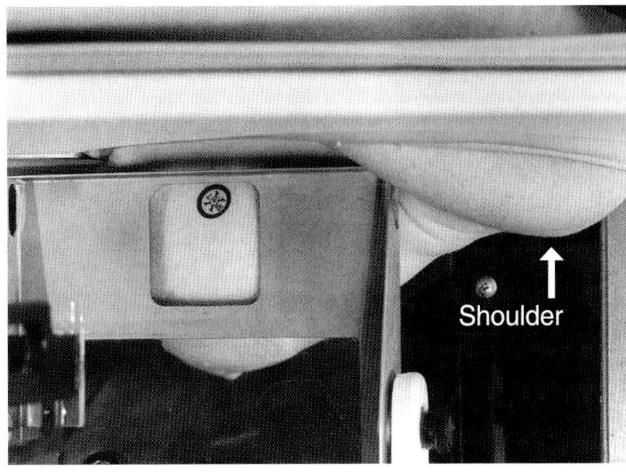

(b)

Figure 6.36 a and b. Shoulder Placement. Placing the patient's shoulder in, or in close proximity to, the table aperture can aid the technologist in accessing posterior abnormalities. Shown here is an LM projection with the shoulder normally placed **(a)**, prohibiting access to this posterior abnormality. Dropping the shoulder **(b) (arrow)** into the table aperture allows access to this abnormality.

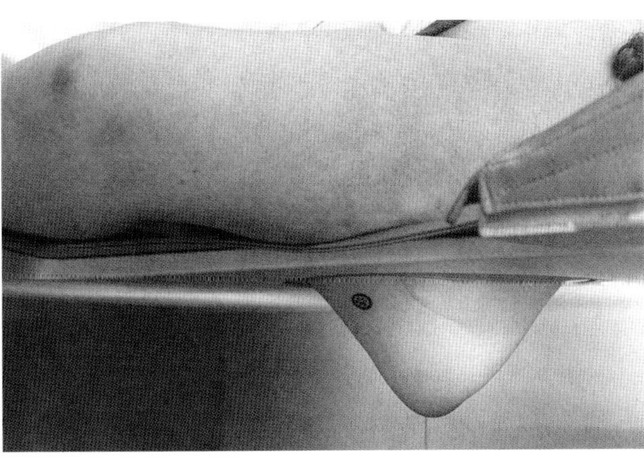

(a)

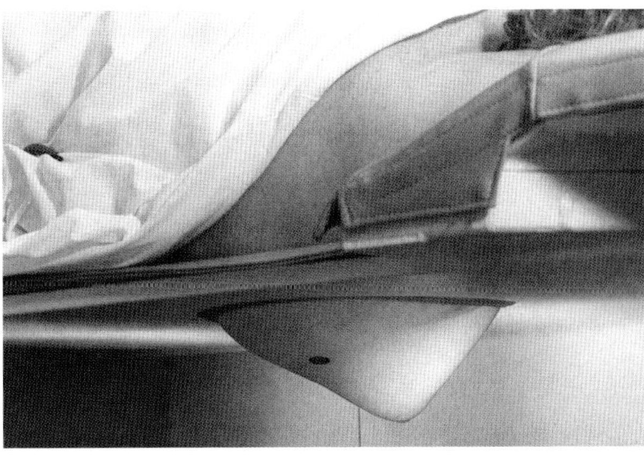

(b)

Figure 6.37 a and b. Utilizing a Steeper Oblique. A close-up of the breast **(a)** illustrates limited access to posterior abnormalities with the patient in the slight RAO position. The close-up **(b)** of the breast illustrates greater posterior access, accomplished by rolling the patient into a steeper oblique, bringing her arm over her head.

Lowering the Arm through the Table Aperture

For very posterior abnormalities, especially in the axilla area, the affected breast and the ipsilateral arm can be lowered through the table opening **(Figure 6.38).** The technologist should extend the arm as much as possible. Some type of support must be provided for both comfort and the reduction of motion. Placing the forearm on an adjustable-height tray provides adequate stabilization. The technologist should demonstrate the abnormality free of the pectoral muscle. Puncture of the pectoral muscle may cause the patient unnecessary discomfort.

Tincture of Benzoin

Applying tincture of benzoin (prior to compression) to the skin that is in contact with the rim of the biopsy window may reduce the breast from slipping from compression.

Subareolar Abnormalities

Complete tissue coverage of the biopsy window with subareolar abnormalities can be difficult, allowing patient and abnormality movement during the procedure. If the breast is large enough, choose a projection that allows nipple rotation upward or downward to cover the biopsy window **(Figure 6.39).** Rotation can also increase stroke margin by bringing more breast tissue behind the abnormality.

If coverage of the biopsy window is not possible, use clay or putty as a wedge filter to enhance imaging. This can be especially helpful when using a digital receptor.

Breast Size

Breast size can impede accessibility and visualization. However, the team should not judge difficulties on the basis of breast size only. A greater volume of breast tissue is often available when the breast is dependent. The suggestions listed below are useful for breasts that provide a challenge.

The Small Breast

In general, the technologist can apply the same methods to the small breast that achieve good results for posterior abnormalities. It is important to gently manipulate the breast and lower as much tissue through the table opening as possible, requesting the patient to relax her torso into the table aperture. Moving the breast support as close as possible to the breast can also increase the volume of available breast tissue.

The Large Breast

Large breasts can present challenges in locating and visualizing the abnormality. The full breast scout can be very helpful in these circumstances. Extra vigilance is necessary when a large breast is of sufficient length to touch or rest on the c-arm. Any c-arm rotation or movement must consider the proximity of the breast to the c-arm, preventing pain or injury.

The stroke margin is rarely an issue with breasts that compress to a thickness greater than 6 cm. However, two problems arise as a result of compression thickness. First, the abnormality of interest is an extended distance away from

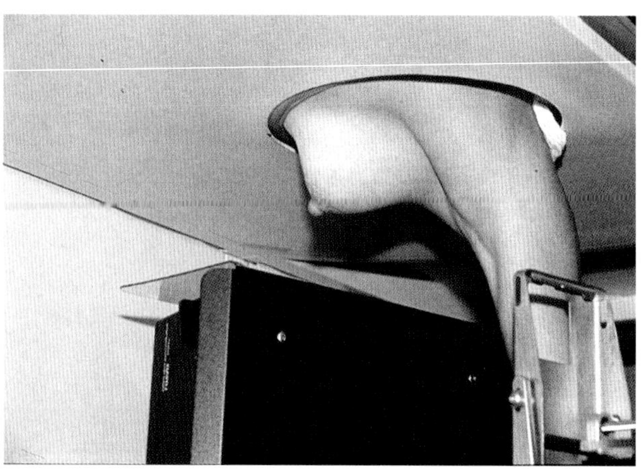

(a)

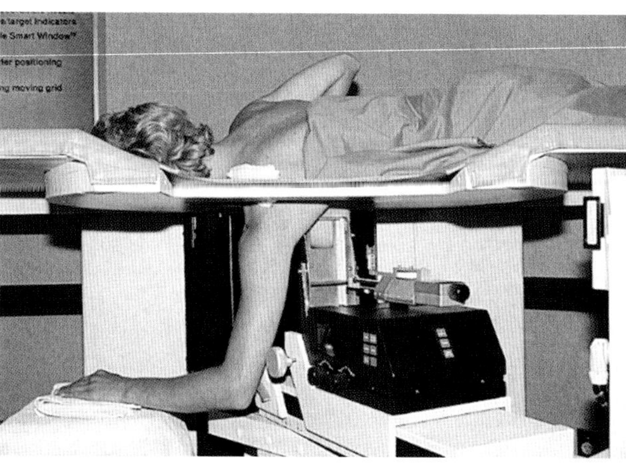

(b)

Figure 6.38 a and b. Positioning for Extremely Posterior Abnormalities in the Axilla. Greater access to posterior abnormalities **(a)** can be achieved by lowering the ipsilateral arm and breast through the table aperture **(b)**.

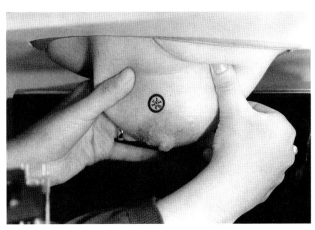

the image receptor, increasing blur. Second, the thickness of the breast creates more scatter, thereby reducing subject contrast. The most effective way to combat these problems is to 1) choose a c-arm projection that makes the breast as thin as possible (maintaining stroke margin), and 2) demonstrate the abnormality in fat. If the breast parenchyma is also dense, overlapping breast structures may inhibit visualization of the abnormality, either on the scout or stereo images. The technologist may use alternative projections. For example, rotating the breast or the c-arm 10-15° can produce visibility on the images where the abnormality was previously occult.

The Thin Breast

The thin breast can pose stroke margin difficulties. If breast compression is marginally close to allowing positive stroke margin, releasing compression slightly may provide the few millimeters necessary to produce a positive stroke margin. Rolling the breast up and toward the breast support may offer increased breast thickness. Alternative projections may also increase the thickness of the compressed breast. For example, positioning the breast in an oblique angle may produce greater thickness than the CC or lateral projections. Another option is to use a biopsy instrument with a smaller stroke, decreasing the necessary stroke margin.

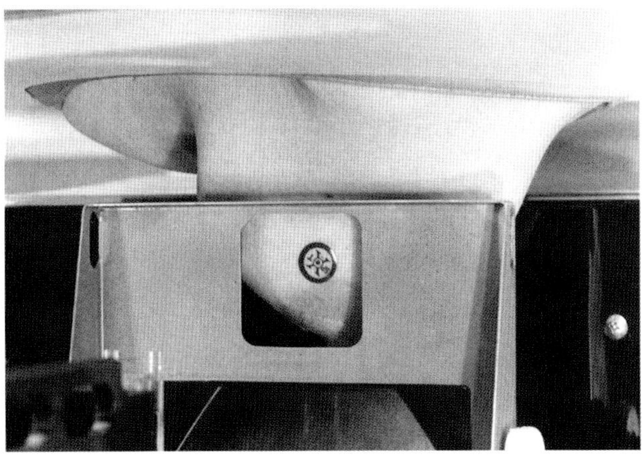

(a)

(b)

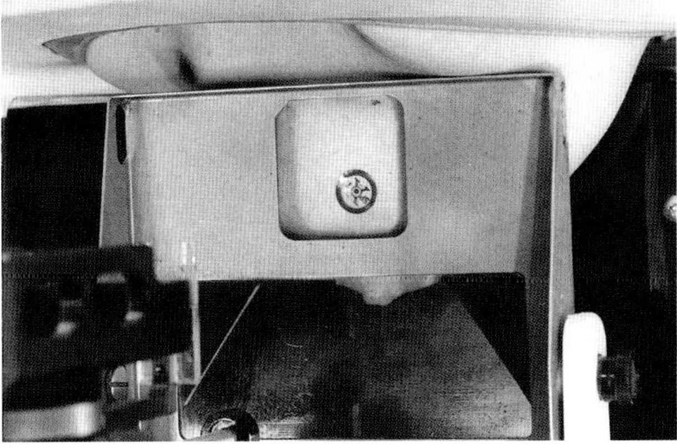

(c)

Figure 6.39 a-c. Nipple Rotation for Subareolar Abnormalities. Leaving the nipple in profile results in incomplete coverage of the biopsy window **(a)**. Rotating the nipple forward **(b)** increases the surface area of the breast, allowing complete coverage of the biopsy window **(c)**.

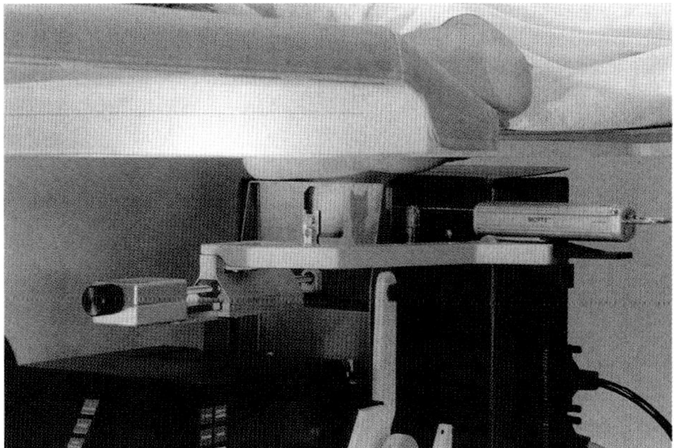

Figure 6.40. Utilizing a Side Arm to Eliminate Negative Stroke Margin. This figure demonstrates positioning of the patient for a side-arm approach. The technologist should position the breast so that the needle traverses the shortest skin-to-abnormality distance.

Side Arm (Orthogonal Arm)

Another alternative solution to negative stroke margin requires the use of an orthogonal arm **(Figure 6.40),** which allows imaging of the abnormality from one perspective and biopsy from another projection.The biopsy team should ensure that the excursion of the needle will not pierce the opposite side of the breast (this is more likely to happen with a subareolar abnormality).

If employing a side arm, the technologist should choose the projection that allows adequate centering in the biopsy window and provides the shortest skin-to-abnormality distance from the side approach. For example, if the abnormality is at 12:00, position the breast for an IL-SM or SL-IM oblique view, rather than the CC, to minimize the amount of breast the needle will have to traverse. A lateral projection may also be appropriate, if it is possible to center the abnormality.

References

1. Eklund, G. W. and Cardenosa, G. 1992. The Art of Mammographic Imaging. *Radiologic Clinics of North America,* 30:1.

Establishing a Successful Breast Needle Biopsy Program

W. Phil Evans, M.D.

7

Introduction

The needle biopsy technique has been in use for many years in the diagnosis of palpable breast abnormalities. In the late 1970s, clinicians at Karolinska Hospital in Sweden began performing fine needle aspiration biopsy (FNA) of mammographically detected impalpable breast abnormalities[1]. With the patient positioned prone on a dedicated biopsy table, stereotactically guided needle placement with an accuracy of +/- 1 mm was accomplished[2]. Using combined evaluation by mammography and cytology of 2,594 abnormalities, 77% were judged benign without the need for surgery[3]. In the group recommended for surgery, 76% were found to have breast cancer. Only one false negative occurred.

The first dedicated prone stereotactic biopsy table in the United States was introduced at the University of Chicago in 1986. Stereotactic FNA biopsy preceding needle localization and surgical biopsy produced a correct malignant diagnosis cytologically in 11 of 12 cases. The needle aspirate was reported to be inadequate in 14 of 84 abnormalities[4].

These efforts led to a similar program at the Baylor-Susan G. Komen Breast Center in 1988, using a stereotactic device that added on to an existing mammography unit. Stereotactic FNA biopsy, or alphanumeric, grid-guided FNA biopsy, was performed on 50 mammographically detected abnormalities prior to needle localization and surgical biopsy[5]. The FNA was done without charge and the results were promising. However, once this preliminary study was completed, the examination was not requested or ordered by any of the usual referring surgeons. Their reasons included: 1) the diagnosis by FNA was not definitive for benign abnormalities, 2) a high insufficient sample rate (20%), and 3) since histology was necessary prior to treatment, the stereotactic FNA merely added another step to the diagnostic procedure.

In 1989, Parker reported on 102 core needle biopsies. Twenty-nine were performed using a prone dedicated stereotactic table, an automated biopsy gun, and a 14-gauge cutting needle[6]. There was 97% agreement for needle biopsy relative to surgery and no inadequate samples. Based on this new information, the Center decided to venture again into breast needle biopsy. This time, however, a different approach was used.

The principal goal was to gain broad support from the largest group of referring physicians—the breast surgeons. A committee consisting of a diagnostic clinician, a medical oncologist, and three surgeons was formed to develop a protocol and guidelines for the core needle biopsy technique. The potential advantages, including reduced morbidity and cost, and definitive diagnosis of benign and malignant abnormalities were emphasized. These advantages would likely attract new patients to the Breast Center, allow additional early cancers to be found, and prompt breast conserving surgery. Concerns about accuracy, especially when abnormalities were diagnosed as "benign," were expressed; therefore, a management protocol was developed to minimize the chance of a stereotactic "miss."

Each potential abnormality would undergo a thorough imaging evaluation prior to needle biopsy. Impalpable breast abnormalities would be classified as either low-intermediate suspicion (LS) or high suspicion (HS) of malignancy (**Figure 7.1**). Based on this categorization, management recommendations could be made prior to biopsy. LS abnormalities with benign needle biopsy results and concordance with the mammographic evaluation would be followed at 6-, 12-, and 24-month intervals following biopsy. HS abnormalities with benign results, discordant LS abnormalities, or

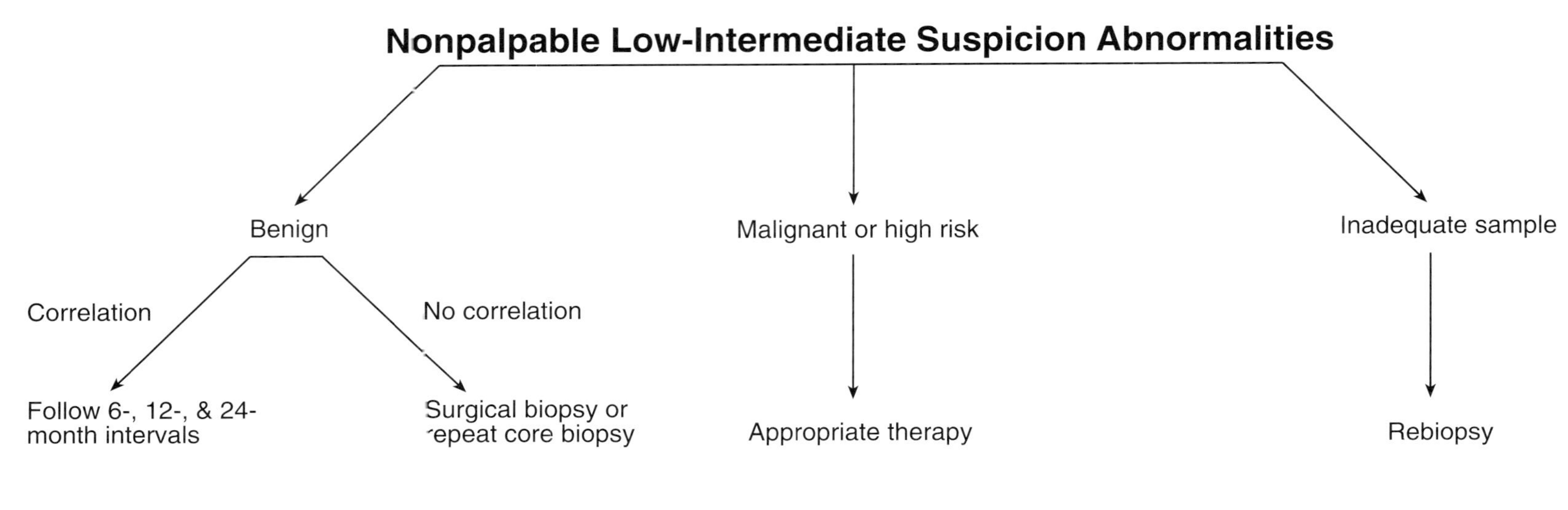

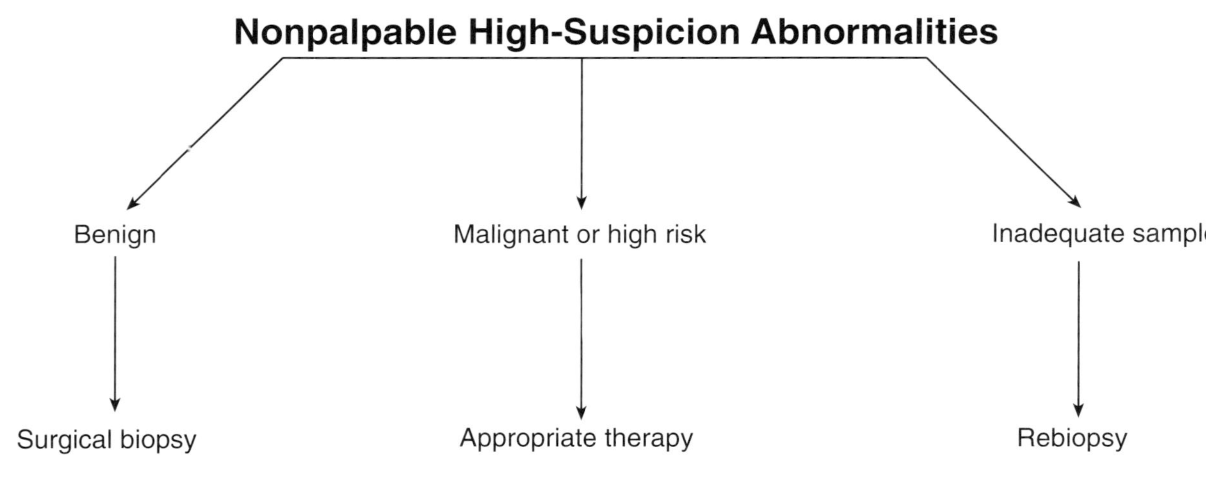

Figure 7.1. Management Flow Chart for Core Needle Biopsy Used at the Susan G. Komen Breast Center, Dallas, Texas.

any abnormality not adequately sampled, would proceed to surgical biopsy. Malignant abnormalities, whether LS or HS, could have definitive therapy based on needle biopsy histology. High-risk abnormalities, including atypical ductal hyperplasia, atypical lobular hyperplasia, lobular carcinoma in situ, or abnormalities where the pathologist requested more tissue would require surgical biopsy.

Since possible hematoma formation could "distort" the clinical surgical impression, surgical consultation and examination would be performed prior to biopsy of any HS abnormality, particularly if the biopsy referral was made directly to the clinician from a primary care physician. The surgeons also requested that the radiologists not biopsy palpable breast abnormalities.

Having had previous experience with stereotactic biopsy techniques, the committee clinician felt that a rapid learning curve would occur, and that the procedure would quickly become part of the breast imaging diagnostic armamentarium. Unlike the prior stereotactic FNA biopsy procedures, the core needle biopsy would not be performed immediately prior to needle localization. In the previous scenario, the radiologist was usually under pressure to get the biopsy and localization completed and the patient to surgery so the "real" biopsy could be done. The core biopsies would be scheduled during the afternoon, allowing the radiologist adequate time to perform the biopsy and obtain satisfactory tissue samples. The tissue was sent to pathology for permanent (not frozen) sections. The radiologist would review the core biopsy cases with the pathologist and notify the patient or the referring physician of the results by telephone.

Moreover, after a few initial cases were performed at no charge, the Center and the clinicians would bill for the procedure using diagnostic radiology and surgical CPT codes. Insurance companies, HMOs, and other payors became more educated with respect to the procedure's potential benefits.

Follow-up of women with benign needle diagnoses and management of the information generated by these biopsies were also considered critically important. Selected items of information were collected with each biopsy and entered into a computerized database. Correlation with surgical biopsies were made and monthly reports were reviewed by the committee chairman. A computerized system also was designed and implemented to send letters to patients and physicians notifying them at the appropriate follow-up time. Breast Center staff members were designated to perform these tasks with the assistance of the clinicians.

The imaging guided core breast biopsy program at the Baylor-Susan G. Komen Breast Center has been in place for over five years (stereotactic beginning in 1990 and ultrasound in 1991). Over 1,000 biopsies have been performed, with the number increasing each year. In reviewing the history of this approach for diagnosis of impalpable breast abnormalities, several important fundamentals emerge that led to establishing a successful breast needle biopsy program.

Fundamentals

Improve the Existing Clinical Situation

If all eligible women in the United States were to follow the American Cancer Society's screening mammography guidelines, approximately one million breast biopsies per year would be recommended for mammographically detected abnormalities[7,8]. If 30% of these biopsies were positive for cancer, 700,000 would return benign results. Surgical biopsies for impalpable breast abnormalities are expensive, costing $2,000-$4,000 in most facilities. Surgical biopsies require needle localization, have an anesthesia risk in many cases, and can create confusing clinical and mammographic pseudo-abnormalities. Although touted as the "gold standard" for breast abnormality diagnosis, surgical biopsies have a reported "miss rate" of from 0.2 to 22%[9-12].

Early detection and diagnosis is the most important factor in breast cancer control. Invasive cancers 1 cm or less can be consistently found through screening mammography[13-15]. Furthermore, these abnormalities are associated with a low incidence of axillary nodal metastases, the most important prognostic factor[16]. Randomized controlled trials have shown up to a 30% reduction in mortality in breast cancer screening programs[17].

The accuracy of imaging guided core needle biopsy with respect to surgical biopsy has been reported by several authors **(Figure 7.2)**[6,18-24]. Based on these studies, it is now relatively clear that experienced operators can obtain adequate samples 99% of the time, with an accuracy equal to surgical biopsy[25]. In most series, misses have occurred with both surgery and stereotactic biopsy. Therefore, to achieve the goal of early breast cancer detection, and to reduce or eliminate the disadvantages of surgical biopsy, imaging guided core needle biopsy is not only a reasonable alternative in diagnosis but a potentially significant improvement.

Achieve Broad-Based Support from the Medical Community

Although some facilities may choose to market directly to the community, most programs will not be successful with-

Author	Needle Gauge	No. of Biopsies	Agreement with Surgical Biopsy
Parker (1990) 18 *	14-18	102	87%
Parker (1991) 19 *	14	102	96%
Dowlatshahi (1991) 20 *	20	250	71%
Dronkers (1992) 21 *	18	53	91%
Elvecrog (1992) 23 **	14	100	94%
Parker (1993) 23 **	14	49	100%
†Gisvold (1994) 24 *	14	104	90%
††Parker (1994) 25 *	14	1,363	99%

Figure 7.2. Core biopsy. Agreement with surgical biopsy.

* Stereotactic
** Ultrasound

† Cases with 5 cores.
†† 23% of core biopsies performed using ultrasound guidance.

out support from referring physicians, especially those with a special interest in breast cancer. This includes breast surgeons, medical oncologists, radiation oncologists, plastic surgeons, and gynecologists. Prior to beginning, the program leader must explain the program and seek the advice of key physicians and third-party payors. He or she should also place emphasis on the technique's advantages, the management and follow-up of benign abnormalities, patient and physician communication, and the collection of appropriate data.

Achieving broad-based support begins with the advocacy of a single person. Thus, the program leader must find one or two physicians who will refer patients for needle biopsy. The best referrer is a busy breast surgeon. In an ideal world, the surgeon would probably prefer to operate only on patients with malignant abnormalities. However, with surgery booked weeks in advance and most biopsies benign, a delay in surgery can result for patients with malignancies. Each benign biopsy also necessitates a follow-up visit, again taking the surgeon's time and decreasing the number of patients seen who have malignant disease. A surgeon with these concerns quickly understands the usefulness of a program that distinguishes benign abnormalities from those requiring surgical therapy.

The success of initial needle biopsies cannot be overemphasized. The accuracy of the biopsy along with patient and physician satisfaction are extremely important. Attend a training program and practice biopsies with phantoms until you and your technologist know the procedure thoroughly. Learn to aspirate cysts using ultrasound guidance before attempting core biopsies. Begin with relatively large abnormalities that you can easily visualize and target mammographically.

Early in the program, requests may be made for biopsy of abnormalities inappropriate to the team's level of experience. These include abnormalities in patients with breast implants, axillary abnormalities, abnormalities seen only on one mammographic view, and tiny clusters (2-3 mm or less) of microcalcifications. Carefully choose the abnormalities to biopsy, and resist the temptation to biopsy difficult abnormalities prematurely. Increase the difficulty as the team gains experience and confidence in its ability to perform the procedure.

Select a Project Leader and Provide the Necessary Resources for Success

Burbank has described the project leader in classical management terms as the biopsy team's "champion[26]." Peters describes a champion as a "dreamer,...a scrounging pragmatist,...and one who takes on activities that have low odds for success but are high-odds matters to him or her precisely because of the passionate attachment[27]." The leader (champion) must also possess several additional qualities. The first is expertise in breast imaging. The program leader must understand the variety of abnormalities to be biopsied and their relative chance of malignancy to be credible with other members of the breast cancer diagnostic team (surgeons, pathologists, etc.). Second, interventional radiology expertise is essential. Although the skills necessary for performing core biopsy are not exceptional, the physician must have the capacity to deal with circumstances that do not always unfold exactly as planned.

An understanding of breast pathology is also important. Core biopsy is a "new world" to some pathologists. The leader must communicate to his or her pathology colleagues expectations of what the histology will exhibit. Ideally, the clinician and pathologist should review all cases together, as this is an excellent learning experience for both.

Finally, as the project leader becomes part of the clinical breast cancer team, there must be a willingness to expand the leader's knowledge of the entire treatment process. The diagnostic core needle biopsy is an important part of patient care, but it must be considered in terms of what is best for the patient. For example, some patients, who experience anxiety when they are told they have a "breast abnormality," insist on surgical excision rather than core biopsy, even though the abnormality may be considered low suspicion. Core needle biopsy for these patients is unnecessary and only adds another procedure to the diagnostic and treatment process.

The project leader must have certain resources to accomplish development. If a physician is in a group radiology practice, one of the most important assets is the support of partners. Internal group issues must be dealt with in an honest and straightforward manner and support achieved before the project leader can successfully deal with external concerns.

Most of the internal opposition will center on one main issue—the time away from the "film reading" practice needed to develop the program. New duties for the project leader include attendance at educational functions to improve breast imaging and interventional skills, organization of the departmental breast diagnostic team, evaluation of biopsied cases with the pathologist, participation in hospital or facility breast cancer case conferences, analysis and verification of data generated by the program, monitoring of outcomes, and the preparation and delivery of educational seminars to potential patients and referring physicians. Initially, a core biopsy case may take from 1-3 hours, a significant commitment for the clinician considering the reimbursement. The radiology group must view the future long-term rewards of the program as greater than the short-term losses.

Other resources include support and training from equipment manufacturers, including software upgrades, a willingness by the pathologists to make specific benign diagnoses from cores of tissue, and overall flexibility from all participants to change the program if some aspect is not proceeding as planned.

Develop A Patient Management, Data Collection, and Follow-Up Protocol Prior to Beginning the Program

The program components above relate to recommendations and events occurring *after* biopsy. The patient management protocol used at the Komen Breast Center (Figure 7.1) has been an important tool for patients and referring physicians, as it demonstrates the management plan for the patient's breast abnormality *before* the biopsy is performed. The protocol provides a logical approach to the procedure using both breast imaging and histologic findings to ensure accuracy. Of over 1,000 biopsies, only 4 known false negatives have occurred. With increasing experience, the number of inadequate samples has been reduced to less than 1%, even with residents and fellows participating in the biopsies. A large data base has also been created, allowing predictions as to any given abnormality's chance of malignancy.

Data collection is an integral part of the program. Literally hundreds of items of information can be collected on each biopsy, but the amount of data collected will be determined by the team's resources. Determining what information the program leader wants is the first step. Basic information includes patient name, identification number, demographics, referring physician, prebiopsy diagnosis (low-intermediate suspicion or high suspicion), abnormality classification (mass or calcifications), abnormality size, biopsy method used (ultrasound or stereotactic), clinician performing the procedure, number of cores obtained, specimen radiography results (if any), needle biopsy results, surgical biopsy results (if any), complications, and results of the 6-, 12-, and 24-month follow-up visits. Other useful data involve procedure time, interpreting pathologist, type of needle and gun, technologist performing the procedure, and any difficulties encountered.

Follow-up of patients with benign biopsies is one of the most demanding yet vital elements of the program. It is possible for any biopsy method (surgical or needle) to miss a cancer. Therefore, for the patient's benefit, follow-up to detect any suspicious change is necessary. Once the biopsy has been performed and data collection procedures are in place, follow-up guidelines can be developed. Some of the guidelines to be established are: *to whom* are follow-up reminder letters sent—patient, the referring physician, or both; *when* are the letters sent—two months before the scheduled follow-up, one month, etc.; *how many* letters are sent before the patient is considered lost to follow-up; and the issue of follow-up in *other facilities*.

At the Komen Center, the first reminder letter is sent to the patient within one month of the expected appointment time. If the patient does not schedule promptly, a second letter is sent to both the patient and the referring physician. If there is still no response, an attempt is made to contact the patient and the referring physician by telephone. Follow-up in other facilities is allowed because it may be more convenient for some patients; however, the patient is requested to have the exam sent to the Center for review and comparison. On occasion an exceptional effort must be made to find a "lost" patient. This includes performing the follow-up exam at no charge or "insurance only," or enlisting a friend or volunteer to bring the patient to the Center. Many times the patient has moved to a new address but can be found through the telephone directory or directory assistance.

As more benign biopsies are performed, the number of patients for follow-up visits increases substantially. An employee, preferably a data manager, whose primary function is to manage the data and recall the follow-up patients, is essential. This person needs not only analytical competence but people skills to deal with patients and doctors' offices to secure follow-up visits.

The recommendations for management of a breast abnormality following needle biopsy, the discussion with the patient, and all follow-up efforts should be clearly documented in the patient's chart. This record can be quite beneficial if a medicolegal situation should occur.

Use Appropriate Billing Codes

Billing categories and CPT codes applicable to core needle biopsy are listed in **Figure 7.3**. They include diagnostic radiology, surgical, and evaluation and management codes. The diagnostic radiology codes have both a technical and professional component. The professional component relates to supervision and interpretation of the procedure. Therefore, in the radiologists's report, an "interpretation" section describing the breast imaging findings is noted separately for each procedure charged. The surgical code relates to the performance of the procedure; thus, a description of how the procedure was accomplished is included in the "procedure" section of the report. The evaluation and management codes relate to the physician's consultation with and examination of the patient, and its complexity. This consultation also requires a separate section in the radiologist's report. The biopsy supply code is a technical component, and like the technical component of other radiologic procedures, it is not noted in the report.

A typical stereotactic biopsy report may be structured and coded as follows:

> LEFT BREAST ABNORMALITY NEEDLE BIOPSY—STEREOTACTIC GUIDANCE
> 8/29/95
> PROCEDURE (19100): Using stereotactic guidance, digital mammography, local anesthesia, the automated biopsy gun, a 14-gauge core needle, and a caudal approach, five cores of tissue were removed from a 1 cm area of microcalcifications at the 6:00 position of the left breast. The cores of tissue were radiographed, placed in formalin, and sent to pathology for histologic evaluation. No immediate complications occurred.
>
> INTERPRETATION (76095): Prefire and postfire stereo images made during the procedure show the needle to be in the proper position and to pass through the abnormality during the biopsy.
>
> SPECIMEN RADIOGRAPH (76098) 8/29/95
> Magnification specimen radiography demonstrates microcalcifications in 3 of the 5 cores.
>
> HISTOLOGY: Nonproliferative fibrocystic change with microcalcifications identified histologically.
>
> CONSULTATION, FOLLOW-UP (99213)
> 8/30/95
> The biopsy site shows minor bruising with no evidence of significant hematoma formation. The histologic findings correlate with mammographic findings. A follow-up left mammogram in six months (February 1996) is recommended. The findings and recommendations were discussed with the patient and her husband. The patient agrees to follow-up and the appointment has been scheduled for February 28, 1996.

Biopsy CPT Codes

Core Biopsy Procedure	CPT Code
Stereotactic localization for needle biopsy, each abnormality	76095
Ultrasound guidance for needle biopsy	79642
Specimen radiograph	76098
Biopsy of breast; needle core	19100
Biopsy tray	99070
Biopsy gun needle	99070
Consultation, initial office visit	99241
Consultation, follow-up visit	99213
Consultation, telephone follow-up	99371

Figure 7.3. Commonly Used Billing Catagories and CPT Codes That Apply to Core Need Biopsy.

Not all practices require patients to return for a follow-up visit to discuss the biopsy findings. Benign results can usually be discussed with the patient by telephone. The physician receives notification through the radiology and pathology reports. When the histology is malignant, or indicates the need for surgical biopsy, the referring physician is contacted first to determine who will communicate with the patient, and to whom the patient will be referred for further therapy.

The typical global charge for stereotactic core biopsy is approximately $1,000 and ultrasound $600-$700.

Monitor and Report Outcomes to the Medical Community

After the biopsy program begins, monitor outcomes on a periodic basis and report to physician colleagues and other members of the medical community. At the Komen Center, the breast imaging staff physicians and a multidisciplinary physician group of breast disease specialists review the results monthly.

In a successful program, the program leader should see the number of core needle biopsies and the percentage of positive needle localizations increase with time. This occurs because core needle biopsy distinguishes benign from malignant abnormalities. The benign abnormalities will be followed with an imaging modality, and needle localization and surgical excision will not be performed. The number of cancers found with needle localization relative to benign abnormalities will increase. Theoretically, with surgical biopsy of most benign abnormalities eliminated, the positive predictive value of the needle localization procedure could reach up to 80%. Overall, the number of needle localizations and surgical biopsies will decrease, unless the program attracts additional patients from other facilities; with most successful programs, this has been a common occurrence.

Furthermore, primary care physicians will begin sending their patients directly to the radiologist for core needle biopsy. If the biopsy is malignant, a surgical referral is made. If benign, the radiologist and primary care physician can follow the patient. This trend will become apparent if a site monitors patient referral sources.

Summary

There will be many obstacles to the development of a successful core needle biopsy program. Most anecdotal examples of extreme concern by surgeons and hospital administrators with respect to the potential loss of revenue have been overstated. Generally, surgeons, as caretaking physicians, want to do what is best for the patient and, in most instances, core needle biopsy has clear advantages over surgical biopsy.

With the inclusion of core needle biopsy in the diagnostic paradigm, the management of nonpalpable breast abnormalities is changing. Radiologists will be asked to perform tasks and roles unfamiliar to them. These include interactions with patients and physicians requiring greater responsibility, new knowledge, and greater visibility for the radiologist. Establishing a successful core needle biopsy program will provide the breast imaging radiologist an expanded clinical role on the breast diagnostic and treatment team.

The author wishes to thank Mollie Standish, B.A., for her invaluable assistance in preparation of this manuscript, and the physicians and technical staff of the Susan G. Komen Breast Center in Dallas, Texas for their outstanding support of the core biopsy program.

References

1. Bolmgren, J., Jacobson, B., Nordenström, B. 1977. Stereotaxic Instrument for Needle Biopsy of the Mamma. *Am J Roentgenol* 129:121.

2. Svane, G., Silfverswärd, C. 1983. Stereotaxic Needle Biopsy of Non-Palpable Breast Lesions: Cytologic and Histopathologic Findings. *Acta Radiol Diagn* 24:283.

3. Azavedo, E., Svane, G., Auer, G. 1989. Stereotactic Fine-Needle Biopsy in 2594 Mammographically Detected Non-Palpable Lesions. *Lancet* 1:1033.

4. Dowlatshahi, K., Jokich, P.M., Schmidt, R., Bibbo, M., Dawson, P.J. 1987. Cytologic Diagnosis of Occult Breast Lesions Using Stereotaxic Needle Aspiration. *Arch Surg* 122:1343.

5. Evans, W.P., Cade, S.H. 1989. Needle Localization and Fine-Needle Aspiration Biopsy of Nonpalpable Breast Lesions with Use of Standard and Stereotactic Equipment. *Radiology* 173:53.

6. Parker, S.H., Lovin, J.D., Jobe, W.E., et al. 1990. Stereotactic Breast Biopsy with a Biopsy Gun. *Radiology* 176:741.

7. Hall, F.M. 1986. Screening Mammography Potential Problems on the Horizon. *N Engl J Med* 314:53.

8. Hall, F.M., Storella, J.M., Silverstone, D.Z., Wyshak, G. 1988. Nonpalpable Breast Lesions: Recommendations for Biopsy Based on Suspicion of Carcinoma at Mammography. *Radiology* 167:353.

9. Yankaskas, B.C., Knelson, M.H., Abernethy, M.L., Cuttino, J.T., Clark, R.L. 1988. Needle Localization Biopsy of Occult Lesions of the Breast: Experience in 199 Cases. *Invest Radiology* 23:729.

10. Homer, M.J., Smith, T.J., Safaii, H. 1992. Prebiopsy Needle Localization: Methods, Problems, and Expected Results. *Radiol Clin North Am* 30:139.

11. Kopans, D.B. 1993. Review of Stereotaxic Large-Core Needle Biopsy and Surgical Biopsy Results in Nonpalpable Breast Lesions. *Radiology* 189:665.

12. Norton, L.W., Zeligman, B.E., Pearlman, N.W. 1988. Accuracy and Cost of Needle Localization Biopsy. *Arch Surg* 123:947.

13. Shapiro, S., Venet, W., Strax, P., Venet, L., Roeser, R. 1982. Ten to Fourteen-Year Effect of Screening on Breast Cancer Mortality. *J Natl Cancer Inst* 69:349.

14. Tabar, L., Fagerberg, C.J.G., Gad, A., et al. 1985. Reduction in Mortality from Breast Cancer After Mass Screening with Mammography. *Lancet* i:829.

15. Seidman, N., Gelf, S.K., Silverberg, E., LaVerda, N,. Lubera, J. A. 1987. The Breast Cancer Detection Demonstration Project: End Result. *Cancer* 37:258.

16. Tabar, L., Fagerberg, G., Duffy, S.W., et al. 1992. Update of the Swedish Two-Country Program of Mammographic Screening for Breast Cancer. *Radiol Clin North Am* 30:187.

17. Shapiro, S., Strax, P., Venet, L. 1971. Periodic Breast Cancer Screening in Reducing Mortality from Breast Cancer. *JAMA* 215:1777.

18. Parker, S.H., Lovin, J.D., Jobe, W. E., et al. 1991. Non-Palpable Breast Lesions: Stereotactic Automated Large-Core Biopsies. *Radiology* 180:403.

19. Dowlatshahi, K., Yaremko, M. L., Kluskens, L. F., Jokich, P. M. 1991. Nonpalpable Breast Lesions: Findings of Stereotaxic Needle-Core Biopsy and Fine-Needle Aspiration Cytology. *Radiology* 181:745.

20. Dronkers, D.J. 1992. Stereotaxic Core Biopsy of Breast Lesions. *Radiology* 183:631.

21. Elvecrog, E.L., Lechner, M. C., Nelson, M. T. 1993. Non-Palpable Breast Lesions: Correlation of Stereotaxic Large-Core Needle Biopsy and Surgical Biopsy Results. *Radiology* 188:453.

22. Parker, S. H., Jobe, W. E., Dennis, M. A., et al. 1993. US-Guided Automated Large-Core Breast Biopsy. *Radiology* 187:507.

23. Gisvold, J. J., Goellner, J. R., Grant, C. S., et al. 1994. Breast Biopsy: A Comparative Study of Stereotaxically Guided Core and Excisional Techniques. *AJR Am J Roentgenol* 162:815.

24. Parker, S., Burbank, F., Tabar, L., et al. (in press) Percutaneous Large Core Breast Biopsy: A Multi-Institutional Experience. *Radiology*.

25. Schmidt, R.A. 1994. Stereotactic Breast Biopsy. *CA Cancer J Clin* 44:172.

26. Burbank, F. 1994. Nine Steps to a New Breast Biopsy Paradigm. *Diagnostic Imag* (May):5.

27. Peters, T. 1987. *Thriving on Chaos*. New York: Harper and Row 298.

Patient Selection and Indications for Breast Needle Biopsy

Gillian M. Newstead, M.D.

8

Introduction

Improved mammographic techniques have resulted in the detection of subtle radiographic abnormalities and the diagnosis of small cancers[1]. A criticism of the widespread use of screening mammography in the United States is the relatively high cost of the identification of each cancer[2,3]. Surgical biopsies represent a large percentage of the induced costs of screening, and nationally 0-90% of these biopsies are benign[4-7]. Although surgical excisional biopsy with prior radiological abnormality localization is a proven safe procedure with low complication rates, recent studies have shown that stereotactic biopsy techniques can play an important role in the management of patients with mammographic screening abnormalities.

Breast needle biopsy can be performed with either fine needle aspiration or with core biopsy. Many institutions have reported sensitivity and specificity of 90% or greater with fine needle aspiration and core biopsy techniques[8-20]. The procedures are especially useful in confirming benignity in abnormalities of low suspicion for malignancy. The need for surgical biopsy or follow-up mammographic studies may thus be avoided. The procedures are simple to perform, have a low complication rate, and are well-tolerated by the patient.

Patient Selection

It is possible to perform fine needle aspiration and/or core biopsy on most patients with nonpalpable mammographically suspicious or indeterminate abnormalities, for which open biopsy would be considered. The decision to perform needle biopsy, however, should not be undertaken until a rigorous imaging work-up has been completed. High-quality mammographic studies, including spot compression views with or without magnification, or additional projections as needed, are essential for complete analysis of the abnormality(ies). It is important to define the mammographic abnormality completely and to determine all of the abnormality characteristics. Assessment of abnormality size, presence or absence of multifocality, and precise location of the abnormality in the breast are important issues in planning the needle biopsy. Ultrasound evaluation of the abnormality may also prove useful, not only to exclude cysts, but also to aid in the assessment of certain abnormalities. Galactography may also be helpful in certain patients with a clinically significant nipple discharge, particularly when the abnormality is mammographically occult, and may also be used in conjunction with stereotactic biopsy to target the abnormality accurately.

Stereotactic needle biopsies are not a substitute for poor imaging and inadequate preprocedure diagnosis. It is not uncommon for a patient to be referred for stereotactic biopsy for an abnormality "seen in one view only." In almost every case, the abnormality can be identified in orthogonal views after careful mammographic evaluation. The additional imaging needed may include spot views of the abnormality in the projection in which the abnormality is seen initially to confirm that a real abnormality is indeed present. Once the presence of a significant abnormality is established, then the abnormality must be found in orthogonal views. Multiple spot views in the appropriate plane of the breast, referable to the nipple or chest wall, may be helpful. In certain patients, ultrasound can help in abnormality localization, particularly in the radiographically dense breast. Therefore, a complete analysis of the mammographic findings and other imaging studies, where appropriate, is essential before making the decision to perform BNB.

There are certain limiting patient and mammographic factors that must be taken into account during the selection of patients for stereotactic biopsy. Patient education directed toward the nature of the procedure, and the reason for this diagnostic option, are most important prior to scheduling stereotactic biopsy. Patient cooperation is key for the successful performance of percutaneous biopsy. Time spent with the patient prior to the procedure to explain the nature of the examination helps to expedite procedure time and improve the success rate. Many patients find that viewing a videotape of the procedure itself is helpful. In general, stereotactic biopsy is well-tolerated by the patient. Those patients with a history of severe back or neck arthritis may find the prone position difficult to maintain and, in some cases, upright stereotactic units may be preferable to use.

A review process for referred patients must be established. It is good policy to review all pertinent patient imaging studies prior to the scheduling of the procedure. Additional imaging may prove necessary and, ideally, should be done ahead of time, along with discussion of the findings with the patient and her physician.

It is important to acquire a medical history. Patients receiving anticoagulant therapy may not be good candidates for a core biopsy unless the medication is adjusted. These patients can often be managed successfully with fine needle aspiration. Similarly, patients requiring prophylactic antibiotics for dental surgery may also require them prior to core biopsy. It is important to discuss these issues with the patient's physician, prior to scheduling the procedure.

Other limiting patient factors include patient weight. The weight limit for any particular prone unit must be taken into consideration. Upright stereotactic units can often be used successfully when patient weight disallows the use of prone stereotactic equipment. The table in **Figure 8.1** provides the major advantages and disadvantages of upright and prone table stereotactic units.

Abnormality Selection

Almost every significant mammographic abnormality is suitable for needle biopsy with a few exceptions. Mammographic abnormalities may be divided into three basic groups: probably benign, possibly malignant, and probably malignant.

Comparison Between Upright and Prone Stereotactic Units			
Advantages		Disadvantages	
Prone Unit	Upright Unit	Prone Unit	Upright Unit
Limitation of patient motion	Multiuse equipment	Single-use equipment	Patient motion
Easy access for different approaches	Preferable for patients with severe neck arthritis	Dedicated room necessary	Vaso-vagal reactions
Easier to perfom core biopsy	Patient weight not an issue	Patient weight may preclude procedure	Limited working room
Patient cannot view procedure	Less expensive	Thin breasts, superficial abnormalities*	Core biopsy more difficult*
Ample working room			
*This may not be a factor if a side arm is available.			

Figure 8.1. A Comparison Between Upright and Prone Stereotactic Units. This table outlines the major advantages and disadvantages of prone and upright SBB units.

Probable Benign Abnormality

These abnormalities can be characterized as exhibiting a mammographic appearance suggestive of, but not pathognomic for, benignity. In some of these cases, needle biopsy may be preferable to a follow-up mammogram, for example, a 6-month interval study. Discussion with the patient and her referring physician is most important. This situation may occur when the patient is very anxious, when there is a strong family history of breast carcinoma, and when a prior mammogram is available. Compliance with 6-month follow-up studies is variable and, in most instances, needle biopsy will provide a confident benign diagnosis, allowing for routine care thereafter.

Possible Malignant Abnormality

Abnormalities that exhibit mammographic characteristics of possible malignancy can be reliably placed in a benign category, or a malignant or possibly malignant category, following successful needle biopsy. Therefore, appropriate management for these patients may be planned. Patients with a confident benign diagnosis can be placed into routine care, eliminating the need for excisional biopsy. The remaining patients will need surgical excisional biopsy for final diagnosis. Any patient with a cytologic/histologic diagnosis of atypia, suspicious, or malignant will need excisional biopsy for final diagnosis.

Probable Malignant Abnormality

Patients with highly suspicious mammographic abnormalities may undergo fine needle and/or core biopsy preoperatively to confirm diagnosis. A positive diagnosis will allow careful surgical planning and therapeutic tumor surgery, rather than an excisional diagnostic biopsy. The demonstration of invasion on the core biopsy may provide additional information for the surgeon. However, the absence of invasion on the core biopsy does not exclude invasion on the final histologic specimen. In those patients where invasion is demonstrated on the core biopsy specimen, an axillary dissection can be planned at the time of the tumorectomy, eliminating the need for a two-step surgical procedure in some patients.

Abnormality Management

Once needle biopsy is determined to be the appropriate procedure, the imaging modality for needle guidance and the method to be used—FNA, core, or both—should be selected. It is useful to characterize the abnormality by degree of suspicion of malignancy, based upon the mammography findings. This is helpful when correlating the biopsy results with the mammographic findings. Significant discordance between the results should prompt re-evaluation with either repeat needle biopsy or excisional biopsy. Very small abnormalities may be preferably evaluated with fine needle aspiration because of the potential risk of removing the entire abnormality with core biopsy. A suggested format for abnormality characterization and biopsy method is shown in **Figure 8.2**.

Other Considerations

Patients with certain mammographic findings, such as suspected radial scar or scattered, nonclustered "indeterminate calcifications," may not be suitable for needle biopsy. The diagnosis of radial scar and its differentiation from tubular carcinoma is often a challenge for the histologist[21]. When the mammographic finding suggests such an abnormality, excisional biopsy is preferred. Scattered calcifications may present a diagnostic problem for the radiologist, particularly when noted in a large area of a breast lobe without focal clustering. The differential diagnosis in these cases includes the possibility of sclerosing adenosis or ductal carcinoma in situ (DCIS). Excisional biopsy is preferred to evaluate the abnormality completely, and perhaps to find significant disease remote from the areas of mammographic calcification.

Needle biopsy is also useful for patients presenting with multiple, separate, discrete mammographic findings. The ability to distinguish benign abnormalities from those requiring further surgical evaluation permits definitive surgery.

Multifocal abnormalities and multiple breast abnormalities can be evaluated with needle biopsy. Preoperative assessment of the extent of malignant disease in the breast allows careful mapping of the carcinoma for the surgeon. Therefore, appropriate surgical management can be planned. Multiple needle biopsies from the primary abnormality and suspected areas of multifocal disease are necessary.

Breast conservation therapy is used increasingly for the treatment of breast cancer. Needle biopsy techniques can be useful for distinguishing postoperative changes from tumor recurrence[22]. These techniques are particularly useful in the breast with significant surgical scarring, and may be used whether the postoperative finding is a soft tissue density or calcifications.

Overview of Abnormality Management

Mammographic Findings	Interventional Procedure		
	FNA	Core	Excisional Biopsy
I. Probably Benign	Benign	No	No
	Insufficient	Yes	Core = benign no
	Atypia	Yes	Yes
	Suspicious	Yes	Yes
	Malignant	Yes	Yes
II. Possibly Malignant	Benign	No	No
	Insufficient	Yes	Core = benign no
	Atypical	Yes	Yes
	Suspicious	Yes	Yes
	Malignant	Yes	Yes
III. Probably Malignant	Benign	Yes	Core = benign yes (or repeat core)
	Insufficient	Yes	Core = benign yes
	Suspcious	Yes	Yes
	Malignant	Yes	Yes

Figure 8.2. Overview of Abnormality Management.This table summarizes three basic abnormality groups and suggests the appropriate biopsy method.

Summary

Needle biopsy of the breast has proved to be an excellent way of reducing the number of benign breast biopsies. Reduction in patient morbidity and anxiety are also important considerations. These nonsurgical techniques can expedite patient diagnosis and treatment (if necessary) and decrease costs[23]. Further research is needed, with long-term follow-up of patients diagnosed with these techniques.

Close communication between the radiologist, referring physician, surgeon, and pathologist is essential for appropriate patient management. The radiologist must assume an increasingly important role in communicating with the patient and her physicians, and can expect an expanded degree of responsibility in the diagnosis and management of breast disease.

Case Studies

The studies appearing on the following pages exemplify the specific indications of FNAC and core biopsy.

Figure 8.3 a-h. Forty-six year old woman with new suspicious calcifications noted in the right breast. Digital mammogram shows a 7 mm cluster of pleomorphic microcalcifications, without a soft tissue mass **(a)**. The calcifications are also shown on an inverted digital image **(b)**. A total of 6 aspirates were obtained from 3 separate areas within the calcific cluster **(c)**. The fine needle aspirate (FNA) was a highly cellular specimen with irregular clusters and small, dyscohesive groups of epithelial cells **(d)** (Diff-Quik® stain, magnification 40x). The small groups contained dyscohesive, intact epithelial cells with nuclear enlargement, but low nucleus to cytoplasm ratios **(e)** (Diff-Quik stain, magnification 400x). A different stain of fixed cells demonstrates the apocrine features of the tumor cells **(f)** (Hematoxylin and Eosin (H&E) stain, magnification 400x). These findings were diagnostic of adenocarcinoma with apocrine features. The corresponding core biopsy contained foci of ductal carcinoma in situ (DCIS), noncomedo cribriform type with apocrine features.The surgical excision specimen contained DCIS, noncomedo and comedo types, and a small focus of infiltrating ductal carcinoma. **Figure 8.3g** shows comedo necrosis in a duct with cribriform pattern of DCIS (H&E stain, magnification 100x). **Figure 8.3h** demonstrates infiltrative ductal carcinoma **(left)** next to cribriform DCIS with apocrine features **(right)** (H&E stain, magnification 40x).

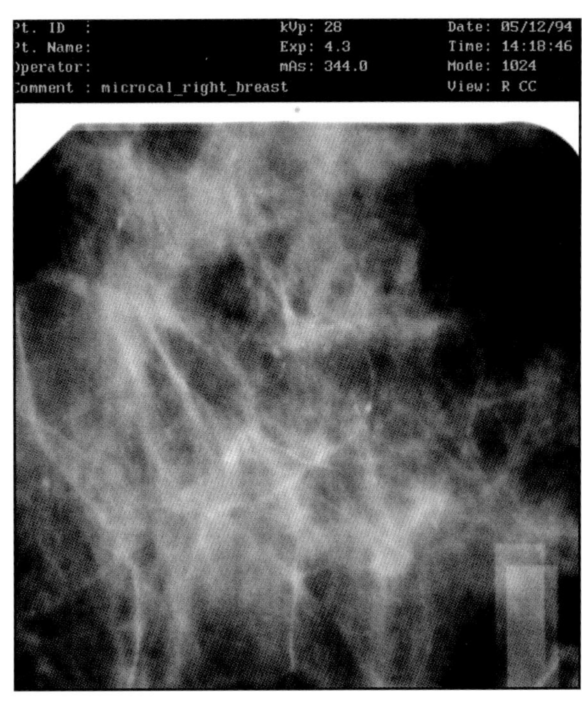

(a)

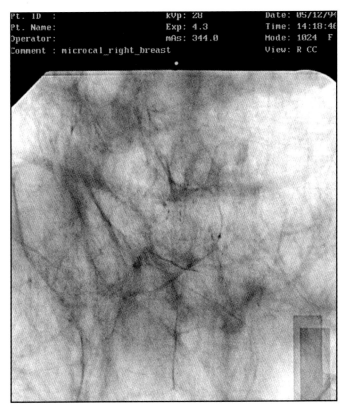

(b)

Figure 8.3 continued.

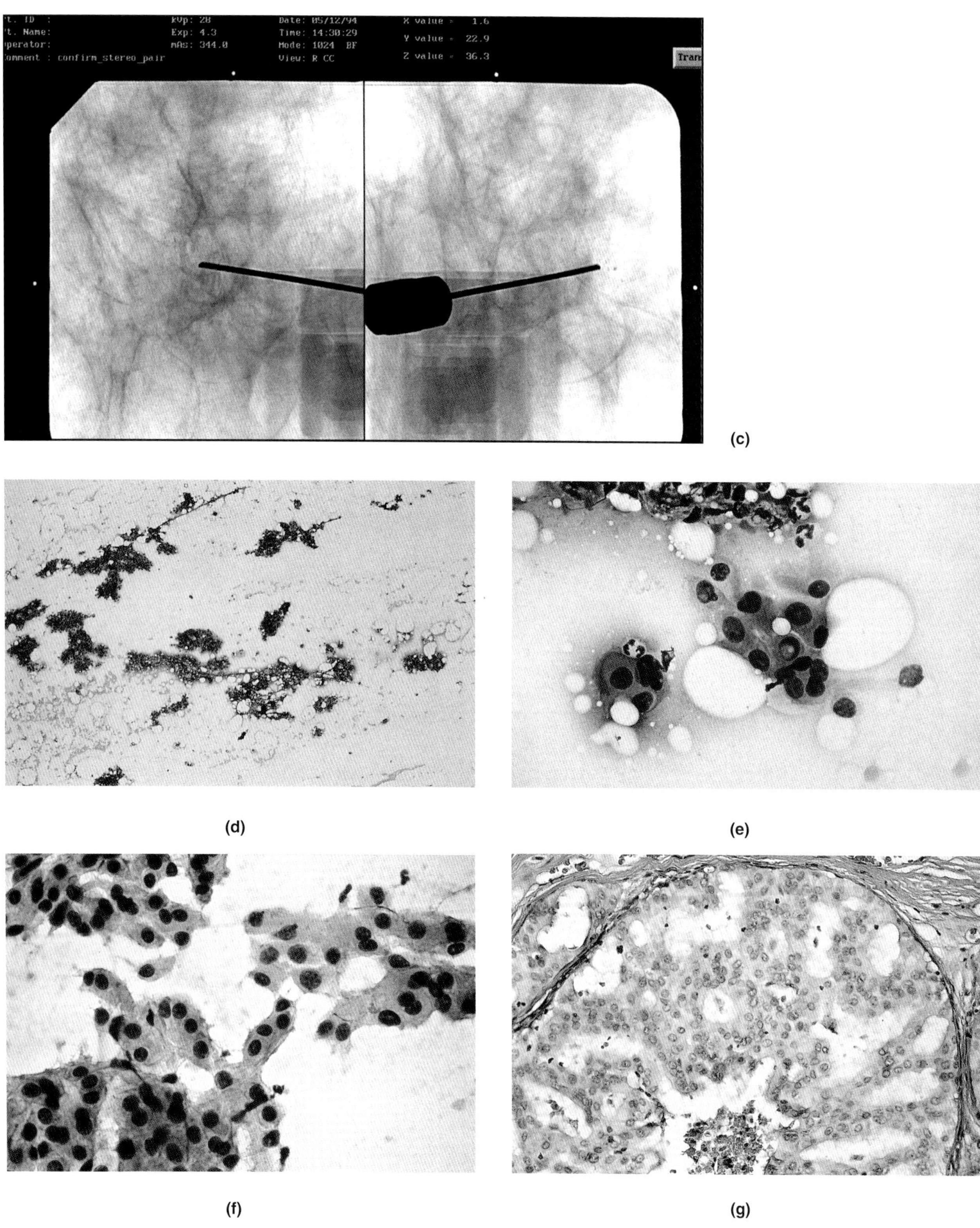

(c)

(d)

(e)

(f)

(g)

Figure 8.3 continued.

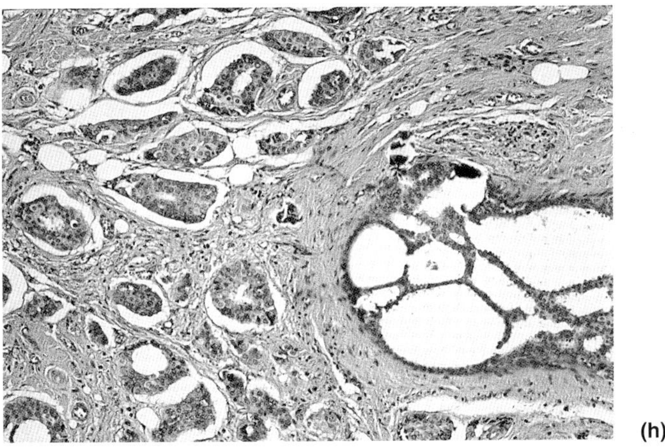

(h)

(a)

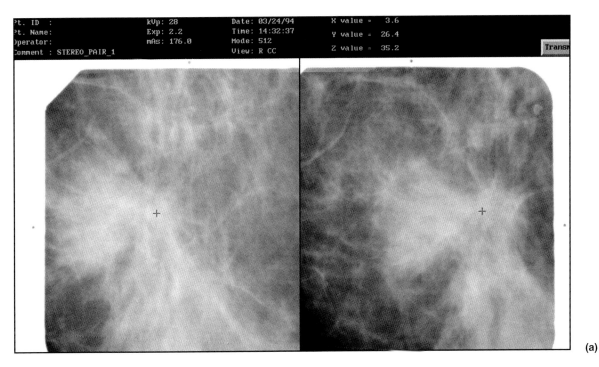

Figure 8.4 a-g. Fifty-four year old woman with a spiculated mass noted on a screening mammogram. Digital stereo mammograms demonstrating a 10 mm spiculated mass, unifocal **(a)**. Stereo digital images following placement of a 22-gauge needle; note the needle deflection in the dense fibrous tissue **(b)**. Postfire core biopsy stereo images, 14-gauge needle, taken following four fine needle aspirations **(c)**. The fine needle aspirates were bloody with few epithelial cells, which had several atypical features. They were in small, irregular groups or sometimes single intact cells **(d) (arrows).** The nucleus to cytoplasm ratios were high, and there was eccentric nuclear placement. These findings are suspicious for adenocarcinoma (Diff-Quik® stain, magnification 400x). The corresponding core biopsies contained portions of tumor with desmoplastic stroma **(e)** (H&E stain, magnification 7x). A significant component of the tumor sample had well-differentiated tubular features and infiltration of adipose tissue was present **(f)** (upper right) (H&E stain, magnification 100x). Other areas of the tumor **(g)** had a single file pattern **(left)**, and cytoplasmic mucin vacuoles imparting a signet-ring cell appearance to the cells **(right)**, indicative of some lobular features (H&E stain, magnification 400x).

Figure 8.4 continued.

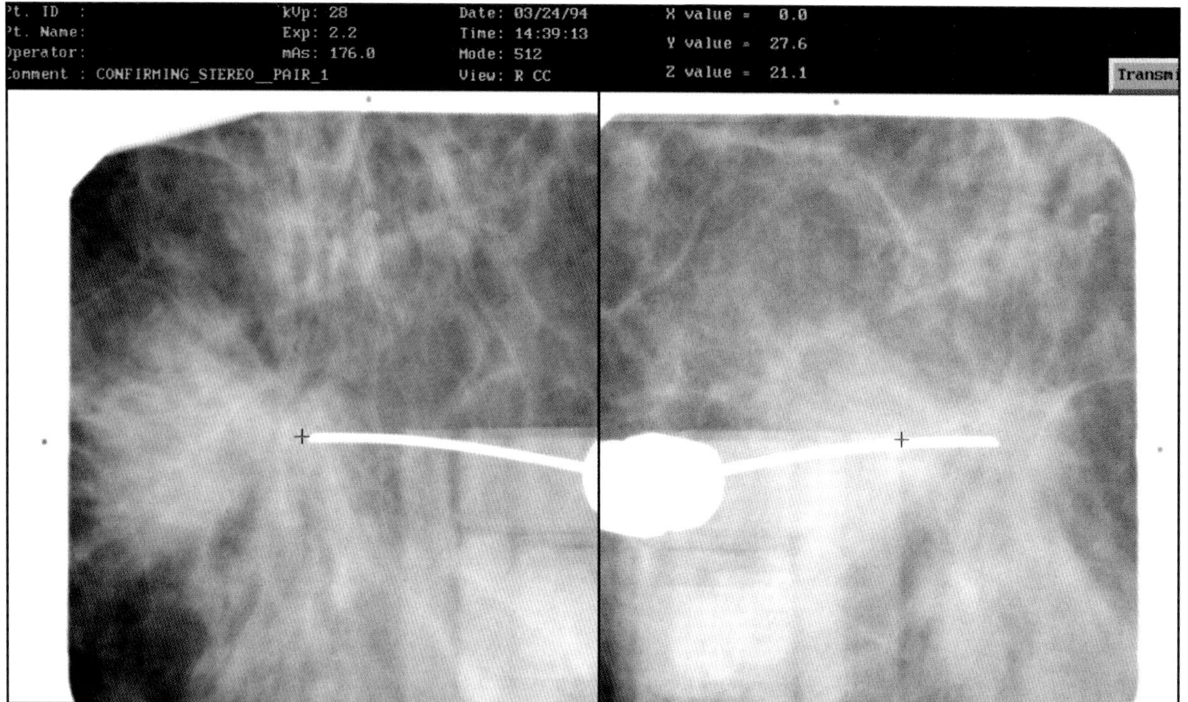

(b)

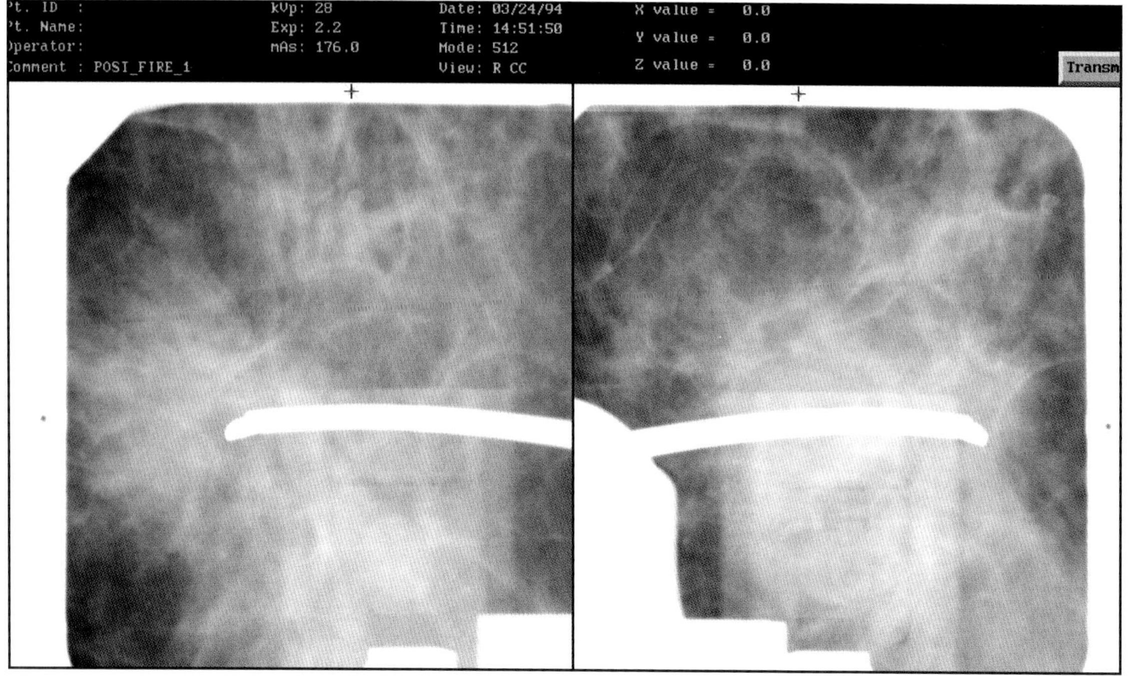

(c)

Figure 8.4 continued.

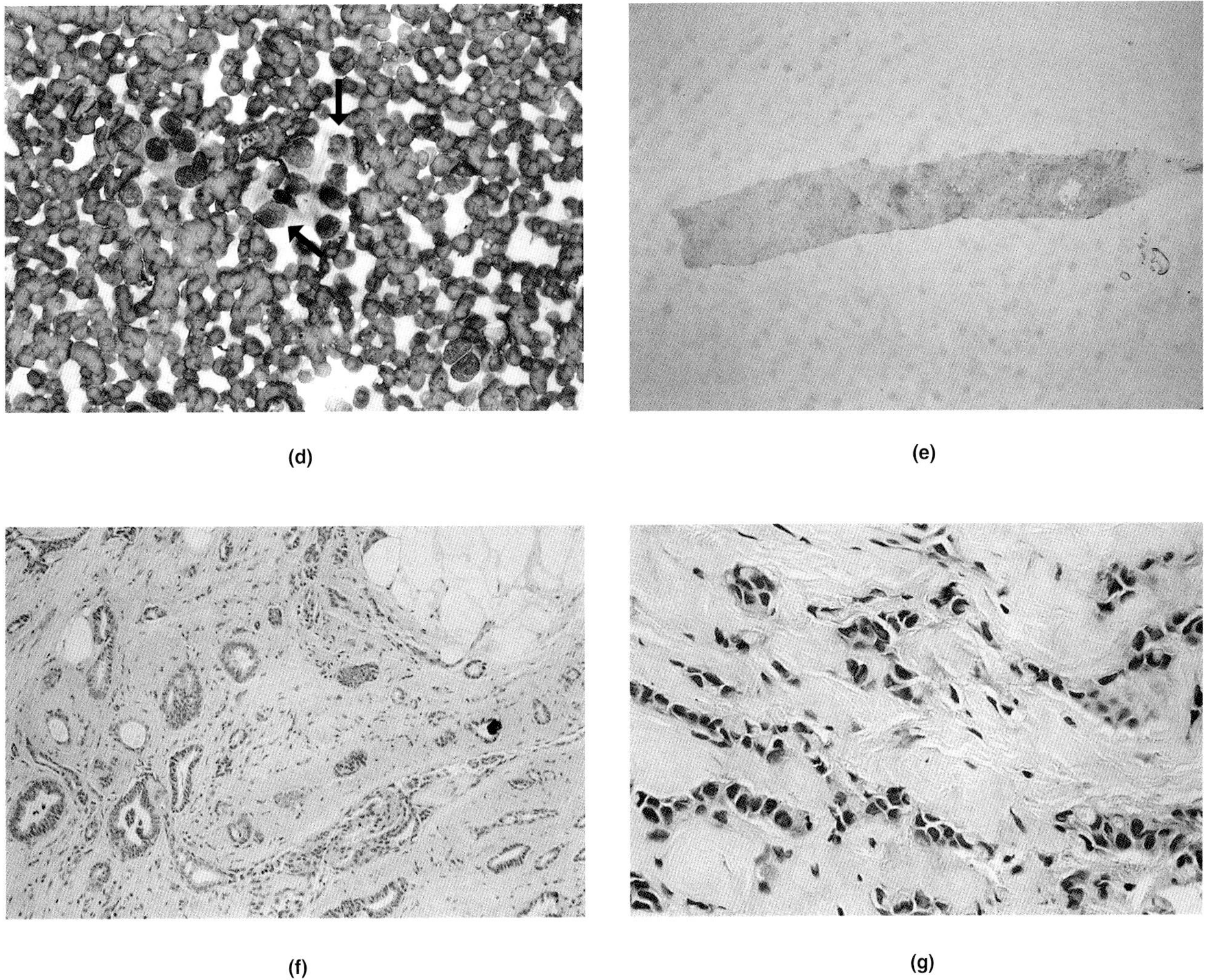

(d) (e)

(f) (g)

Figure 8.5 a-d. Fifty-two year old woman with a 12 mm mass noted in the subareolar region in the left breast. There was no history of a significant nipple discharge. A smoothly outlined mass in the subareolar region with some adjacent benign calcifications is noted on digital stereo mammograms **(a).** Three aspirates were obtained from two different regions within the nodule **(b)**. The FNA contained cohesive, flat, branched sheets of ductal epithelial cells in a background of proteinaceous fluid, a few stripped nuclei, and smaller, fragmented epithelial groups **(c)** (H&E stain, magnification 100x). The epithelial sheets contain myoepithelial cells **(d)** (Diff-Quik® stain, magnification 400x). The branched epithelial sheets in this subareolar nodule are consistent with a subareolar papilloma.

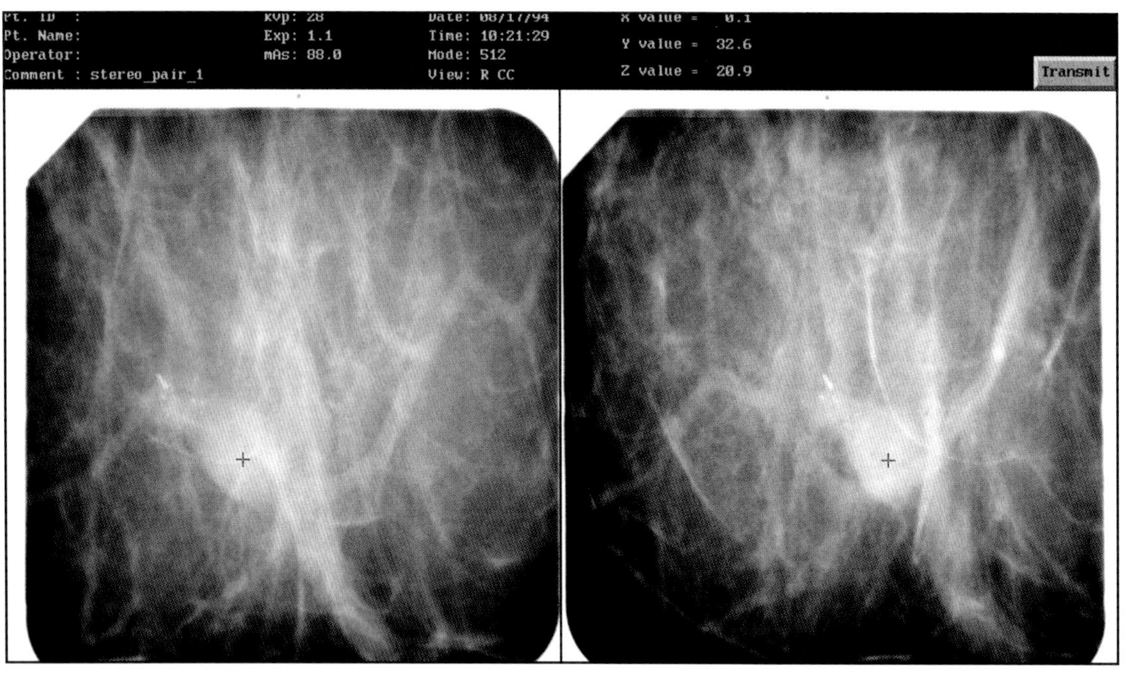

(a)

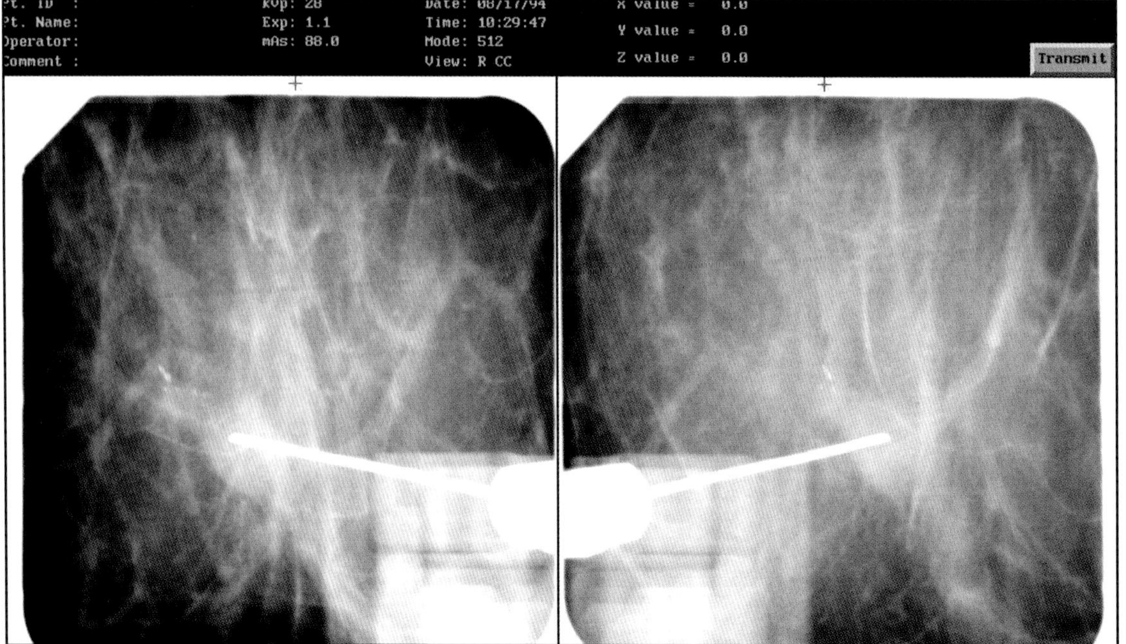

(b)

Figure 8.5 continued.

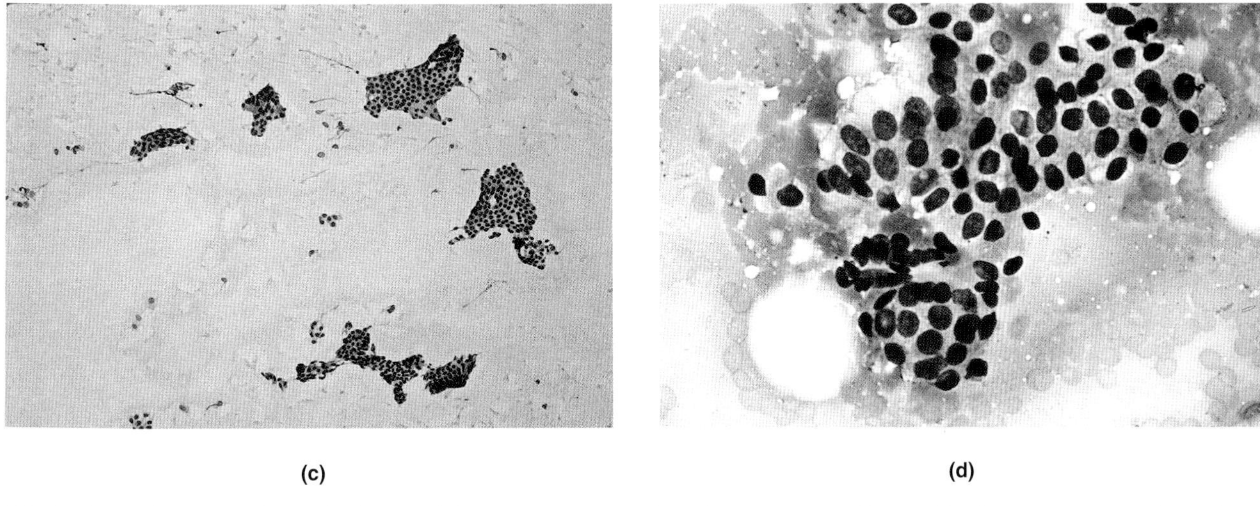

(c) (d)

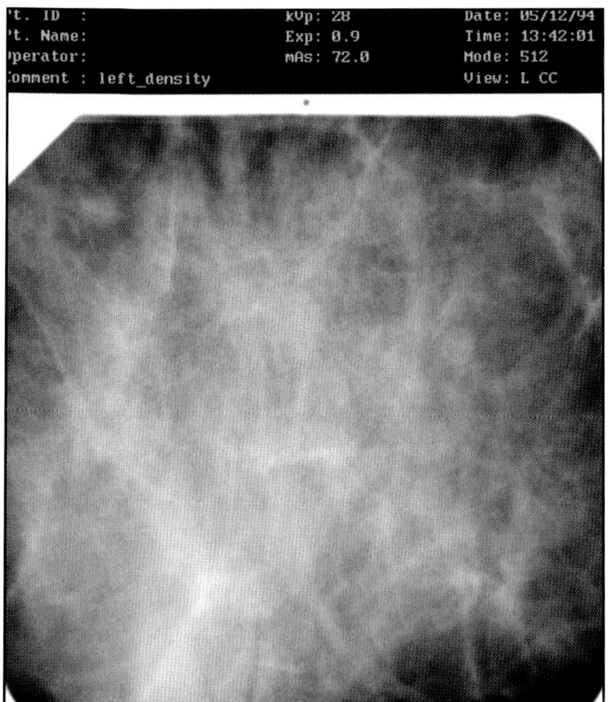

(a)

Figure 8.6 a-c. Forty-two year old woman with a subtle new area of architectural distortion noted on a screening mammogram. Digital scout image demonstrates a 7 mm area of distortion with some spiculation; no calcifications are present **(a)**. Four aspirates were obtained using a 22-gauge needle **(b)**. The FNAs contained benign, cohesive epithelial groups as well as rare, single, small epithelial cells with eccentric nuclear placement **(c)**. Rare, intact, single epithelial cells are suspicious for adenocarcinoma (Diff-Quik® stain, magnification 400x).

Figure 8.6 continued.

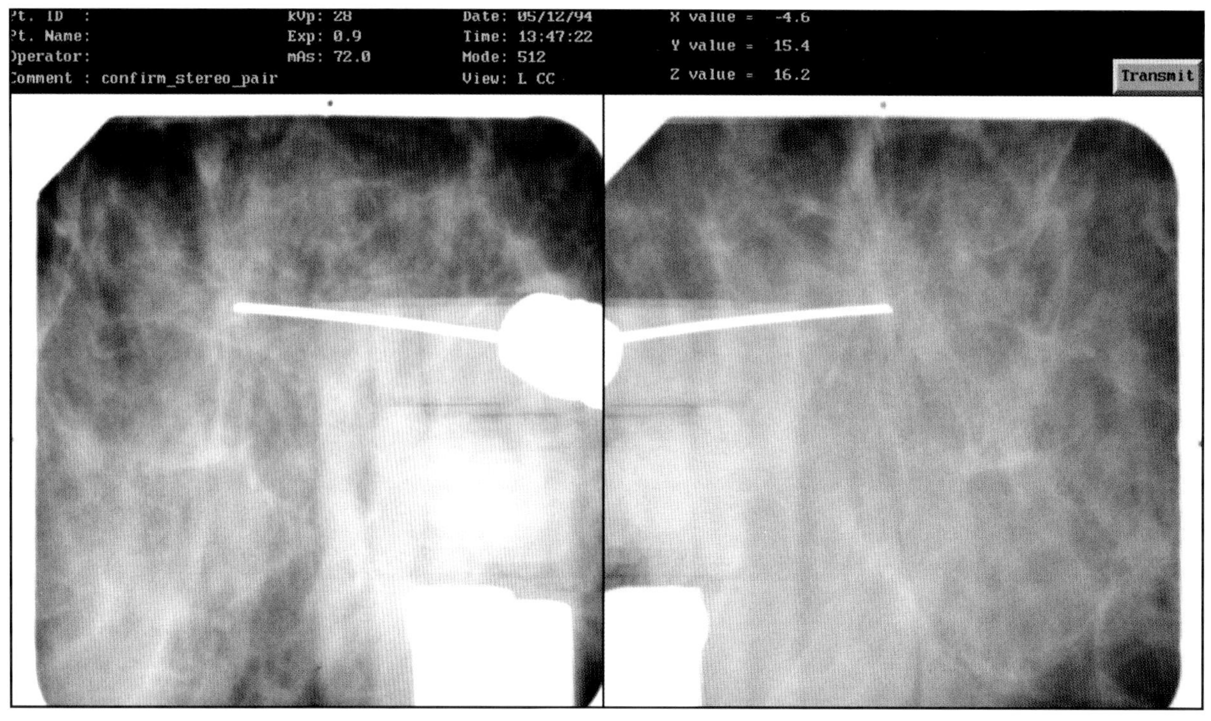

(b)

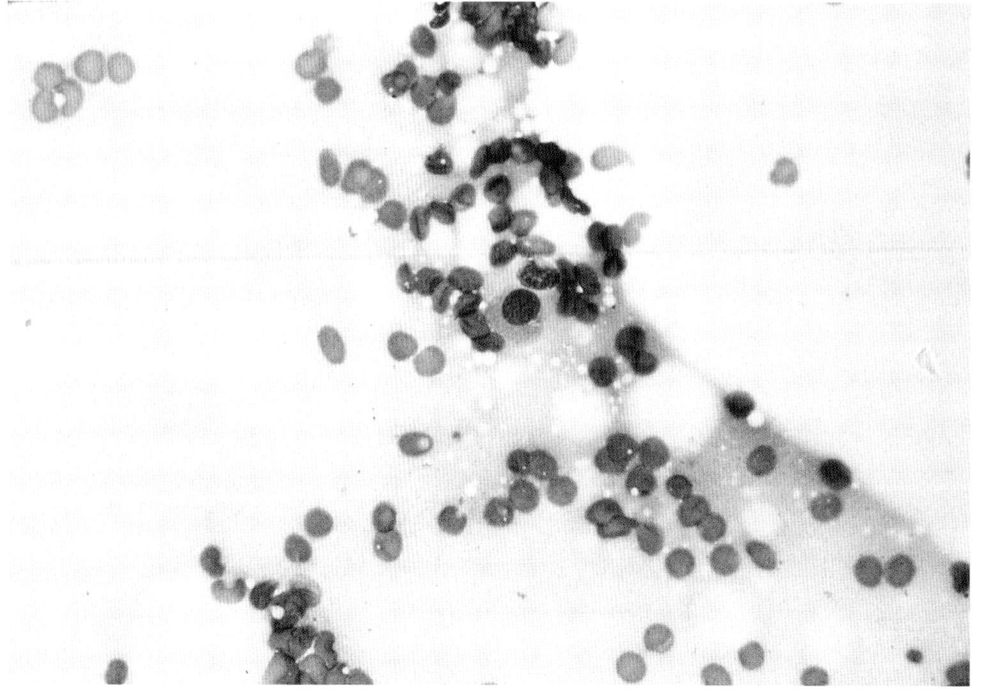

(c)

Figure 8.7 a-g. Sixty-two year old woman with a 12 mm area of malignant calcifications noted in the lateral aspect of the right breast on a screening mammogram. Scout digital mammogram shows a single cluster of pleomorphic calcifications **(a)**. Two 4 mm adjacent benign nodules were also present. Six aspirates (22-gauge needle) from three areas within the cluster were obtained. The FNAs of the left mammary microcalcification contained numerous intact, single, atypical epithelial cells in a background of necrotic and calcific debris. Some of these cells have large cytoplasmic vacuoles **(c)** (Diff-Quik® stain, magnification 400x). These findings were diagnostic of adenocarcinoma.The FNAs of the two adjacent right breast nodules contained apocrine epithelial cells and proteinaceous secretions and fluid, consistent with cystic change **(d)** (Diff-Quik® stain, magnification 400x). The surgical excision of the carcinoma contained ductal carcinoma in situ of solid and comedo types, with two tiny foci of infiltrating lobular carcinoma. **Figure 8.7e** shows the solid pattern of DCIS adjacent to a focus of infiltrating lobular carcinoma **(left)** (H&E stain, magnification 40x). **Figure 8.7f** shows comedo type DCIS with calcification (H&E stain, magnification 100x). **Figure 8.7g** shows a lobule with atypical lobular hyperplasia (H&E stain, magnification 400x).

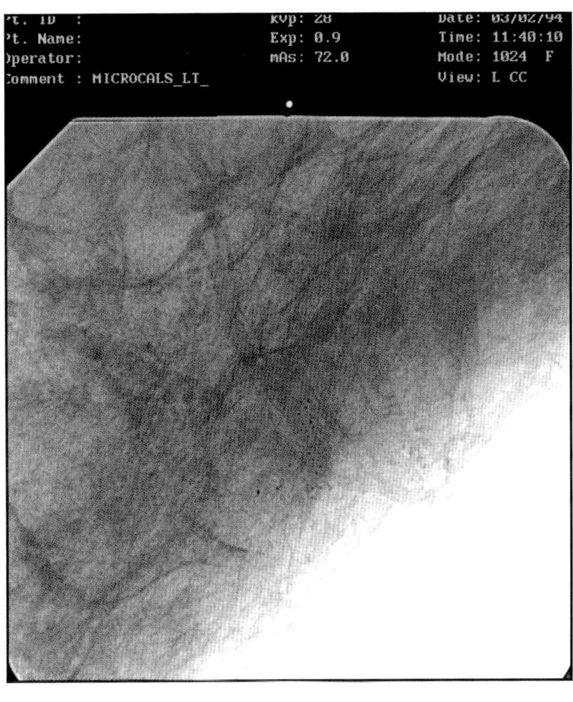

(a)

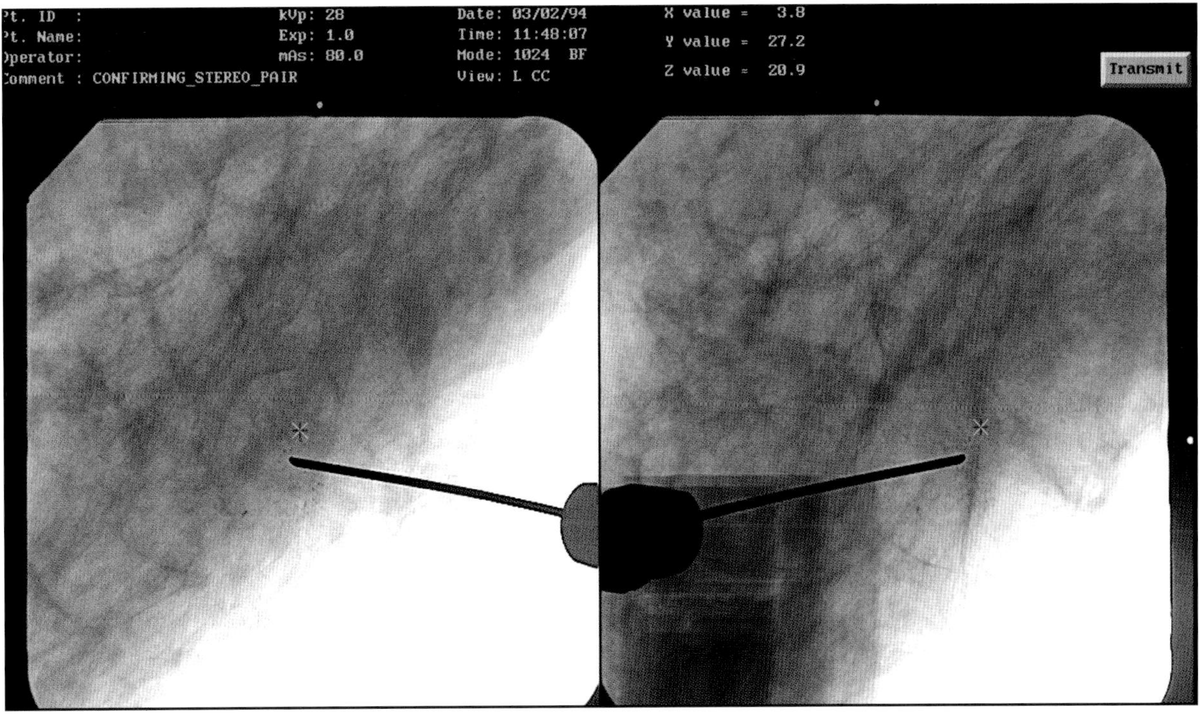

(b)

Figure 8.7 continued.

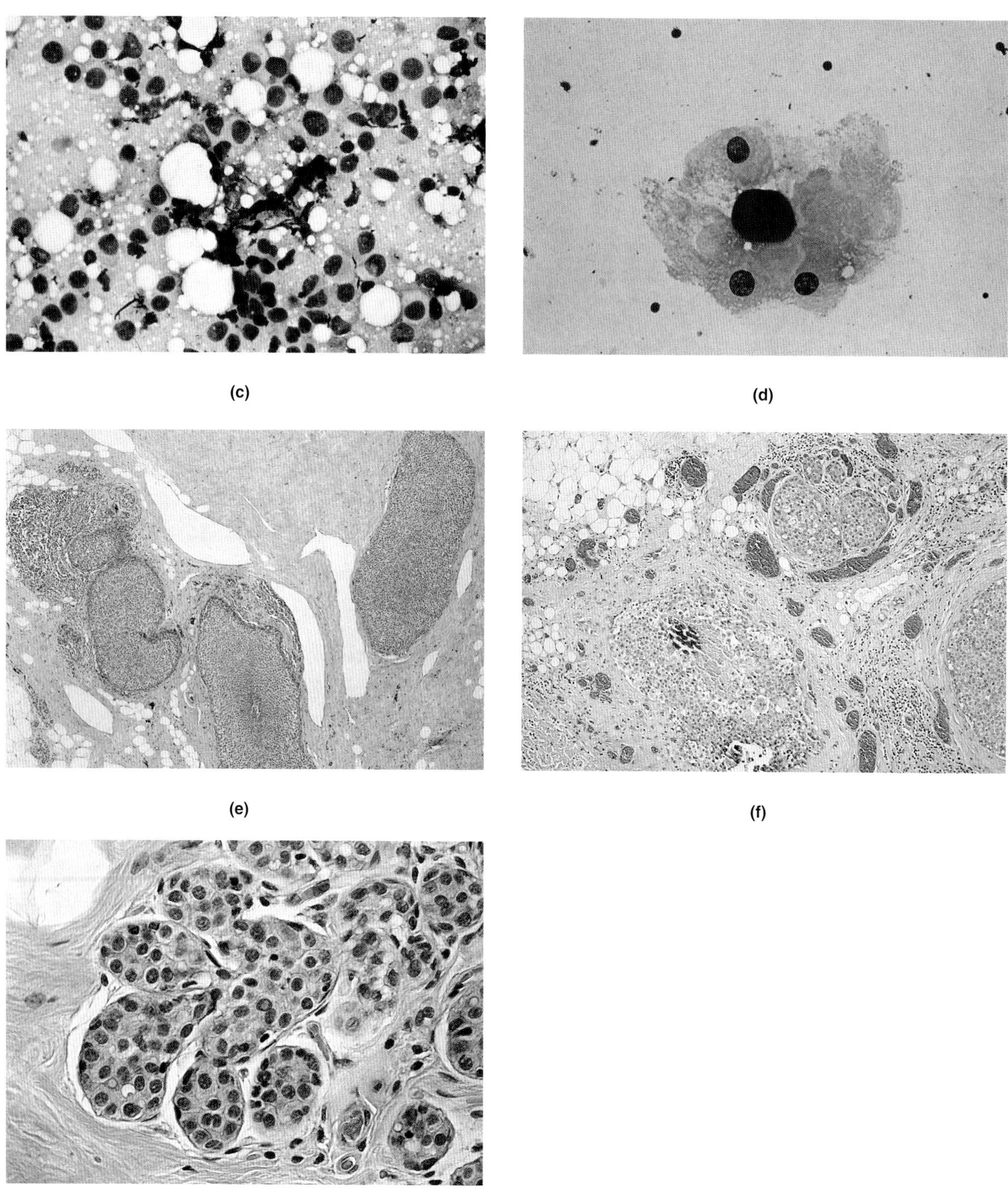

(c) (d) (e) (f) (g)

Figure 8.8 a-c. Fifty-one year old woman with a smoothly outlined nodule noted in the central right breast **(a) (arrow)**. Ultrasound of this abnormality demonstrated a solid mass **(b)**. A stereotactic core biopsy (14-gauge needle) revealed findings consistent with a fibroadenoma. A mammogram performed six months later demonstrated significant enlargement of the mass from 20 mm to 30 mm **(c) (arrow)**, and an excisional biopsy was recommended to evaluate for possible phyllodes tumor. Final histology at excisional biopsy was infarcted phyllodes tumor.

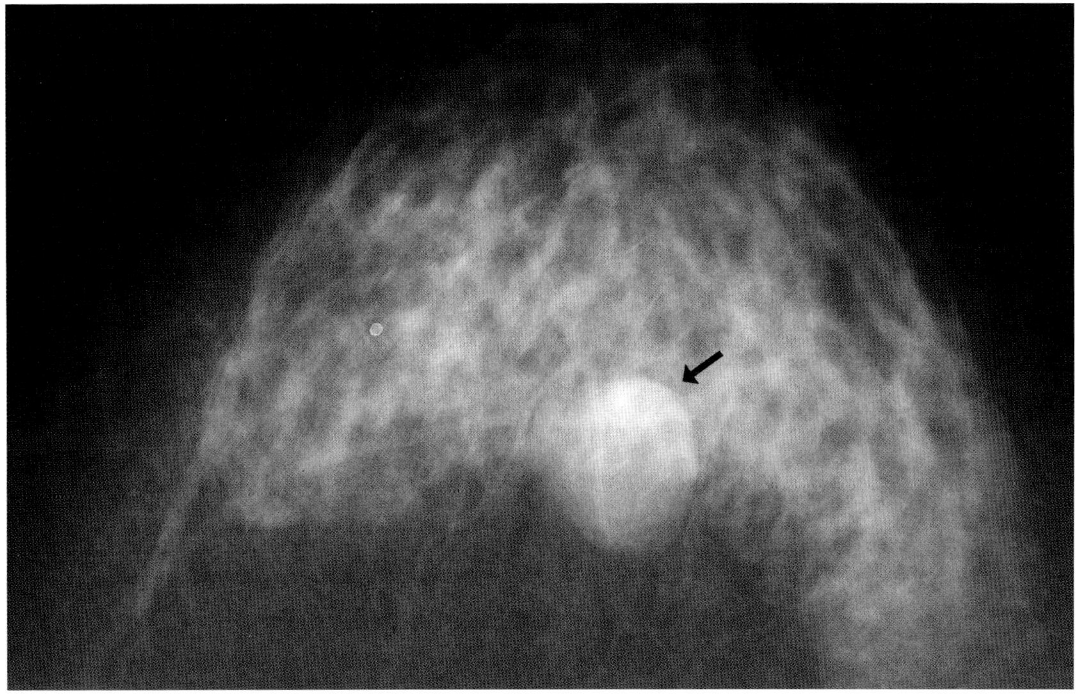

(a)

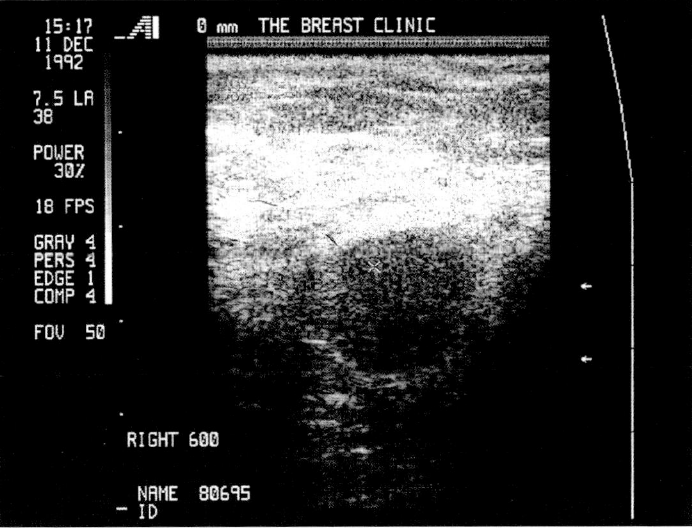

(b)

Figure 8.8 continued.

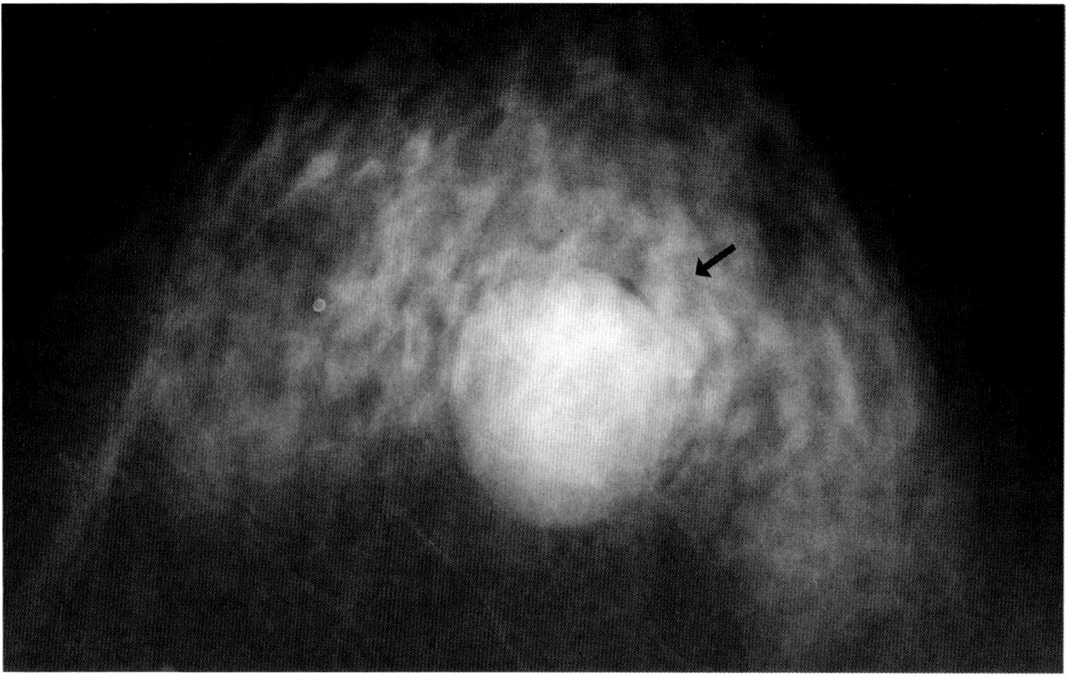

(c)

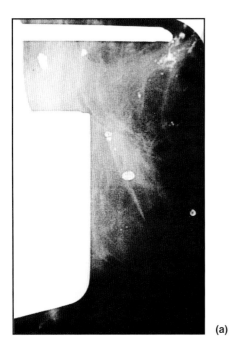

(a)

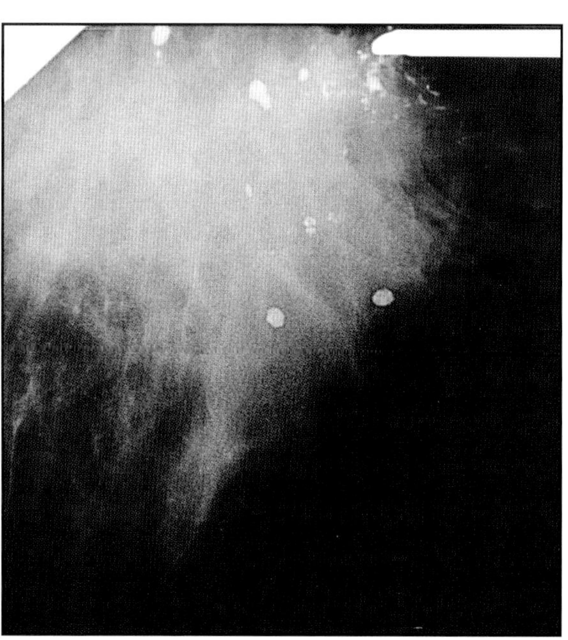

(b)

Figure 8.9 a and b. Thirty-nine year old woman with a history of carcinoma of the right breast (8 mm invasive ductal carcinoma NOS) treated 40 months previously with segmental excision and whole breast irradiation. Follow-up mammograms demonstrated very dense breast tissue with extensive scarring **(a)**. Current mammogram demonstrates new calcifications, which were thought to represent fat necrosis. Core biopsy confirmed the presence of fat necrosis without malignancy **(b)**.

Figure 8.10 a-c. Fifty-nine year old woman with four adjacent spiculated masses noted on a screening mammogram. There were no physical findings. No associated microcalcifications were noted. The largest spiculated mass measured 15 mm **(a)**. A digital scout mammogram taken prior to stereotactic FNA/Core biopsy showed two additional foci of spiculation **(b)**. Each spiculated mass was evaluated separately and confirmed the presence of a multifocal invasive carcinoma **(c)**. Four spiculated invasive ductal carcinomas were found at final histology with bridging between them.

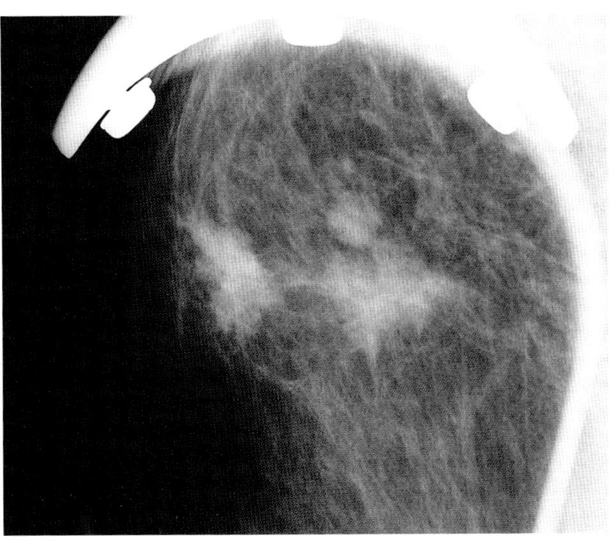

(a)

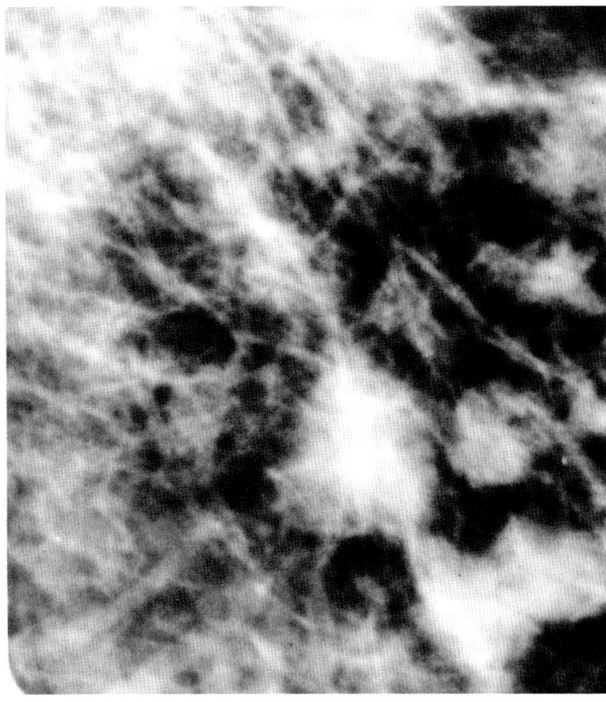

(b)

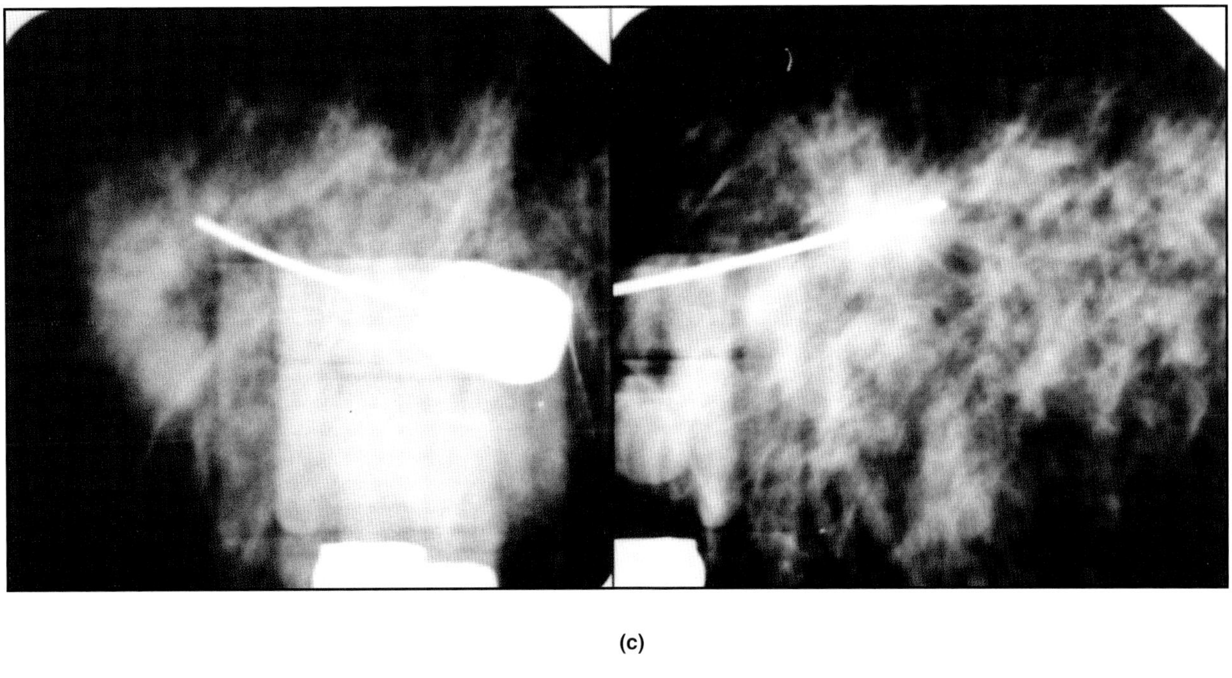

(c)

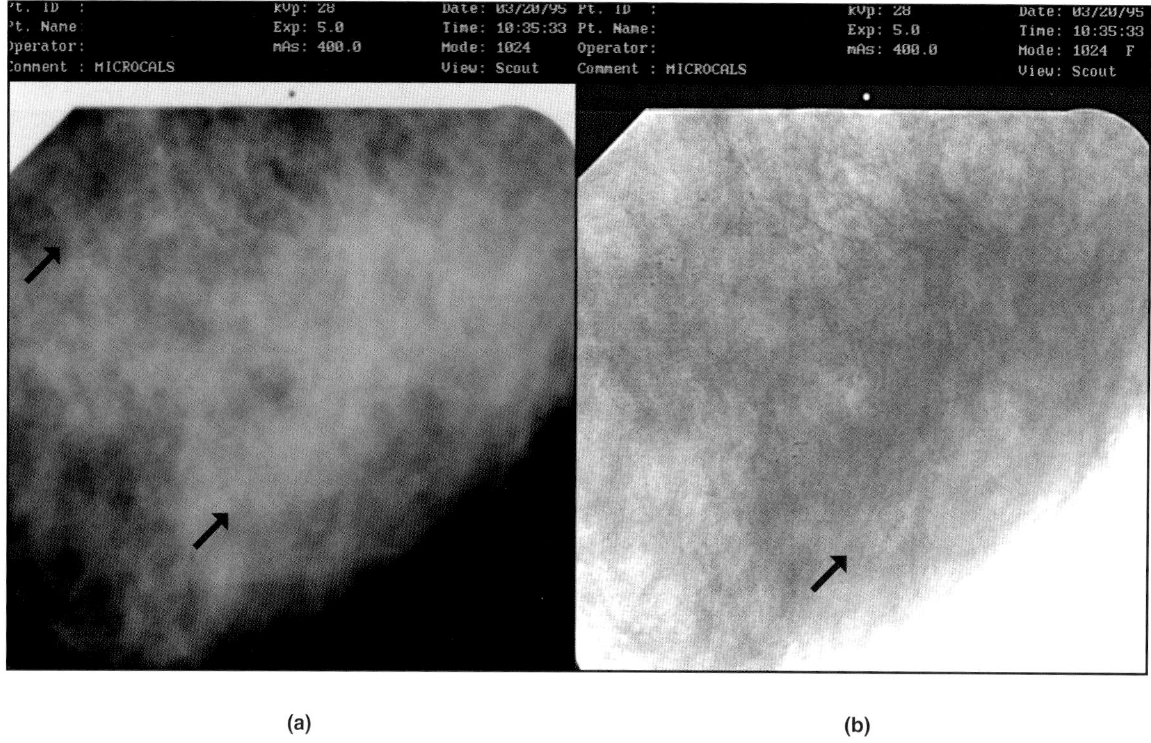

(a) (b)

Figure 8.11 a-f. Thirty-two year old woman, ten weeks postpartum, presented for a second opinion consultation. Pertinent history was that during her seventh month of pregnancy, she had noticed a lump in her left breast. Physical examination at that time revealed an approximately 20 mm hard mass. FNA was done revealing adenocarcinoma. Surgical excision of the carcinoma was performed at 32 weeks without an imaging evaluation. Excisional biopsy revealed a 15 mm invasive carcinoma with minimal associated in situ carcinoma, high nuclear grade, comedo type. Clear histologic margins were reported. Axillary dissection was negative for metastatic disease. Physical examination revealed a well-healed scar and no palpable breast masses. Mammographic examination showed four separate areas of suspicious calcifications located near the surgical site, within very dense breast tissue. Digital mammogram taken prior to stereotactic biopsy shows focal areas of calcification **(a, arrows; b, inverted image)**. Fine needle aspiration of each area of calcification was performed **(c, d, e)** and showed each cluster to represent adenocarcinoma. Core biopsy was also performed and invasive tumor was noted at one site **(f)**. The extent of residual malignancy, shown by stereotactic biopsy, precluded a breast conservation procedure and mastectomy was performed.

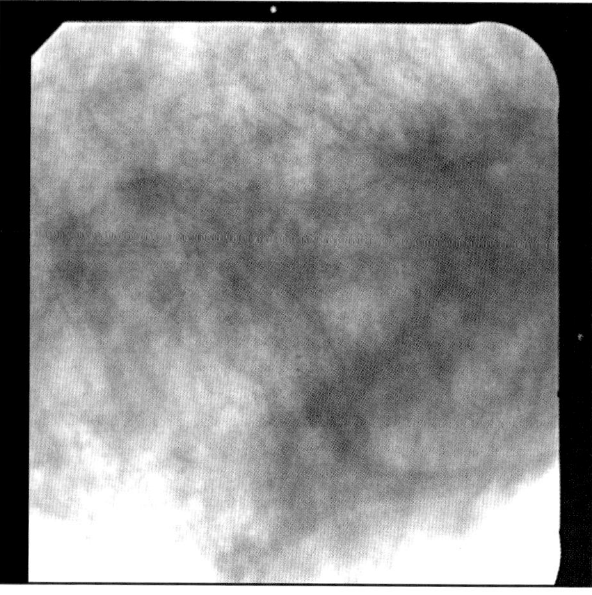

(c)

Figure 8.11 continued.

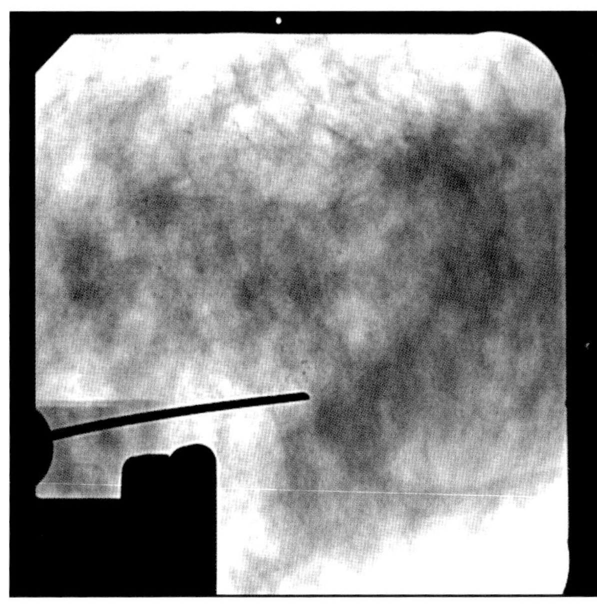

(d)

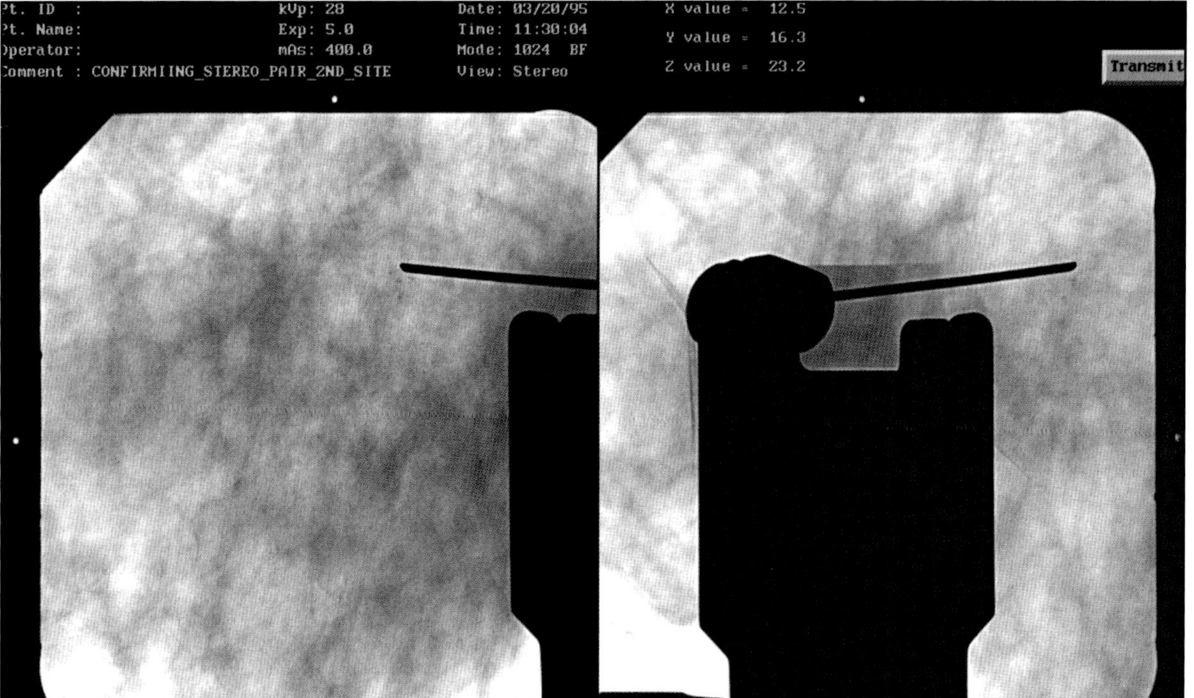

(e)

Figure 8.11 continued.

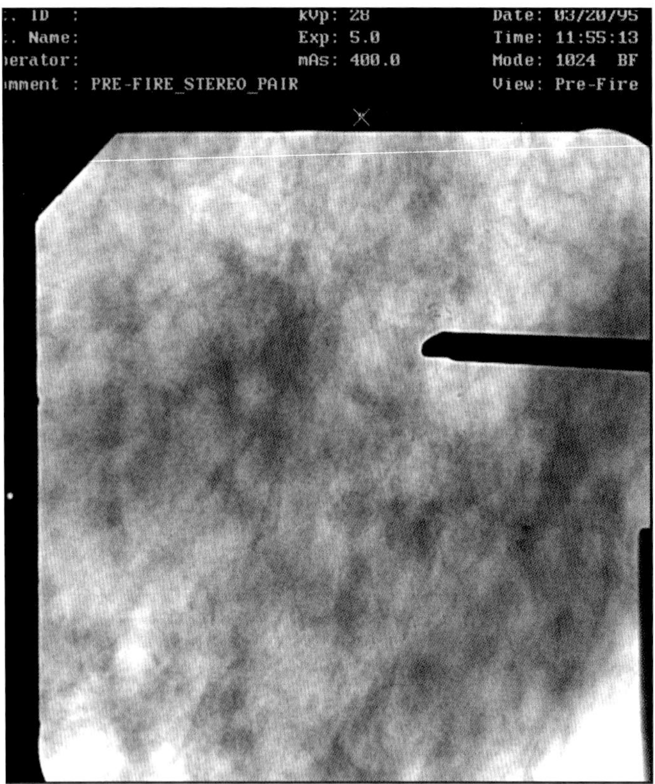

(f)

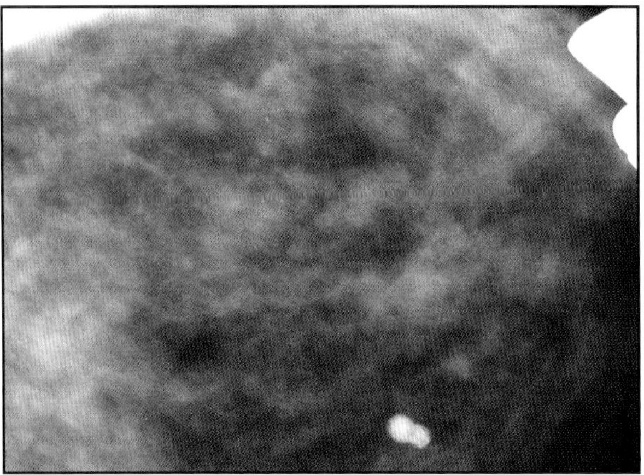

(a)

Figure 8.12 a-f. Fifty-six year old woman with 6-month history of sero-sanguinous nipple discharge. There were no palpable masses or other symptoms. Mammographic examination reveals new pleomorphic faint calcifications in the central right breast **(a)**. Galactography showed irregular mucosal abnormalities within the ducts at the site of the mammographic calcifications. The findings were suspicious for intraductal carcinoma **(b)**. FNA **(c)** and core biopsy showed adenocarcinoma, papillary type. Needle localization and excisional biopsy were performed. The excised surgical specimen is shown **(d).** Final histology revealed papillary carcinoma and comedo carcinoma in-situ **(e and f)**.

Figure 8.12 continued.

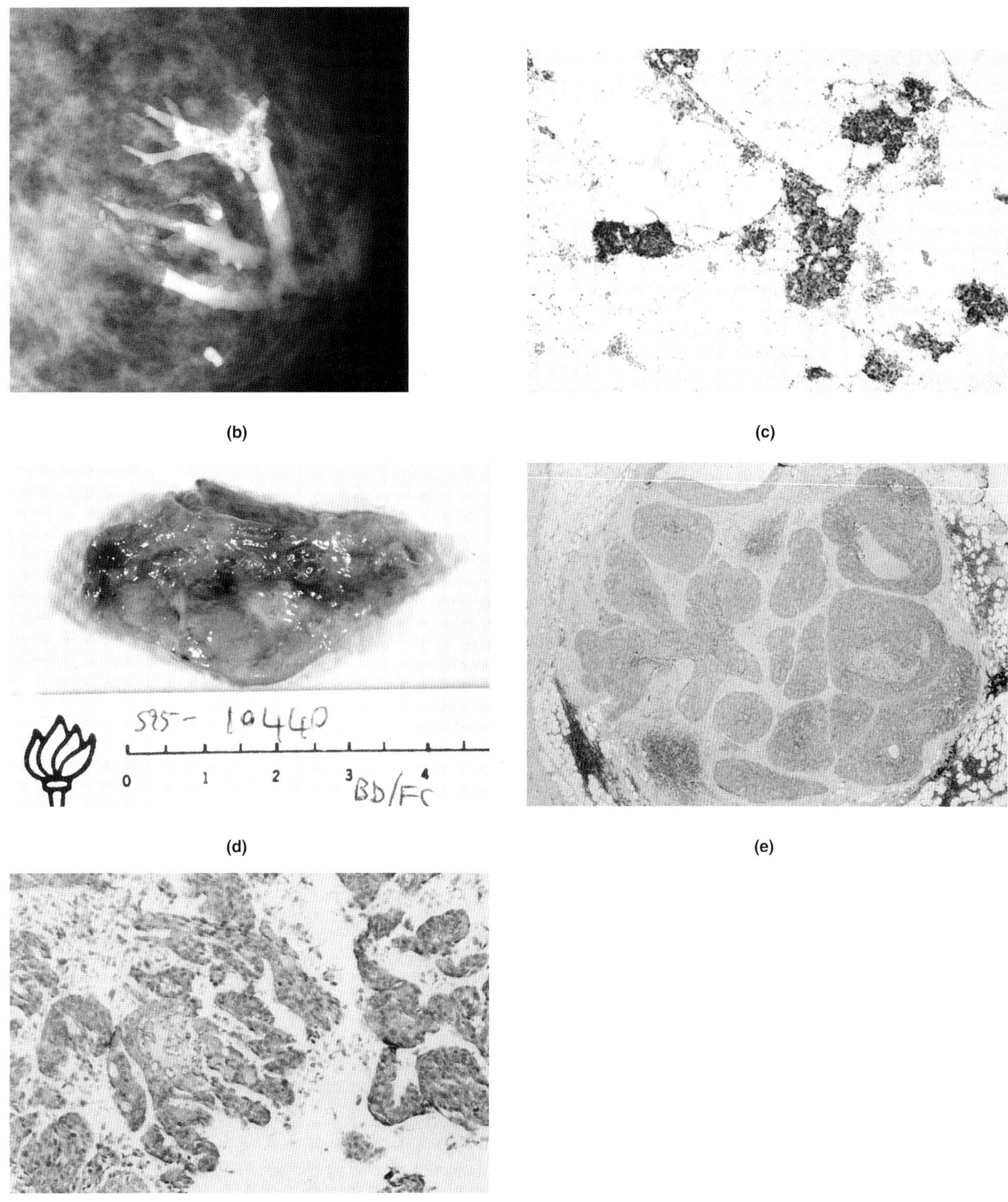

(b)

(c)

(d)

(e)

(f)

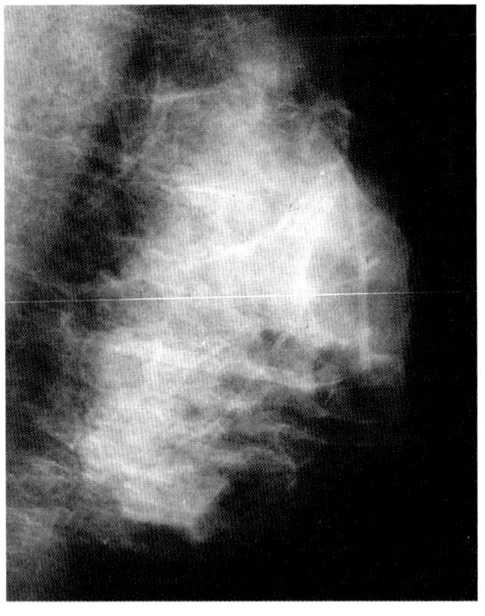

(a)

Figure 8.13 a-e. Forty-four year old woman with multiple calcifications in the right breast on screening mammogram. Most of the calcifications are noted to be scattered and most likely benign in nature, MLO view **(a)**, CC view **(b)**. A small cluster of calcifications with a granular appearance are noted centrally, and magnification views indicated calcifications of more concern for malignancy **(c)**. Multiple core biopsies of the scattered calcifications revealed sclerosing adenosis. Core biopsy of the small cluster of calcifications with specimen radiography was performed **(d and e)** and histology showed in situ carcinoma. The patient underwent needle localization and excisional biopsy of the small calcific cluster, confirming the diagnosis of in situ carcinoma of a mixed solid and comedo type.

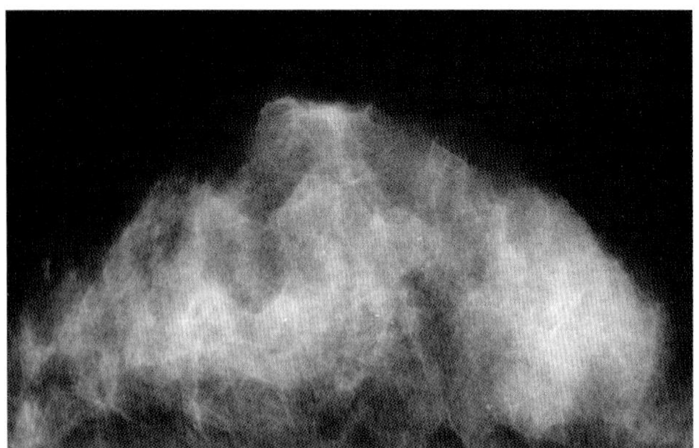

(b)

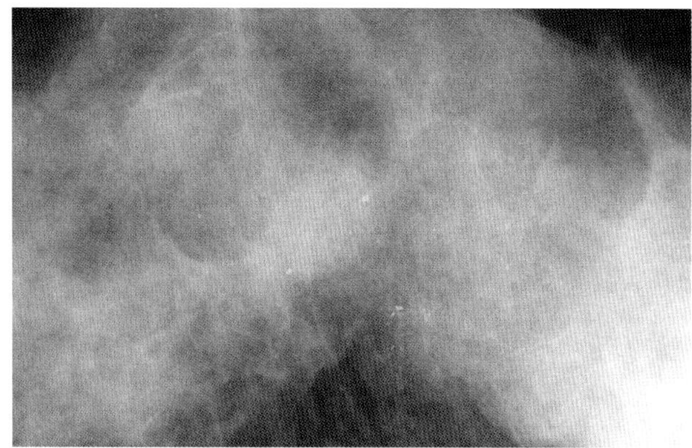

(c)

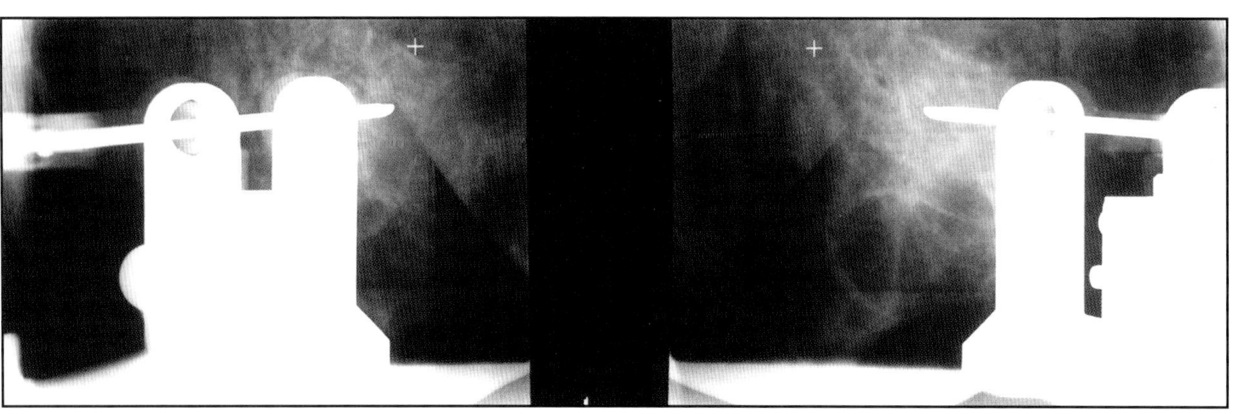

(d)

Figure 8.13 continued.

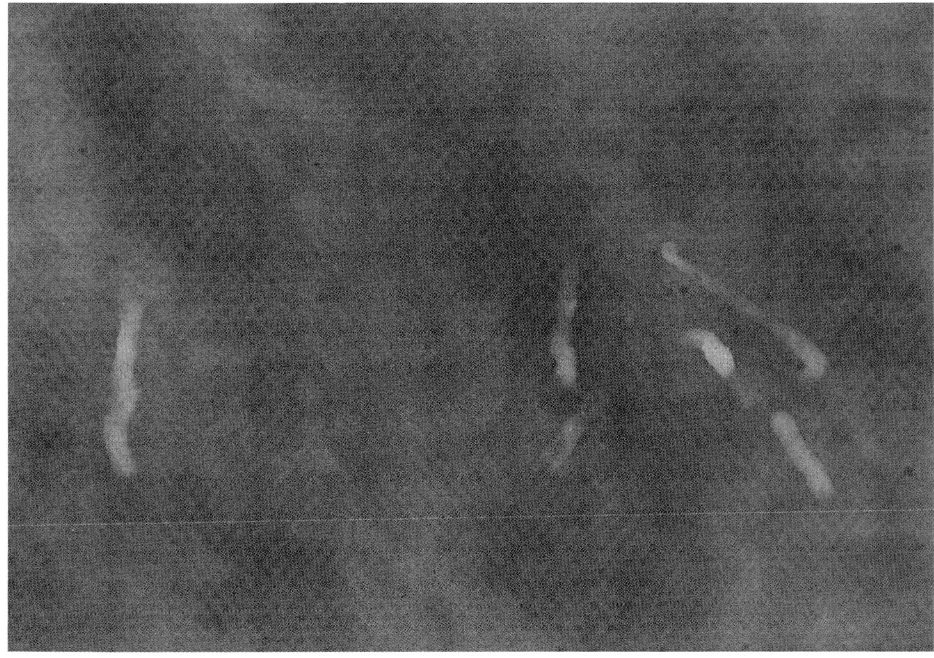

(e)

References

1. Tabar, L., Fagerberg, C.J.G., Gad, H., et al. 1985. Reduction in Mortality from Breast Cancer After Mass Screening with Mammography. *Lancet* 1:829-832.

2. Eddy, D.M. 1989. Screening for Breast Cancer. *Annals of Internal Medicine* 111:389-399.

3. Hall, F. 1986. Screening Mammography: Potential Problems on the Horizon. *NEJM* 31:53-55.

4. Norton, L., Zeligman, B., Pearlman, N. 1988. Accuracy and Cost of Needle Localization Breast Biopsy. *Arch Surg* 123:947-950.

5. Leinster, S.J., Whitehouse, G.H., McDicken, I. 1987. The Biopsy of Impalpable Lesions of the Breast. *Surgery, Gynecology, and Obstetrics* 164 (3):269-71.

6. Leis, H.P. Jr., Cammarata, A., LaRaja, R., Higgins, H. 1985. Breast Biopsy and Guidance for Occult Lesions. *International Surgery* 70 (2):115-8.

7. Tersegno, M.M. 1993. Mammogrpahy Positive Value and True-Positive Biopsy Rate. *AJR* 160 (3):660-1.

8. Azavedo, E., Auer, G., Svane, G. 1989. Stereotactic Fine Needle Biopsy in 2,394 Mammographically Detected Nonpalpable Breast Lesions. *Lancet* 1:1033-1036.

9. Dowalatshahi, K., Gent, H. Schmidt, R. 1989. Nonpalpable Breast Tumors: Diagnosis with Stereotaxic Localization and Fine-Needle Aspiration. *Radiology* 170: 426-433.

10. Dronkers, D. 1992. Stereotaxic Core Biopsy of Breast Lesions. *Radiology* 183:631-634.

11. Evans, P., et al. 1992. Fine-Needle Aspiration Cytology and Core Biopsy of Nonpalpable Breast Lesions. *Current Opinion in Radiology* 4:V:130-138.

12. Fajardo, L., Davis, J., Wiens, J., Trego, D. 1994. Mammography-Guided Stereotactic Fine-Needle Aspiration Cytology of Nonpalpable Breast Lesions: Prospective Comparison with Surgical Biopsy Results. *AJR* 162:815-820.

13. Gisvold, J., Goeliner, J., Grant C., et al. 1994. Breast Biopsy: A Comparative Study of Stereotaxically Guided Core and Excisional Techniques. *AJR* 193-91-95.

14. Jackerman, R., Nowels, K., Shepard, M., et al. 1994. Stereotaxic Large-Core Needle Biopsy of 450 Nonpalpable Breast Lesions with Surgical Correlation in Lesions with Cancer or Atypical Hyperplasia. *Radiology* 193:91-95.

15. Jackson, V.P. 1990. Mammographically Guided Fine-Needle Aspiration Cytology of Nonpalpable Lesions. *Current Opinion in Radiology* 2 (5):741-5.

16. Jackson, V.P. 1992. The Status of Mammographically Guided Fine Needle Aspiration Biopsy on Nonpalpable Breast Lesions. *Radiologic Clinics of North America* 30 (January) (1):155-66.

17. Kopans, D. 1993. Review of Stereotaxic Large-Core Needle Biopsy and Surgical Biopsy Results in Nonpalpable Breast Lesions. *Radiology* 189: 665-666.

18. Parker, S.H., Lovin, J., Jobe, W. 1991. Nonpalpable Breast Lesions: Stereotactic Automated Large-Core Biopsies. *Radiology* 180:403-407.

19. Parker, S. H., Lovin, J., Jobe, W., et al. 1990. Stereotactic Breast Biopsy with a Biopsy Gun. *Radiology* 176:741-747.

20. Parker, S.H., Burbank, F., Jackman, R.J., et al. 1994. Percutaneous Large-Core Breast Biopsy: A Multi-Institutional Study. *Radiology* 193:359-364.

21. Torre, A., Lindholm, K., Lingren, A. 1994. Fine Needle Aspiration Cytology of Tubular Breast Carcinoma and Radial Scar. *Acta Cytol* 38 (November/December) 6.

22. Mitnick, J., Vasquez, M., Plesser, K., et al. 1993. Distinction Between Postsurgical Changes and Carcinoma by Means of Stereotaxic Fine-Needle Aspiration Biopsy After Reduction Mammaplasty. *Radiology* 188:457-462.

23. Lindfors, K., Rosenquist, J. 1994. Needle Core Biopsy Guided with Mammography: A Study of Cost Effectiveness. *Radiology* 190:217-222.

Pathological Interpretation of Core Biopsy

Andrea E. Dawson, M.D.

9

Introduction

The implementation of screening mammography in the United States has led to increased detection of small breast tumors (less than 1 cm) and in situ carcinomas. These early breast cancers have an excellent prognosis with increased long-term survival rates[1]. However, the number of breast biopsies performed for nonpalpable breast abnormalities has led to a high cost for identifying each cancer, particularly in younger women. Benign disease is found in 60-90% of the open biopsies performed for mammographic abnormalities[2]. Relatively noninvasive methods, such as fine needle aspiration cytology (FNAC) and stereotactic core needle biopsy (SCNB) for the evaluation of mammographically detected breast abnormalities have an important role in the cost-effective and timely management of breast disease.

FNAC in conjunction with various localizing techniques was initially reported to improve the specificity of mammography, providing an alternative to either follow-up or open surgical biopsy[3-5]. FNAC gained widespread acceptance, first in Scandinavia, followed by increasing utilization of the technique in the United States. The reported sensitivity and specificity rates are high for cytologic assessment of both palpable and nonpalpable breast abnormalities[6-8]. However, reported limitations of FNAC include difficulties in interpretation if an experienced cytopathology laboratory is not available, and lack of specificity in some diagnostic categories, such as differentiation of invasive from in situ carcinomas[5,9,10]. Despite these limitations, FNAC has gained acceptance as a cost-effective, rapid method of evaluating breast abnormalities[6].

Stereotactic breast biopsy originated in Sweden using FNAC[4]. More recently, stereotactic core needle biopsy has been implemented for the diagnosis of mammographically detected abnormalities. Parker et al.[11-13] compared stereotactic large core biopsy diagnoses with surgical follow-up biopsy. The agreement between core biopsy and surgical biopsy histologic diagnoses in these reports are excellent, ranging from 87 to 100%. These studies report occasional false negative diagnoses for malignancy in both the needle core biopsy and surgical biopsy, but only rare false positive results for malignancy have been reported for SCNB. In everyday practice, where the experience of the pathologist interpreting SCNB may vary, there may be diagnostic limitations not yet appreciated from the reported studies.

In some institutions, FNAC followed by core biopsy is performed on all abnormalities not shown to be cysts[14]. Dowlatshahi et al. compared the results of 250 stereotactic FNACs and 250 SCNBs of mammographically detected nonpalpable breast abnormalities suspicious for malignancy[15]. For the diagnosis of palpable masses greater than 1 cm, the core biopsy was superior to stereotactic FNAC. Stereotactic FNAC was better in this series for diagnosing malignant microcalcifications. In 13 of 29 SCNBs (45%) and only in 3 of 29 stereotactic FNACs (10%) there were false negative diagnoses for malignancy. Others have found that SCNB, with the appropriate number of samples, has best diagnosed ductal carcinoma in situ, which often presents as microcalcifications[16]. Dowlatshahi and colleagues concluded that SCNB and FNAC complement each other in the diagnosis of suspicious breast abnormalities and advocated both stereotactic FNAC and SCNB for these abnormalities.

Although good to excellent histologic correlation has been reported between SCNB and surgical biopsy[11-15,17-19], the diagnostic difficulties in the pathologic interpretation of SCNB have yet to be described. In general, the morphologic findings of SCNB are similar to those that have been well-described for the surgical pathology of the breast. Therefore, it might be expected that the diagnostic problems are also similar, with additional difficulties relating to the smaller specimen size. The focus of this chapter will be on the technical considerations of SCNB and the potential pitfalls in the diagnosis of common breast abnormalities.

Technical Considerations

Many factors are involved in producing good SCNB specimens. Among these are operator experience, nature of the abnormality, accuracy of needle placement, and number of samples obtained[20].

Variation exists in the literature concerning the size of the core needle used for SCNB. Biopsy gun needles used in these studies ranged from 14 to 20-gauge[15,17]. Although the effect of needle size on the specimen has not been evaluated in detail from a pathologic viewpoint, Parker et al. conclude that the larger 14-gauge needle provides more specific and sensitive results[11]. Others suggest that multiple passes with a 14-gauge needle may be unacceptable for patient comfort and complications[20]. In our experience, difficulties in interpretation of SCNB arise when the core biopsy is fragmented and hemorrhagic (**Figure 9.1**). In these cases, isolated cells or clusters of cells may be called atypical and therefore may lead to an uncertain diagnosis. However, the correlation between fragmented biopsies and needle core size has not been demonstrated.

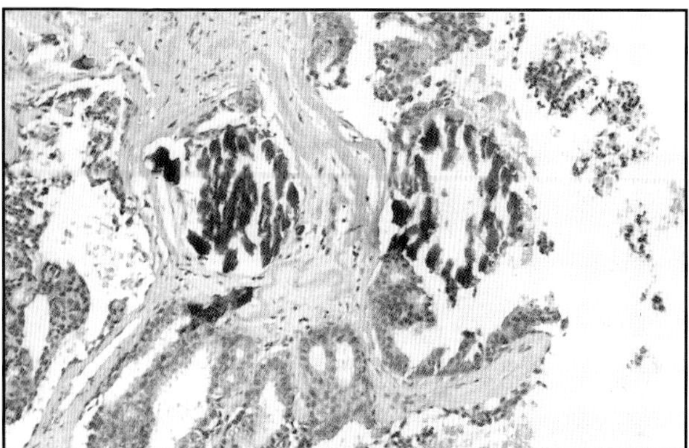

Figure 9.1. SCNB with Fragmentation, Hemorrhage and Isolated Proliferative Epithelial Cells. In this core biopsy, the differential diagnosis is proliferative fibrocystic change versus low grade carcinoma in situ (micropapillary or cribriform type). Additional core biopsies or an open surgical biopsy should be performed to further evaluate the abnormality. H&E stain, magnification 200x.

A second technical problem may occur when a suspicious abnormality is missed or only partially sampled. Sampling error or false negative SCNB results can be the result of a "miss" of the abnormality by SCNB, or the abnormality may be present in the specimen but the histologic sections do not go deep enough into the tissue block to demonstrate the pathology. To prevent some of these problems the following approaches can be taken. If the clinician is performing a biopsy for calcifications, the specimen core can be imaged to confirm the presence of microcalcifications[16]. When the pathologist is given the information that SCNB was done to sample calcifications, then a diligent search for microcalcifications should be performed, including extra sections and core biopsy specimen radiography, if necessary. We have had a few cases where the initial sections of SCNB revealed benign breast tissue, but further sections (at the request of the clinician) to find the calcifications revealed ductal carcinoma in situ or a small infiltrating carcinoma (**Figure 9.2**). Although sampling error can never be completely resolved, close collaboration between the clinician and pathologist interpreting the abnormality is required to reduce the number of false negative diagnoses. This collaborative approach has been advocated by many for FNAC, and it is equally important for the approach to SCNB[20, 21].

The third problem that we have encountered in the interpretation of SCNB is occasional artifactual distortion of the tissue. This mainly occurs in abnormalities that are fibrotic and may have proliferative epithelial changes. The epithelium may be crushed during the biopsy procedure, making it difficult to render a definitive diagnosis (**Figure 9.3**). If the epithelium is stripped or fragmented away from the basement membrane, it may be difficult to determine if this epithelium is derived from a hyperplastic process or from carcinoma in situ. Despite the limitations discussed above, in the majority of cases, a definitive pathologic diagnosis can be made on a technically well-performed SCNB.

There are a wide variety of benign, borderline, and malignant abnormalities that can present as a mammographic abnormality. It is beyond the scope of this chapter to discuss each one in detail. However, it is essential that the pathologist and clinician have a good understanding of the differential diagnosis based on the mammographic, clinical and pathologic findings, and the implication of the diagnosis for patient management.

The approach to SCNB should be similar to that used for FNAC (**Figure 9.4**). If the radiologic/clinical picture and

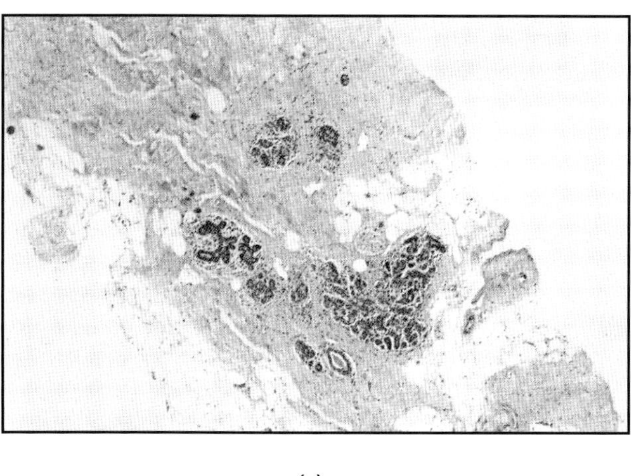

(a)

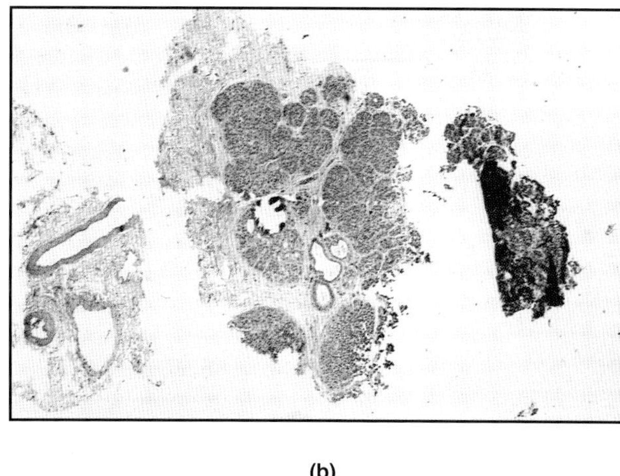

(b)

Figure 9.2 a and b. Carcinoma In Situ Detected on Further Sections. The initial sections of this core biopsy showed benign tissue **(a)**. When extra sections were done to find the calcifications, ductal carcinoma in situ was diagnosed **(b)**. H&E stain, magnification 200x.

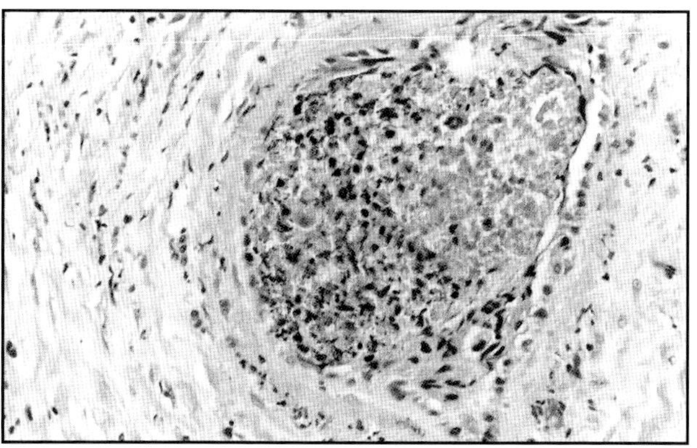

Figure 9.3. Crushed Ductal Epithelium. This illustrates the difficulties that can be encountered when the epithelium is distorted by SCNB. This case had carcinoma in situ on open biopsy. H&E stain, magnification 400x.

pathologic findings do not correlate, the patient should have further work-up and/or close follow-up. In the next sections, the most commonly encountered specific benign **(Figure 9.5)** and malignant entities **(Figure 9.6)** will be discussed in regard to differential diagnosis, pitfalls, and approach to patient management.

Benign Abnormalities

Fibrocystic Changes

Fibrocystic changes are a common etiology of both mammographic nonpalpable and palpable breast abnormalities. The histologic manifestations of fibrocystic changes are heterogeneous and can include: cysts, fibrosis, apocrine metaplasia, sclerosing adenosis, and epithelial hyperplasia[22]. The diagnostic characteristics of fibrocystic changes are easily recognized on SCNB, allowing for a specific diagnosis to be made **(Figure 9.7)**. Microcalcifications can be identified in fibrocystic changes, reassuring the clinician that the appropriate area has been sampled[23] **(Figure 9.8)**. Sclerosing adenosis is a proliferation of the lobular acini with surrounding sclerosis that is seen frequently in fibrocystic changes. If the sclerosing adenosis is florid, it may be mistaken for an infiltrating carcinoma, in particular, if it is seen in a small core biopsy specimen **(Figure 9.9)**.

Proliferative breast disease (moderate epithelial hyperplasia or greater) has been shown to correlate with increased risk for the subsequent development of invasive carcinoma[24,25]. The degree of epithelial hyperplasia allows stratification into nonproliferative and proliferative breast disease[22]. The criteria for the diagnosis of proliferative breast disease (moderate to florid to atypical ductal hyperplasia) are defined from histologic sections and have not been readily applied to cytologic specimens. Although criteria for the cytologic diagnosis of proliferative breast disease are being defined[26], the usefulness of FNAC for identifying women at increased risk has not been well-established. Theoretically, the well-known histologic criteria for diagnosing epithelial hyperplasia can be applied to SCNB to provide a relatively noninvasive method of identifying women who need close follow-up.

There may be limitations to the diagnosis of fibrocystic changes and, in particular, the degree of proliferative breast

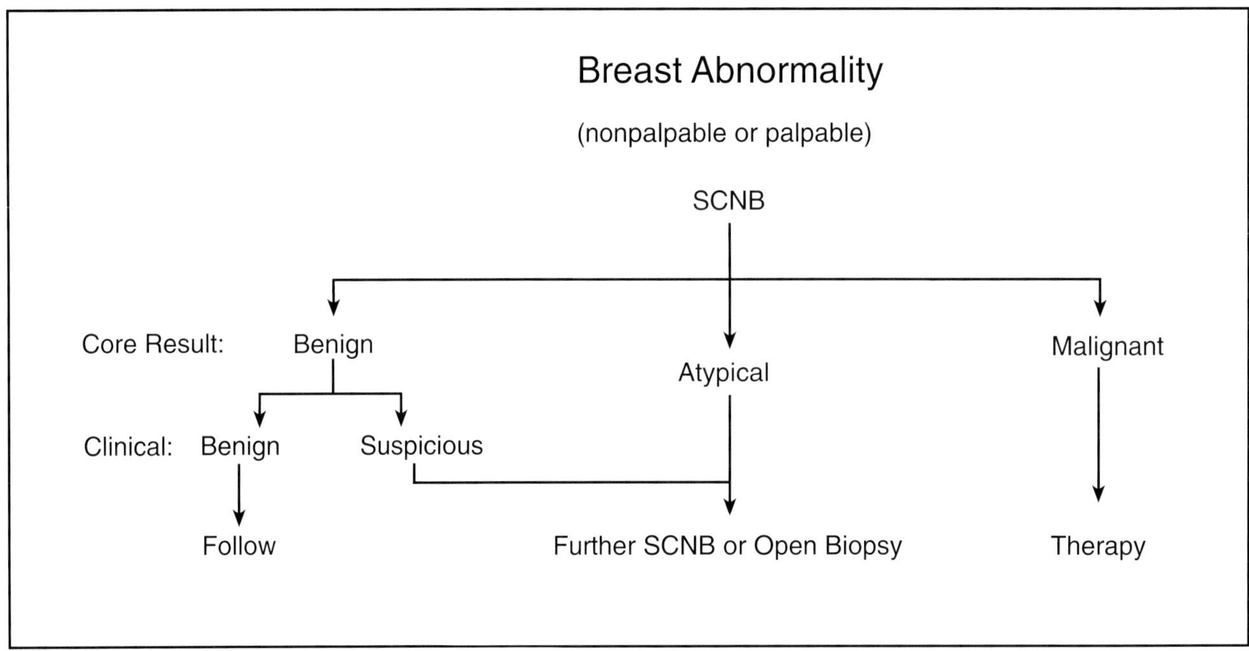

Figure 9.4. Approach to Stereotactic Core Biopsy. This chart illustrates the management of a breast abnormality based on the pathologic diagnosis and mammographic/clinical impression.

Stereotactic Core Needle Biopsy: Common Benign Abnormalities

Diagnosis	Hallmark of Abnormality	Significance*	Differential**
Fibrocystic Changes:			
Nonproliferative	Mild ductal hyperplasia	No increased risk	
Proliferative	Moderate to atypical hyperplasia	Increased risk	Carcinoma in situ
Fibroadenoma	Benign biphasic stromal neoplasm	No increased risk	Phyllodes tumor
Papilloma	Fibrovascular cores, single cell layer	Indeterminate risk	Intracystic papillary CA
Radial Scar	"Pseudoinfiltrative," ducts, fibrosis	Indeterminate risk	Invasive cancer

*The significance refers to the known increased risk for development of subsequent invasive breast cancer.
**The differential diagnosis can be wide for many of these abnormalities, however, the most common differential that would be considered is listed.

Figure 9.5 Stereotactic Core Needle Biopsy: Common Benign Abnormalities.

Stereotactic Core Needle Biopsy: Common Malignant Abnormalities

Diagnosis	Hallmark of Abnormalities	Prognosis*	Differential**
In situ:			
Comedo DCIS	High grade nuclei, necrosis	High grade	Invasive cancer
Noncomedo DCIS	Micropapillary, cribriform	Low grade	Atypical ductal hyperplasia
Lobular CIS	Uniform, small nuclei	Low grade	Lobular hyperplasia
Invasive:			
Ductal	Variable, well to poorly differentiated	Variable	
Lobular	Bland, uniform cells	Intermediate	
Tubular cancer	Open, angulated ducts	Good	Radial scar
Mucinous cancer	Mucin, bland cells	Good	Mucocele-like abnormality

*Prognosis for in situ cancers refers to the risk of developing subsequent invasive cancer. High-grade abnormalities have a much higher risk than low-grade abnormalities. The prognosis for invasive cancer is related to survival rates.
** The differential diagnosis can be extensive, but only common abnormalities encountered in the differential are listed.

Figure 9.6 Stereotactic Core Needle Biopsy: Common Malignant Abnormalities.

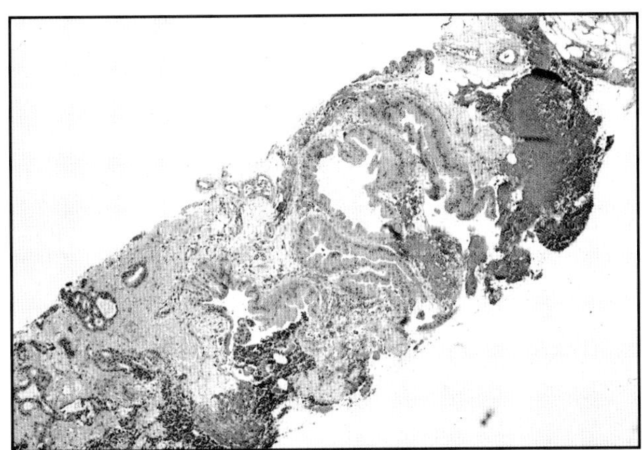

Figure 9.7. SCNB with Fibrocystic Changes. There is abundant apocrine metaplasia in this core biopsy. H&E stain, magnification 100x.

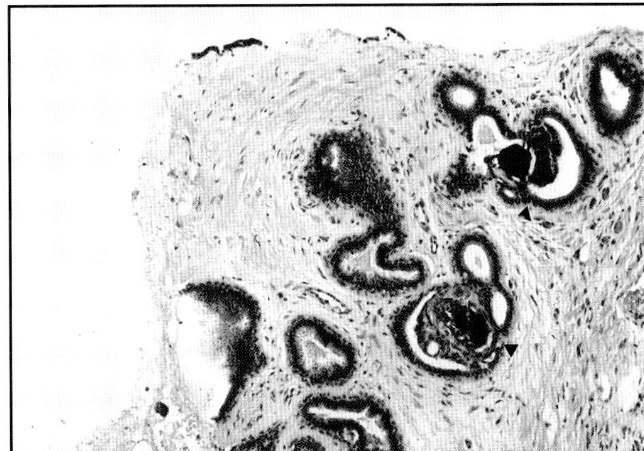

Figure 9.8. Fibrocystic Changes and Microcalcifications. Microcalcifications are easily identified in this core biopsy with fibrocystic changes **(arrowheads)**. H&E stain, magnification 200x.

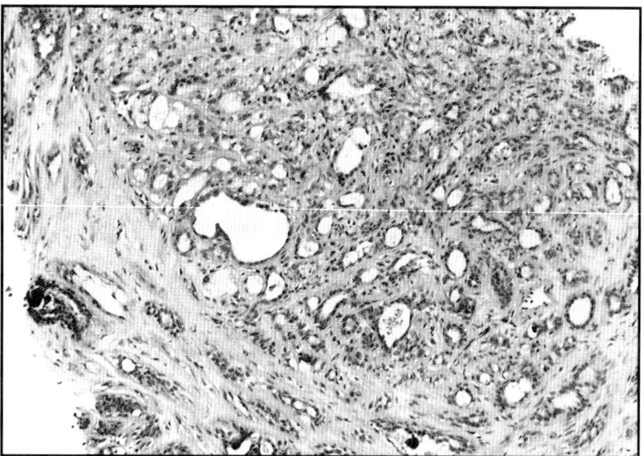

Figure 9.9. Sclerosing Adenosis. There is a proliferation of lobular acini with sclerosis, diagnostic of sclerosing adenosis. H&E stain, magnification 200x.

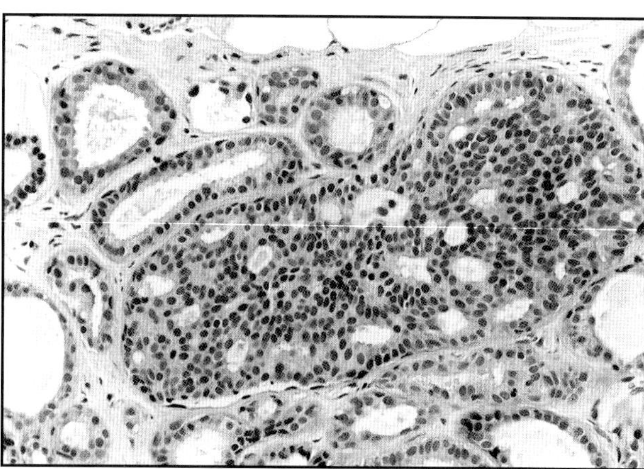

Figure 9.10. Proliferative Epithelial Changes in SCNB. The differential diagnosis in a case such as this includes atypical hyperplasia versus carcinoma in situ. Also note microcalcifications. H&E stain, magnification 200x.

disease with SCNB. The first limitation is one of sampling. Fibrocystic changes can be found in areas adjacent to infiltrating cancers. Thus, the clinician must be confident that the area of suspicion on the mammogram is well-sampled. The second limitation involves interpretation. It has been shown that although the criteria for the diagnosis of proliferative breast disease are well-defined, there can be significant observer variability in the diagnosis[27]. We have noted that the diagnosis of atypical ductal hyperplasia can be problematic on SCNB, secondary to the small sample and artifactual distortion of the core tissue as result of the technique. The diagnosis of atypical ductal hyperplasia on SCNB may underdiagnose a carcinoma in situ **(Figure 9.10)**.

Alternatively, a diagnosis of carcinoma in situ based on abnormal architecture in one to two ductal spaces may result in an over diagnosis of atypical ductal hyperplasia or lesser abnormality. As has been suggested for FNAC[28], when a diagnosis of atypia is made on SCNB, it may be prudent to recommend either close clinical follow-up, an additional SCNB, or a diagnostic surgical biopsy, depending on the clinical situation.

Fibroadenoma

Several studies of SCNB have reported technical difficulties with core biopsy of fibroadenomas. This has been attributed in some instances to a "shift" in the abnormalities when the needle is inserted, since these benign tumors are characteristically firm and mobile[11]. When a good representative core sample is obtained, the diagnostic features of fibroadenoma can be easily recognized. The histologic features consist of a stromal proliferation that can range from myxoid to cellular, which compresses adjacent ductal epithelial structures to a varying degree[29]. If the boundary between the fibroadenoma and normal breast tissue is included in the SCNB, the well-circumscribed nature of the abnormality can be easily recognized **(Figure 9.11)**. Difficulties in diagnosing fibroadenoma by SCNB arise in cases where the stroma is extremely hyalinized and the characteristic biphasic stromal and epithelial features are not observed.

Another diagnostic dilemma occurs when the stromal element is hypercellular and the differential diagnosis includes a phyllodes tumor. Phyllodes tumors are benign stromal breast tumors that may recur if not entirely resected **(Figure 9.12)**. The malignant counterpart of this abnormality is a malignant cystosarcoma phyllodes tumor. The distinction between benign and malignant phyllodes tumors can be difficult and is based on an assessment of stromal nuclear atypia and tumor mitotic activity[29].

SCNB is limited by its small sample size in distinguishing between fibroadenoma, benign phyllodes tumor, and malignant cystosarcoma. The recognition of increased stromal cellularity in a stromal neoplasm of the breast may warrant consideration of this differential diagnosis and a further excisional surgical biopsy.

Papillomas

Intraductal papillomas are benign abnormalities that often occur in a subareolar location. They have prominent

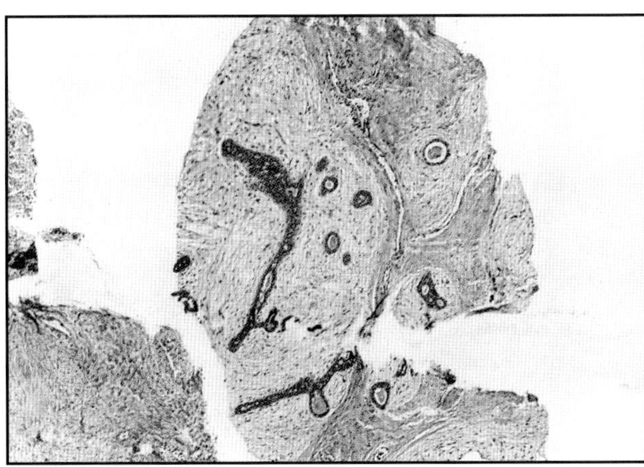

Figure 9.11. Core Biopsy of a Fibroadenoma. This abnormality was difficult to interpret on fine needle aspiration cytology but the diagnosis of fibroadenoma was made on SCNB. H&E stain, magnification 400x.

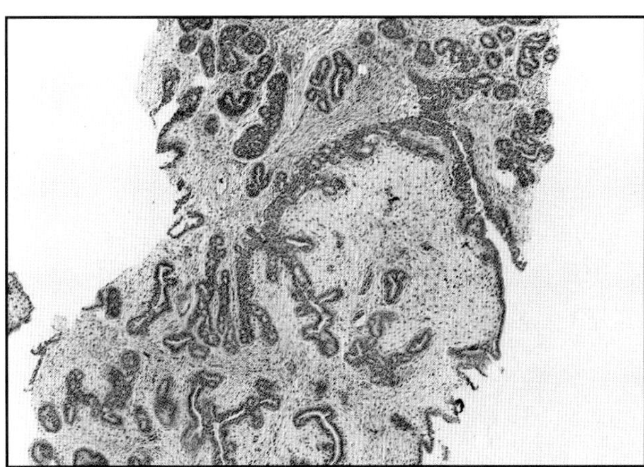

Figure 9.12. Core Biopsy of a Cellular Stromal Abnormality. Although not diagnostic on SCNB, open surgical biopsy revealed a benign phyllodes tumor. H&E stain, magnification 100x.

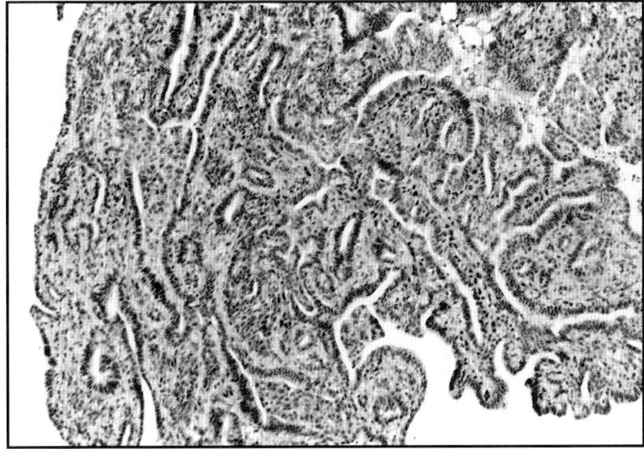

Figure 9.13. SCNB of a Papilloma. The SCNB shows diagnostic well-defined fibrovascular cores and a single-cell epithelial layer, even though the biopsy is fragmented. H&E stain, magnification 100x.

fibrovascular cores lined by a benign two-cell ductal epithelial layer (**Figure 9.13**). Apocrine metaplasia can often be seen in an intraductal papilloma. The differential diagnosis of a papilloma includes a noninvasive or intracystic papillary carcinoma, which tends to occur in older women and has a good prognosis.

The histologic features that allow intracystic papillary cancer to be distinguished from intraductal papilloma are the presence of a homogeneous cell pattern, architectural features of carcinoma in situ, hyperchromasia of the nuclei, and an absence of apocrine metaplasia[30]. In FNAC, intraductal papilloma and intracystic papillary cancer are difficult to distinguish due to overlapping features[31]. SCNB experience with this particular abnormality has not been reported, however, it is reasonable to expect that SCNB would be more specific than FNAC since the differential diagnosis is based on histologic and architectural criteria.

Malignant Abnormalities

Carcinoma In Situ

With widespread screening mammography, there has been an increase in the detection of carcinoma in situ of the breast[32]. The accurate diagnosis of infiltrating versus in situ carcinoma, and even the precise subtype of in situ carcinoma, is critical for decision making in patient management[33, 34]. One of the limitations of FNAC has been the inability to reliably distinguish invasive from in situ carcinomas[10]. SCNB has the advantage of being able to identify the architectural features of invasive cancer in the core. A limitation of SCNB is sampling error; for example, an in situ cancer may be adjacent to a focus of invasion that has not been sampled by the core. Carcinoma in situ with early stromal invasion can be difficult to diagnose and can be over or underdiagnosed with SCNB. We have seen examples of early invasion diagnosed on a small SCNB specimen with no invasive cancer in the open surgical biopsy or lumpectomy specimen. Retrospective review of the core revealed that distortion of the ducts involved with ductal carcinoma in situ led to the false positive diagnosis of invasive cancer.

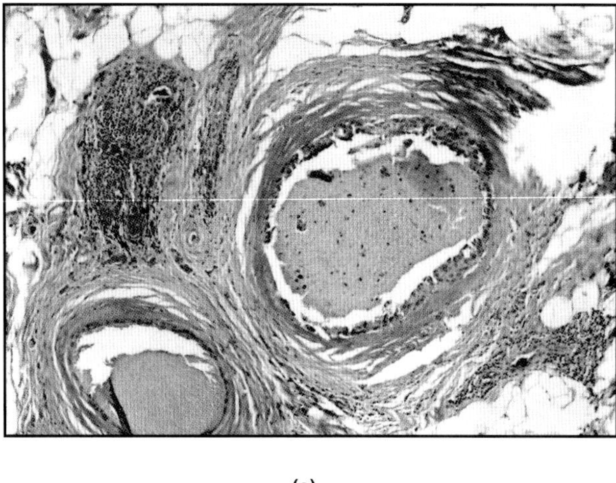

(a)

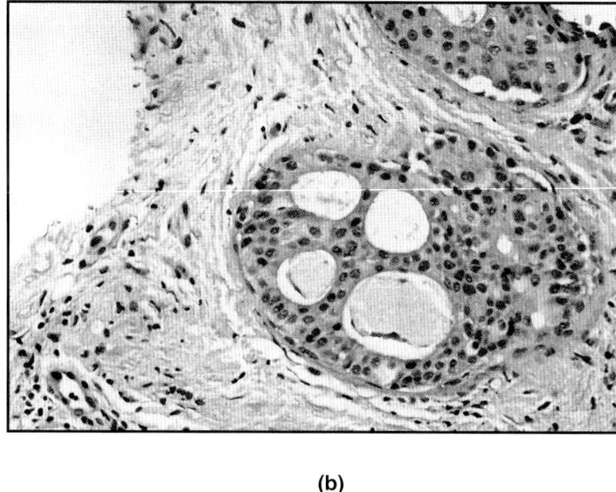

(b)

Figure 9.14. Ductal Carcinoma In Situ. Comedo ductal carcinoma in situ with central necrosis is present in this SCNB **(a)**. Noncomedo ductal carcinoma in situ with a punched out cribriform pattern is seen **(b)**. H&E stain, magnification 400x.

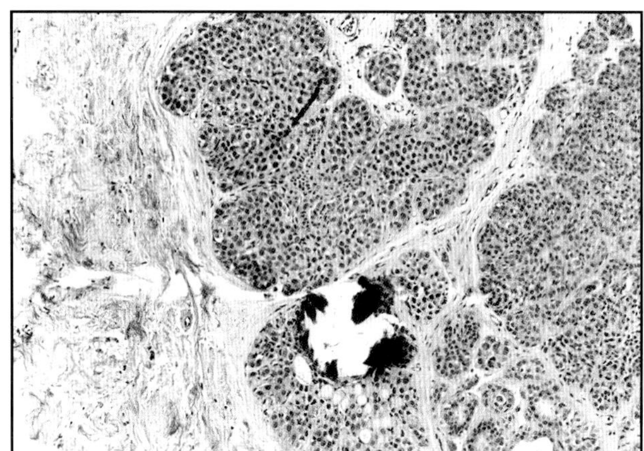

Figure 9.15. Lobular Carcinoma In Situ. The uniform cells of lobular carcinoma in situ expand the lobular unit. Microcalcification is present. H&E stain, magnification 400x.

The subtype of carcinoma in situ is playing an increasingly important role in the management of patients[34]. Comedo ductal carcinoma in situ (C-DCIS) is a more aggressive subtype with high grade nuclear features and abundant central necrosis **(Figure 9.14a)**. Noncomedo ductal carcinoma in situ (NC-DCIS) includes the subtypes of micropapillary and cribriform carcinoma in situ, which have bland nuclear features and either delicate micropapillary configurations or punched out cribriform spaces **(Figure 9.14b)**. This low grade cancer may have atypical ductal hyperplasia in the differential diagnosis.

Lobular carcinoma in situ is a distinct subtype of in situ cancer, which is treated more conservatively than ductal carcinoma in situ[35]. Classically, lobular carcinoma in situ consists of a population of small, relatively uniform cells that expand the lobular units **(Figure 9.15)**. The cells may vary from this "classic appearance" with variations in size, shape, and cytoplasm. Ductal carcinoma in situ may be in the differential diagnosis when the cells are more pleomorphic and, in rare cases, when necrosis and calcification are present in lobular carcinoma in situ. The heterogeneity of lobular, ductal, and mixed carcinoma in situ abnormalities may be difficult to distinguish on an SCNB sample. This is important to recognize only in that the SCNB diagnosis may not correlate exactly with the open surgical biopsy, when the abnormality is heterogeneous and only small regions have been sampled.

Infiltrating Carcinomas

Infiltrating ductal carcinomas are the most common type of invasive breast carcinoma. Although the histologic appearance often varies from patient to patient, the diagnosis is usually straightforward. FNAC has a high rate of accuracy for the diagnosis of invasive carcinoma, with the main limitation being the distinction between invasive and in situ cancer. The diagnosis of invasive cancer can easily be made with SCNB, assuming the appropriate area has been sampled. Difficulties in diagnosis based on SCNB may arise when a complex sclerosing abnormality or radial scar-like abnormality has been biopsied **(Figure 9.16)**. These abnormalities often have a "pseudoinfiltrative" appearance, which can often only be distinguished in the context of the architecture of the entire abnormality. There is controversy as to whether an abnormality thought to be a radial scar can be adequately sampled and correctly diagnosed by SCNB[14]. If the diagnosis is uncertain on SCNB, it is recommended in most cases to proceed to surgical biopsy for a definitive diagnosis.

Infiltrating lobular carcinomas are the next most common invasive cancer of the breast[35]. These cancers can have a deceptively bland histologic and clinical appearance. The diagnosis of invasive lobular carcinoma can be problematic for both FNAC and SCNB due to sampling problems. If the appropriate abnormal tissue is sampled, SCNB offers the advantage of being able to identify the uniform bland cells infiltrating through adjacent breast parenchyma **(Figure 9.17)**. Invasive cancers can also have mixed lobular and ductal histologic features; therefore, a discrepancy may exist between the core biopsy and the final pathologic diagnosis of the lumpectomy or mastectomy specimen. Since these subtypes of invasive cancers are managed in a similar fashion, the difference in diagnosis is not important clinically.

Special Types of Infiltrating Carcinomas

There are several histologic subtypes of invasive carcinoma that fall into the category of "good prognosis" or low malignant potential cancers. Included in this category are tubular carcinomas, mucinous (colloid) cancers, papillary carcinomas, and medullary carcinomas. Tubular carcinomas present by mammography as small spiculated abnormalities and most likely represent an early, well-differentiated ductal carcinoma[36]. The histologic appearance is distinctive with infiltrative open angulated ducts, bland nuclear features, and cytoplasmic apocrine "snouts"**(Figure 9.18)**. The differential diagnosis of tubular carcinoma includes a radial scar or complex sclerosing abnormality with a "pseudoinfiltrative appearance." Infiltration into adjacent adipose tissue and the presence of one cell layer in the ducts are often clues that help to differentiate tubular carcinoma from these benign abnormalities.

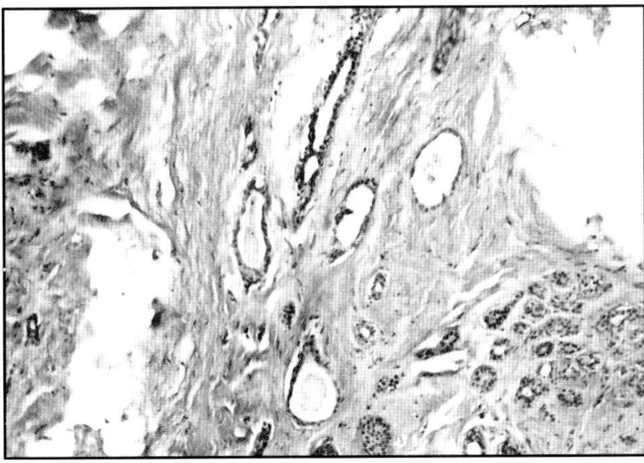

Figure 9.16. Radial Scar-like Abnormality in a Core Biopsy. Epithelial proliferation is present with extensive sclerosis. Angulated, distorted epithelial groups can be difficult to differentiate from invasive cancer. H&E stain, magnification 400x.

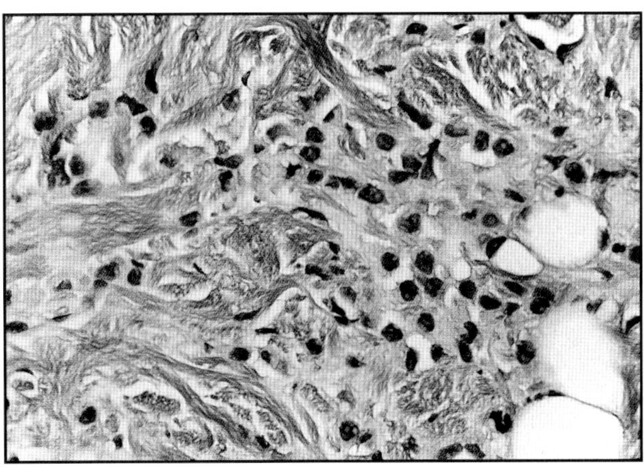

Figure 9.17. Invasive Lobular Carcinoma. Lobular carcinoma cells infiltrating through fibrotic stroma can be difficult to detect due to their bland appearance. SCNB may be better than FNAC for diagnosis of this cancer since the invasiveness of the bland cells is apparent. H&E stain, magnification 400x.

Mucinous or colloid carcinomas in their pure form are also associated with a better prognosis. These tumors are present in older women and often have a soft, gelatinous consistency. Histologically, they are distinctive with clusters of bland epithelial cells floating in large pools of extravasated mucin[37] **(Figure 9.19)**. If a mucinous carcinoma has a mixed component of infiltrating ductal carcinoma, the abnormality then takes on the prognosis of the worse component (ductal carcinoma). Although the diagnosis of mucinous carcinoma can easily be made on SCNB, the biopsy may miss the infiltrating ductal component. Therefore, it is important that the entire abnormality be evaluated in the surgical biopsy specimen before an assessment of patient prognosis is made based on the histologic subtype.

Medullary carcinomas are another subtype of tumor with a better prognosis, having a distinct histologic appearance and a well-circumscribed pushing border. They may be con-

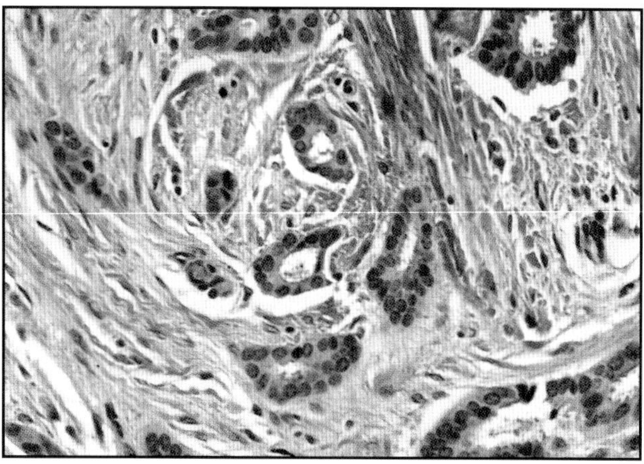

Figure 9.18. Tubular Carcinoma. This core biopsy had infiltrative open ducts, diagnostic of tubular carcinoma. H&E stain, magnification 200x.

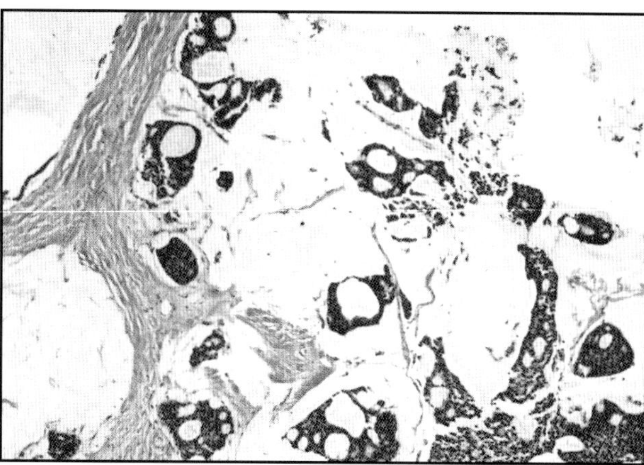

Figure 9.19. Mucinous or Colloid Carcinoma. Pools of mucin and clusters of malignant epithelial cells allow the diagnosis of mucinous or colloid carcinoma on this SCNB. H&E stain, magnification 200x.

fused clinically with fibroadenomas. However, an SCNB with tumor cells demonstrating high grade nuclear features forming syncytial aggregates and lymphocytes will suggest the diagnosis[38].

Special Studies in Breast Cancer

In addition to providing adequate tissue for the diagnosis of breast cancer and other benign abnormalities, special studies performed on paraffin-embedded tissue can aid in both predicting prognosis and determining patient management. One distinct advantage of SCNB over FNAC is that sections from the core specimen can be used for special studies, such as steroid receptor analysis and flow cytometry. Although the feasibility of performing these studies on cytologic material has been demonstrated, they are not widely utilized because of the small number of tumor cells and other technical considerations[39,40]. This chapter cannot address all of the potential studies that can be performed on paraffin-embedded tissue that include molecular diagnostic techniques, but it will illustrate a few examples where there is a defined clinical utility for the test.

Steroid Receptors

The presence or absence of estrogen and progesterone receptors in breast cancer has become an important guide to therapeutic decision making[41]. Traditionally, these steroid receptors were assayed by methods that require a substantial amount of tumor. More recently, immunocytochemical techniques that visualize the presence of receptor on the formalin-fixed, paraffin-embedded tissue has been accepted, based on the results of several studies showing it to be equal to the more traditional assays[42]. Immunocytochemical techniques may offer an advantage in the histologic section, that is, the presence of receptor on the actual tumor cells can be evaluated. In addition, false positive results due to positive steroid receptors on the adjacent normal breast tissue are eliminated.

Immunocytochemical techniques can be successfully applied to SCNB. Limited tumor sampling may lead to false negative results in some cases, since tumor cells may exhibit variability in the staining pattern of estrogen and progesterone receptors. In patients with advanced breast cancer, it may be particularly important to assess the estrogen and progesterone receptor status prior to preoperative chemotherapy. SCNB is ideally suited for this purpose and prevents the need for an excisional biopsy prior to therapy.

Using similar immunocytochemical techniques, other potential markers of prognosis can be assessed on SCNB, such as the oncogene, Her2neu, and the tumor suppressor gene, p53. In advanced breast cancer patients, data exists suggesting that the expression of the intrinsic multidrug resistance gene, p-glycoprotein (p-gp) correlates with response to therapy[43]. This may be important information to obtain before preoperative chemotherapy. In select cases, we have demonstrated p-glycoprotein expression immunocytochemically in the SCNB.

DNA analysis by flow cytometry can be performed on paraffin-embedded tissue, and in many institutions is routinely performed on all breast cancer specimens. This provides information about the DNA content of the tumor and the S-phase estimate, or proliferative rate, of the tumor. The S-phase estimate has been correlated with prognosis and is used to guide clinical management in many patients[44]. Lovin et al. have reported the results of flow cytometric studies on the SCNB of 135 patients, and have compared these findings to the flow cytometry of their surgical biopsies. They concluded that with SCNB, there was sufficient tissue for both accurate histologic diagnosis of breast disease and flow cytometric measurements of ploidy and S-phase[45].

Summary

Studies to date have demonstrated excellent results for SCNB compared with open surgical biopsy[11-13, 15, 17]. This chapter has focused on the major pitfalls and limitations of SCNB that may be encountered in a routine surgical pathology practice. A better understanding of the diagnostic limitations enables clinicians to be aware of clinical and pathological situations when a definitive diagnosis cannot be made. In our own institution, the agreement between SCNB and subsequent follow-up biopsies or mastectomy has been very good. It also appears that the SCNB can provide adequate material for ancillary studies that may be useful in predicting patient prognosis or determining appropriate patient management[45]. Both SCNB and FNAC will likely play an increasing role in the management of breast disease, offering patients accurate, cost-effective, relatively noninvasive diagnostic tests as an alternative to open biopsy.

References

1. Feig, S.A. 1988. Decreased Breast Cancer Mortality Through Mammographic Screening: Results of Clinical Trials. *Radiology* 167:659-665.

2. Hall, F.M., Storela, J.M., Silverstone, D.Z., Wyshak, G. 1988. Nonpalpable Breast Lesions: Recommendations for Biopsy Based on Suspicion of Carcinoma at Mammography. *Radiology* 167:353-358.

3. Fajardo, L.L., Davis, J.R., Weins, J.L., Trego, D.C. 1990. Mammographically-Guided Stereotactic Fine Needle Aspiration Cytology of Non Palpable Breast Lesions: Prospective Comparison of Surgical Biopsy Results. *American Journal of Radiology* 155:977-981.

4. Svane, G. and Silfversward, C. 1983. Stereotaxic Needle Biopsy of Non-Palpable Breast Lesions. *Acta Radiologica Diagnosis* 24:283-288.

5. Sullivan, D.C. 1994. Needle Core Biopsy of Mammographic Lesions. *American Journal of Radiology* 162:601-608.

6. Frable, W.J. 1993. Fine Needle Aspiration Biopsy. *Hum Path* 14:9-28.

7. Logan-Young, W.W., Hoffman, N.Y., Janus, J.A. 1992. Fine-Needle Aspiration Cytology in the Detection of Breast Cancer in Non-Suspicious Lesions. *Radiology* 184:49-53.

8. Hann, L., Ducatman, B.S., Wang, H.H., Fein,V., McIntire, J.M. 1989. Nonpalpable Breast Lesions: Evaluation by Means of Fine-Needle Aspiration Cytology. *Radiology* 171:373-376.

9. Giard, R.W.M., Hermans, J. 1989. The Value of Aspiration Cytology. *Radiology* 171:373-376.

10. Wang, H.H., Ducatman, B.S., Eick, D. 1989. Comparative Features of Ductal Carcinoma In-Situ and Infiltrating Ductal Carcinoma of the Breast on Fine Needle Aspiration Biopsy. *American Journal of Clinical Pathology* 92:736-742.

11. Parker, S.H., Lovin, J.D., Jobe, W.E., Luethke, J.M, Hopper, K.D., Yakes, W.F. and Burke, B.J. 1990. Stereotactic Breast Biopsy with a Biopsy Gun. *Radiology* 176:741-747.

12. Parker, S.H., Lovin, J.D., Jobe, W.E., Burke, B.J., Hopper, K.D., Yakes, W.F. 1991. Non Palpable Breast Lesions: Stereotactic Automated Large-Core Biopsies. *Radiology* 180:403-407.

13. Parker, S.H., Jobe, W.E., Dennis, M.A., Stavros, A.T., Johnson, K.K., Yakes, W.F., Truell, J.E., Price, J.G., Kortz, A.B. and Clark, D.G. 1993. US-Guided Automated Large-Core Breast Biopsy. *Radiology* 187:507-511.

14. Schmidt, R.A. 1994. Stereotactic Breast Biopsy. *CA Cancer J Clin* 44:172-191.

15. Dowlatshahi, D., Yaremko, M.L., Kluskens, L.F., Jokich, P.M. 1991. Non Palpable Breast Lesions: Findings of Stereotaxic Needle-Core Biopsy and Fine Needle Aspiration Cytology. *Radiology* 181:745-750.

16. Liberman, L., Evans, W.P. 3rd, Dershaw, D.D., et al. 1994. Radiography of Microcalcifications in Stereotaxic Mammary Core Biopsy Specimens. *Radiology* 190:223-225.

17. Grisvold, J.J., Goellner, J.R., Grant, C.S., Donohue, J.H., Sykes, M.W., Karsell, P.R., Coffey, S.L., Jung, S. 1994. Breast Biopsy: A Comparative Study of Stereotaxically Guided Core and Excisional Techniques. *American Journal of Radiology* 162:815-820.

18. Dronkers, D.J. 1992. Stereotaxic Core Biopsy of Breast Lesions. *Radiology* 183:631-634.

19. Elvecrog, E.L., Lechner, M.C., Nelson, M.T. 1993. Non Palpable Breast Lesions: Correlation of Stereotaxic Large-Core Needle Biopsy and Surgical Biopsy Results. *Radiology* 188:453-455.

20. Jackson, V.P., Reynolds, H.E. 1991. Stereotaxic Needle Core Biopsy and Fine Needle Aspiration Cytologic Evaluation of Non-Palpable Breast Lesions. *Radiology* 181:633-634.

21. Hermansen, C., Poulsen, H.S., Jensen, J., Langfeldt, B., Steenskov, V., Frederiksen, P., Jensen, O.M. 1987. Diagnostic Reliability of Combined Physical Examination, Mammography and Fine Needle Puncture ("Triple-Test") in Breast Tumors. A Prospective Study. *Cancer* 60:1866-1871.

22. Page, D.L., Anderson, T.J., Rogers, L.W. 1987. Epithelial Hyperplasia. In: Page, D.L., Anderson, T.J. *Diagnostic Histopathology of the Breast*. New York: Churchill Livingstone 120-156.

23. Meyer, J.E., Lester, S.C., Frenna, T.H., White, F.V. 1993. Occult Breast Calcifications Sampled with Large-Core Biopsy Confirmation with Radiography of the Specimen. *Radiology* 188:581-582.

24. Dupont, W.D. and Page, D.L. 1985. Risk Factors for Breast Cancer in Women with Proliferative Breast Disease. *New England Journal of Medicine* 312:146- 151.

25. Dupont, W.D., Parl, F.F., Hartmann, W.H., Brinton, L.A., Winfeld, A.C., Worrell, J.A., Schuyler, P.A., Plummer, W.D. 1993. Breast Cancer Risk Associated with Proliferative Breast Disease and Atypical Hyperplasia. *Cancer* 71:1258-1265.

26. Dawson, A.E., Mulford, D.K., Sheils, L.A. 1995. The Cytopathology of Proliferative Breast Disease. Comparison to Ductal Carcinoma In Situ. *Am J Clin Pathol* 103:438-442.

27. Rosai, J. 1991. Borderline Epithelial Lesions of the Breast. *Am J Surg Pathol* 15:599-603.

28. Mulford, D.K., Dawson, A.E. 1994. Atypia in Fine Needle Aspiration Cytology of Nonpalpable and Palpable Mammographically Detected Breast Lesions. *Acta Cytol* 38:9-17.

29. Tavassoli, F.A. 1992. Biphasic Tumors. In: Tavassoli, F.A. *Pathology of the Breast*, Appleton & Lange 425-465.

30. Page, D.L., Anderson, T.J. 1987. Papilloma and Related Lesions. In: Page, D.L., Anderson, T.J. *Diagnostic Histopathology of the Breast,* New York: Churchill Livingstone 104-119.

31. Dawson, A.E. and Mulford, D.K. 1994. Benign Versus Malignant Papillary Neoplasms of the Breast. Diagnostic Clues in Fine Needle Aspiration Cytology. *Acta Cytol* 38:23-28.

32. Schnitt, S.J., Silen, W., Sadowsky, N.L., Connolly, J.L., Harris, J.R. 1988. Ductal Carcinoma In-Situ (Intraductal Carcinoma) of the Breast. *New England Journal of Medicine* 318:898-903.

33. Lennington, W.J., Jensen, R.A., Dalton, L.W., Page, D.L. 1994. Ductal Carcinoma In-Situ of the Breast. Heterogeneity of Individual Lesions. *Cancer* 73:118-124.

34. Bellamy, C.O.C., McDonald, C., Salter, D.M., Chetty, U. and Anderson, T.J. 1993. Noninvasive Ductal Carcinoma of the Breast: The Relevance of Histologic Categorization. *Hum Pathol* 24:16-23.

35. Tavassoli, F.A. 1992. Lobular Neoplasia. In: Tavassoli, F.A. *Pathology of the Breast*. Appleton & Lange 263-291.

36. Parl, F.F., Richardson, L.D. 1983. The Histological and Biological Spectrum of Tubular Carcinoma of the Breast. *Hum Pathol* 14: 694-698.

37. Rasmussen, B.B., Rose, C., Christensen, I. 1987. Prognostic Factors in Primary Mucinous Carcinoma of the Breast. *Am J Clin Pathol* 87:155-160.

38. Ridolfi, R.E., Rosen, P.P., Post, A., et al. 1977. Medullary Carcinoma of the Breast. A Clinical Pathological Study with 10 Year Follow-up. *Cancer* 40:1365-1385.

39. Coombes, R.C., Powles, T.J., Berger, U., Wilson, P., McClelland, R.A., Gazet, J.C., Trott, P.A., Ford, H.T. 1985. Prediction of Endocrine Response in Breast Cancer by Immunocytochemical Staining of Fine Needle Aspirates. *Br J Surg* 72:991-993.

40. Greenebaum, E., Koss, L.G., Sherman, A.B., Elequin, F. 1984. Comparison of Needle Aspiration and Solid Biopsy Technics in the Flow Cytometric Study of DNA Distributions of Surgically Resected Tumors. *Am J Clin Pathol* 82:559-564.

41. Clark, G.M., McGurie, W.L. 1988. Steroid Receptors and Other Prognostic Factors in Primary Breast Cancer. *Sem Oncol* 15 (Suppl. 1):20.

42. Wilbur, D.C., Willis, J., Mooney, R.A., Fallon, M.A., Moynes, R. and di Sant'Agnese. 1992. Estrogen and Progesterone Receptor Detection in Archival Formalin-Fixed, Paraffin Embedded Tissue from Breast Carcinoma: A Comparison of Immunohistochemistry with the Dextran-Coated Charcoal Assay. *Mod Pathol* 5:79-84.

43. Ro, J., Sahin, A., Ro, J.Y., Fritsche, H., Hortobabyi, G. and Blick, M. 1990. Immunohistochemical Analysis of P-Glycoprotein Expression Correlated with Chemotherapy Resistance in Locally Advanced Breast Cancer. *Hum Pathol* 21:787-791.

44. Clark, G.M., Dressler, L.G., Owens, M.A., Pounds, G., Oldaker, T., McGuire, W.L. 1989. Prediction of Relapse or Survival in Patients with Node-Negative Breast Cancer by DNA Flow Cytometry. *New Engl and Journal of Medicine* 320:627-633.

45. Lovin, J.D., Sinton, E.B., Burke, B.J., Reddy, V.B. 1994. Stereotaxic Core Breast Biopsy: Value in Providing Tissue for Flow Cytometric Analysis. *American Journal of Radiology* 162:609-612.

Pathological Interpretation of Fine Needle Aspiration Cytology

Shahla Masood, M.D.

10

Introduction

Breast cancer continues to be a medical and social challenge and is associated with significant physical and psychological impairment. This has led to a multidisciplinary effort for early detection and better management of patients with breast cancer.

In recent years, mammography has made a significant contribution in the early diagnosis of breast cancer. The mammographic detection of in situ abnormalities and cancers less than 1 cm in size has resulted in better overall survival[1,2].

Although mammography is available to detect occult breast abnormalities, it suffers from relatively low specificity. Only up to one third of mammographically suspicious abnormalities are found to be malignant[3,4]. Thus, it is essential to obtain tissue diagnoses for all suspicious abnormalities noted at mammography[5]. These occult abnormalities, which are most amenable to cure, offer the greatest dilemma for the physician because they are nonpalpable and therefore, difficult to clinically localize for diagnostic biopsy.

Percutaneous needle localization biopsy procedure, introduced in 1974, provided a means of overcoming this problem[6]. This approach is now the most widely used method for accurately and safely sampling clinically occult breast abnormalities[1, 2, 5,7-11]. Nevertheless, the positive predictive value of mammography ranges from 14%-38%[3,4]. Many women who undergo unnecessary surgical biopsies for benign breast disease can benefit from less invasive alternatives.

Fine needle aspiration biopsy (FNAB) has proven to be a safe, accurate, and reliable diagnostic procedure in the evaluation of patients with palpable breast abnormalities[11-15]. Therefore, it is logical to assume that under appropriate radiological guidance, FNAB can be applied to the study of nonpalpable breast abnormalities.

The advantages of this modality are multiple. Women are given the opportunity to have their occult breast abnormalities examined without significant morbidity and the associated cost.

Cytomorphology of Nonpalpable Breast Abnormalities

With increasing use of screening mammography, more cases of high-risk proliferative breast disease and carcinoma in situ are being detected. This is exemplified by the incidence of ductal carcinoma in situ (DCIS). As a palpable mass, DCIS accounted for less than 3% of breast cancers[16,17]. As detected by mammography, this incidence has increased to 30%[18]. Thus, it is important to define the cytomorphology of these entities and to use the same terminology for breast FNAB that is commonly used in diagnostic histopathology, as this information has significant clinical implications[19-21].

Cytomorphology of Ductal Carcinoma In Situ (DCIS)

Cytomorphology of DCIS varies according to different histologic patterns. Aspirates from noncomedo type DCIS may present with variable cellularity, and show clusters and isolated atypical epithelial cells with no accompanying myoepithelial cells. This is in contrast with atypical

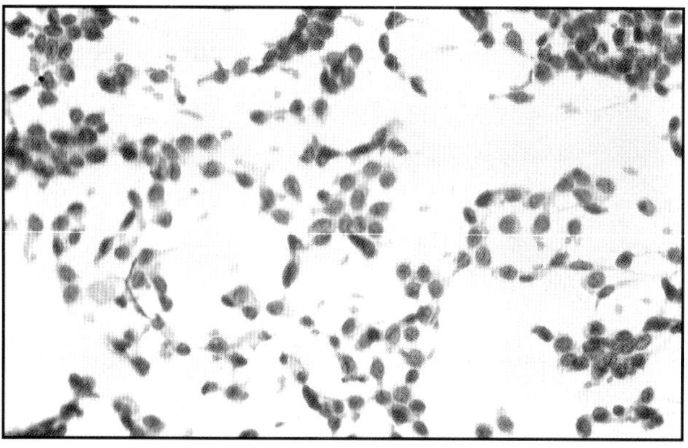

Figure 10.1. Noncomedo Carcinoma. Loosely cohesive clusters of monotonous appearing epithelial cells. Papanicolaou stain, magnification 100x.

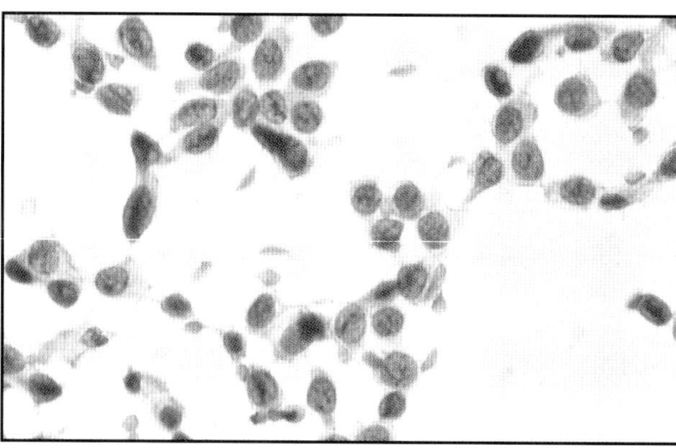

Figure 10.2. Noncomedo Carcinoma. Groups of epithelial cells forming a cribriform pattern. No myoepithelial cells are present. Papanicolaou stain, magnification 200x.

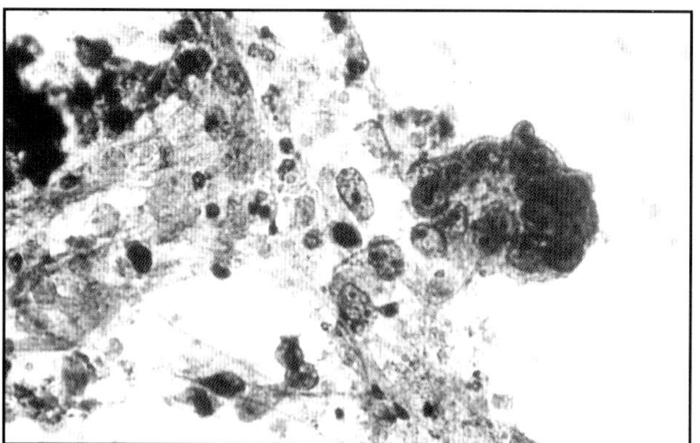

Figure 10.3. Comedocarcinoma. Clusters of highly atypical cells in a necrotic background. Papanicolaou stain, magnification 200x.

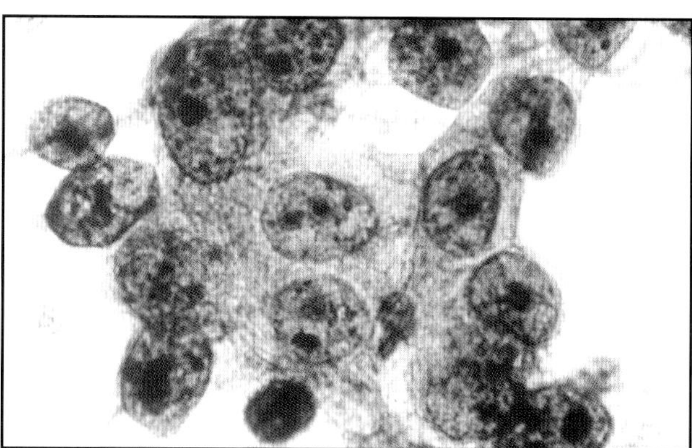

Figure 10.4. Comedocarcinoma. Pleomorphic population of neoplastic cells with evidence of individual cell necrosis. Papanicolaou stain, magnification 400x.

hyperplasia, where the myoepithelial cells appear as a part of the cellular aggregate. The cell clusters may have a solid, cribriform or papillary pattern. Microcalcified particles, foamy histiocytes, and isolated myoepithelial cells may be seen in the background **(Figures 10.1 and 10.2)**. Aspirates of comedocarcinoma are usually cellular with loosely cohesive clusters of pleomorphic populations of malignant cells in a necrotic background with individual cell necrosis and mitosis **(Figures 10.3 and 10.4).** Comedo DCIS is more likely to be diagnosed as positive on FNAB than is noncomedo DCIS. Noncomedo carcinoma, tubular carcinoma, and well-differentiated ductal carcinoma may show overlapping features with atypical ductal hyperplasia.

The features seen in in-situ breast abnormalities may also be seen in invasive carcinomas and are not exclusive. In our experience, we have not been able to define a cytomorphological criteria to distinguish in situ from invasive abnormalities. Similar observations have also been made by others[22-25].

Nevertheless, associated with specific clinical presentation and mammographic findings, it may be possible to maximize the utility of FNAB and to suggest the correct diagnosis. This includes the recognition of cytological features of mucinous, medullary, sarcomatoid, and small cell carcinomas that usually present as an invasive abnormality. Fixed nipple, skin retraction, ulceration and inflammatory carcinoma, and/or evidence of metastasis associated with neoplastic epithelial cells in breast aspirates indicate the presence of advanced carcinoma. Intracystic papillary carcinoma presents as a cystic abnormality by mammography or sonography. The aspirates are cellular and show three-dimensional cell clusters with small or large papillae and scattered single epithelial cells (**Figures 10.5 and 10.6**).

The recommended treatment for DCIS in palpable breast abnormalities is generally similar to invasive ductal carcinoma[26], so this separation may not be critical. However, this distinction becomes essential for nonpalpable breast abnormalities, as a considerable percentage of these are small, in situ, and may not require mastectomy[27]. In these circumstances, assessment of tumor invasion utilizing core or surgical biopsy is indicated.

Cytmorphology of Lobular Carcinoma In Situ (LCIS)

Lobular carcinoma in situ is often an incidental finding on the pathological study of tissue removed from palpable breast abnormalities, or by a needle localization of a mammographic abnormality[28,29]. In published series, LCIS has been found in 0.8-3.6% of breast biopsy specimens. A similar incidence has been reported for LCIS discovered by mammographic localization of nonpalpable breast abnormalities (1-2%)[30,31]. It is important to distinguish between LCIS and infiltrating lobular carcinoma (ILC), since the management of these two entities is quite different. LCIS is now considered only a marker for the subsequent development of breast cancer, with bilateral mastectomies or close observation as management. In contrast, the treatment of ILC is similar to other invasive cancers.

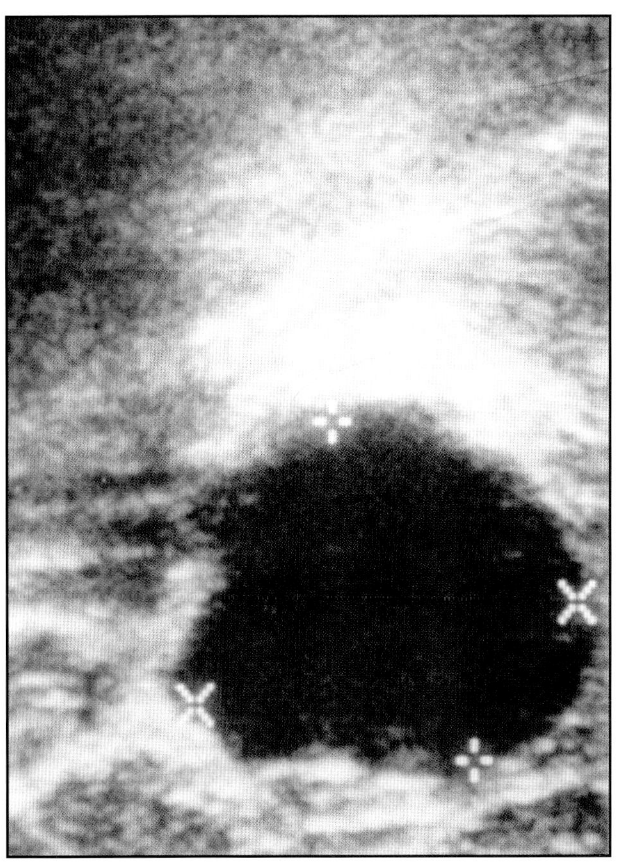

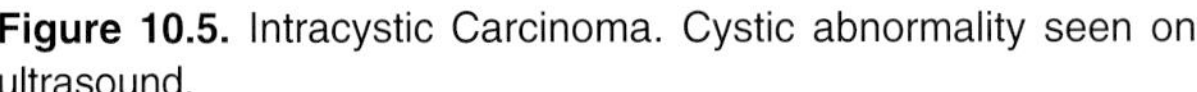

Figure 10.5. Intracystic Carcinoma. Cystic abnormality seen on ultrasound.

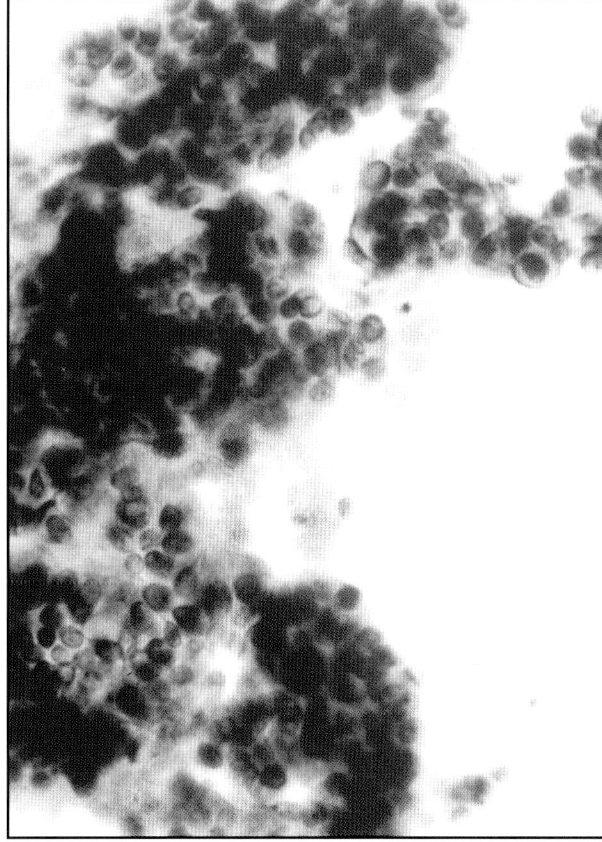

Figure 10.6. Intracystic Carcinoma. Clusters of neoplastic epithelial cells in a hemorrhagic background. Diff-Quik® stain, magnification 200x.

We are in agreement with the observation of Kline and Kline, Salhany and Page, and Sneige that the cytomorphological distinction between atypical lobular (ALH), LCIS, and infiltrating lobular carcinoma (ILC) may be difficult[32-34]. Aspirates of LCIS and ALH may show loosely cohesive groups of small uniform cells with eccentric regular nuclei and occasional intracytoplasmic lumina. The nuclei are hyperchromatic with fine chromatin clumping and occasional inconspicuous nucleoli. Occasionally, small cell groups forming "cell balls," conforming to acini of lobular neoplasia may be seen **(Figures 10.7 and 10.8)**. Aspirates of ILC show overlapping features but are more cellular and contain more atypical single cells. Characteristic cytomorphological findings in ILC include a low to moderate cell yield. The smears show a relatively uniform population of small to medium-sized cells. The cells have scanty, ill-defined cytoplasm with increased nuclear cytoplasmic ratio, and tend to occur vaguely in small groups, sometimes with a cord or "single file" arrangement. The cytoplasm may contain sharply punched out vacuoles. Occasionally, signet ring forms may be seen **(Figures 10.9 and 10.10)**.

We believe that the cellular aspirates that contain significant numbers of small uniform cells characteristic of ILC should be diagnosed accordingly, and followed by definite therapy. However, patients whose aspirates are scanty in cellularity should undergo an excisional biopsy to establish the diagnosis.

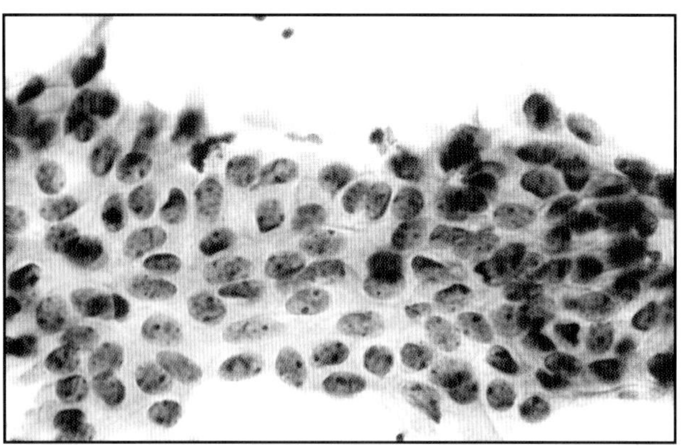

Figure 10.7. Lobular Neoplasia. Monotonous bland appearing epithelial cells. Papanicolaou stain, magnification 200x.

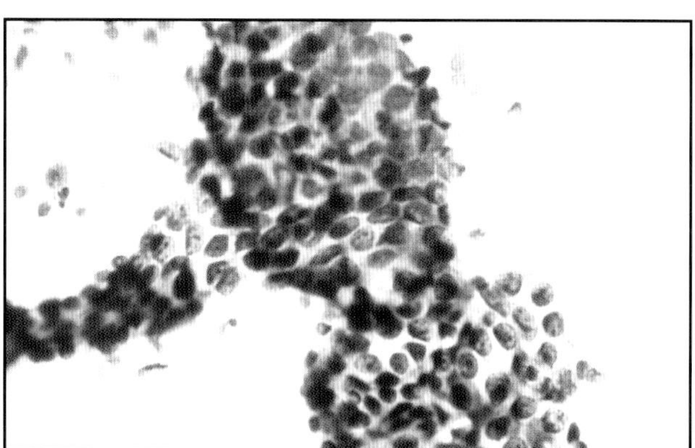

Figure 10.8. Lobular Neoplasia. "Cell balls" conforming to acini. Papanicolaou stain, magnification 200x.

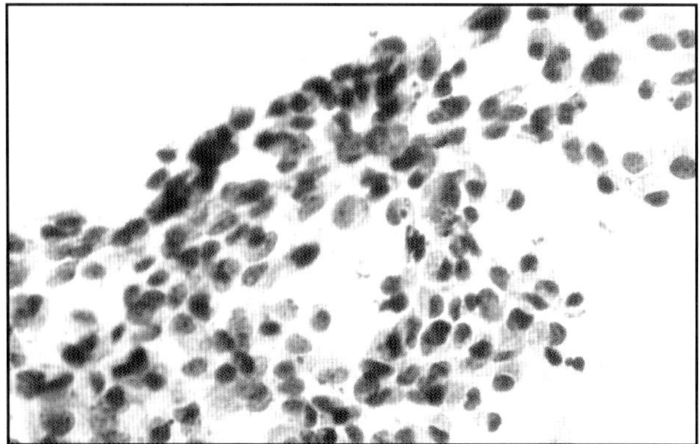

Figure 10.9. Infiltrating Lobular Carcinoma. Loosely arranged uniform-appearing epithelial cells with eccentric nuclei. Papanicolaou stain, magnification 200x.

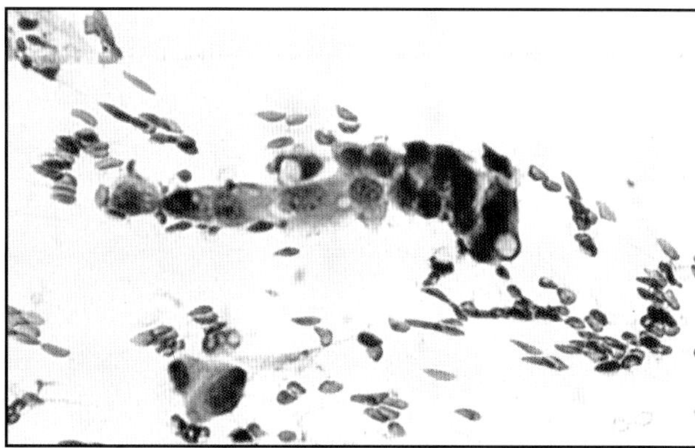

Figure 10.10. Infiltrating Lobular Carcinoma. Signet rings and chain of small cells in "single file" pattern. Papanicolaou stain, magnification 200x.

Cytomorphology of Proliferative Breast Disease (PBD)

Fibrocystic change, the most commonly diagnosed benign breast disease, reflects a spectrum of changes that range from normal physiologic alterations in the breast to proliferative changes approximating in situ carcinoma. Similarly, this spectrum of changes is associated with variable risk for subsequent development of breast cancer[19-21].The histology of these entities is already well-characterized[35-37]. The use of the same diagnostic terminology for breast fine needle aspirates would also offer a significant advantage, if it can be accurately applied.

In a prospective study utilizing mammographically directed FNAB of nonpalpable breast abnormalities, we assessed the reliability of a cytologic grading system to define the cytologic features of proliferative and nonproliferative breast disease, and to separate hyperplasia from neoplasia[38,39]. Using a cytologic grading system, we evaluated these aspirates for cellular arrangement, degree of cellular pleomorphism and anisonucleosis, presence of myoepithelial cells and nucleoli, and status of chromatin pattern (**Figure 10.11**). Based on the given range of scores to each defined entity, we found a high degree of concordance between the results of cytology and corresponding histology (**Figures 10.12 and 10.13**).

By far, the most important aspect of our study is the ability of the cytological grading system to define the continuous changes in breast abnormalities and to separate hyperplasia from neoplasia. This is also the first study to advocate the use of the same diagnostic terminology in cytology that is used in histology. Since then, this concept has been further studied and challenged by others[22, 40-45].

Nonproliferative Breast Disease

The cell yield in these aspirates is variable and depends on the nature of the abnormality. In noncystic abnormalities, the aspirate is scanty or moderate. Frequently, the aspirate consists of clusters of monotonous, small, uniform-appearing epithelial cells arranged in monolayered sheets with a honeycomb pattern. Foam cells, apocrine cells, single naked cells, and fragments of stromal cells are frequently observed. The cells have regular nuclei with fine chromatin pattern. Nucleoli are not commonly seen. Myoepithelial cells are easily identified (**Figures 10.14 and 10.15**). Occasionally, only fragments of adipose and fibrous tissue may be present. This finding is not inconsistent with benign sclerotic abnormalities of the breast.

Proliferative Breast Disease without Atypia

Proliferative breast disease differs from nonproliferative breast disease by its higher cell yield and most unique cellular arrangement. The cellularity is moderate to high, depending on the degree of proliferative epithelial changes. There are increased numbers of tightly cohesive groups of ductal epithelial and myoepithelial cells with some overriding of the nuclei, occasional loss of polarity, and some variability in the nuclear size. Micronucleoli may be seen. Cytological atypia is inconspicuous. Apocrine cells, histiocytes, and occasional naked nuclei are the accompanying cells in these aspirates (**Figures 10.16 and 10.17**).

Proliferative Breast Disease with Atypia (Atypical Hyperplasia)

The cellular aspirates are frequently rich and composed of multiple clustering of epithelial cells. The crowded clusters of cells show conspicuous loss of polarity and overriding of the nuclei. Nucleoli are present and display an irregular and coarse chromatin pattern. Variation in nuclear size and cellular pleomorphism are also present. Within the crowded atypical epithelial cells, there is morphological evidence of myoepithelial cell differentiation (**Figures 10.18 and 10.19**).

Diagnostic Dilemma

Controversy remains in the ability of cytology to diagnose different spectrum of fibrocystic change. Fibroadenoma can occasionally simulate proliferative breast disease with or without atypia or papillary abnormalities. Aside from mammographic appearance, the key to correct diagnosis is the presence of "antler horn clusters," flat monolayered sheets, and fragments of fibromyxoid stroma[46]. It should also be remembered that proliferative changes, and even cancer, can arise within a fibroadenoma, and the diagnosis of one is not always mutually exclusive of the other[47].

Radial scar, a special type of proliferative breast disease, forms an impalpable but mammographically detected abnormality that mimics cancer radiologically, grossly and microscopically[48,49]. Cytologic specimen of a radial scar is frequently obtained via a stereotactic FNAB[49,50]. The smears are cellular and contain uniform cells arranged in small groups and round or angular clusters. There is a tendency for the cells to form tubules. Branching sheets are uncommon but single cells are frequently observed. The cells have distinct cytoplasmic borders and are evenly spaced.

Cytologic Criteria Grading System for Interpretation of Mammographically Guided Fine Needle Biopsies

Cellular Arrangement	Cellular Pleomorphism	Myoepithelial Cells	Anisonucleosis	Nucleoli	Chromatin Clumping	Score
Monolayer	Absent	Many	Absent	Absent	Absent	1
Nuclear overlapping	Mild	Moderate	Mild	Micronucleoli	Rare	2
Clustering	Moderate	Few	Moderate	Micro and/or rare macro-nucleoli	Occasional	3
Loss of cohesion	Conspicuous	Absent	Conspicuous	Predominately micronucleoli	Frequent	4

From Masood, S., et al. 1990. Prospective Evaluation of Radiologically Directed Aspiration Biopsy of Nonpalpable Breast Lesions. *Cancer* 66:1480-1487. (Reproduced with permission)

Figure 10.11

Cytologic Findings Compared with Histologic Diagnosis in 100 Mammographically Suspicious Cases

Cytology	No. of Cases	Nonproliferative Breast Disease	Proliferative without Atypia	Proliferative with Atypia	Carcinoma In Situ LCIS	Carcinoma In Situ DCIS	Invasive Cancer
Insufficient	9	7	2	-	-	-	-
Nonproliferative breast disease	34	29	4	-	1*	-	-
Proliferative without atypia	17	-	15	2	-	-	-
Proliferative with atypia	23	-	-	21	1*	1*	-
Carcinoma	17	-	-	-	-	5	-
Total	100	36	21	23	2	6	12

LCIS: Lobular Carcinoma In Situ; DCIS Ductal Carcinoma In Situ.
*FALSE-NEGATIVE CYTOLOGIC INTERPRETATIONS
From Masood, S., et al. 1990. Prospective Evaluation of Radiologically Directed Aspiration Biopsy of Nonpalpable Breast Lesions. *Cancer* 66: 1480-1487. (Reproduced with permission)

Figure 10.12

Concordance Between Cytologic Evaluation vs Histologic Diagnosis in 100 Mammographically Guided Fine Needle Aspirates

Diagnosis	No. of Cases	Concordance %
Nonproliferative breast disease	29/34	85
Proliferative breast disease without atypia	15/17	88
Proliferative breast disease with atypia	21/23	91
Cancer	17/20	85

Adapted from Masood, S., et al. 1990. Prospective Evaluation of Radiologically Directed Aspiration Biopsy of Nonpalpable Breast Lesions. *Cancer* 66:1480-1487.

Figure 10.13

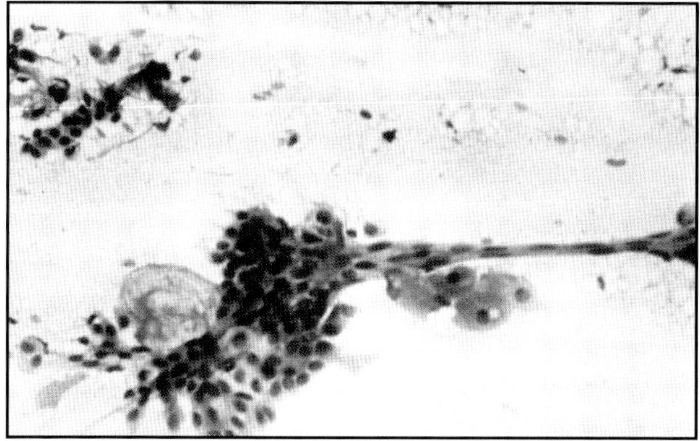

Figure 10.14. Nonproliferative Breast Disease. Scanty cellular smear with cluster of epithelial cells with a few apocrine cells. Papanicolaou stain, magnification 100x.

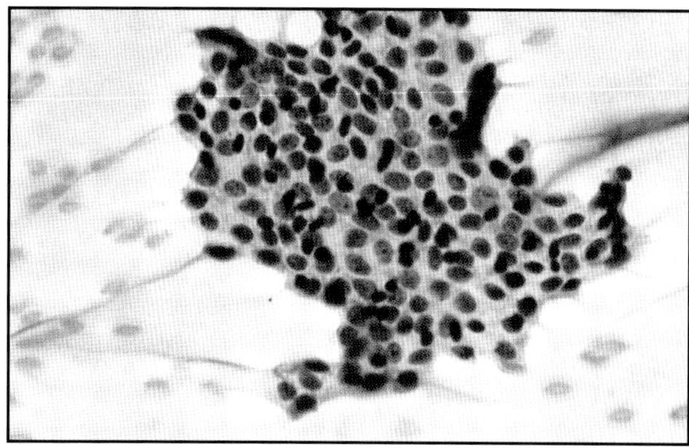

Figure 10.15. Nonproliferative Breast Disease. Monolayered appearance of ductal epithelial cells. Papanicolaou stain, magnification 200x.

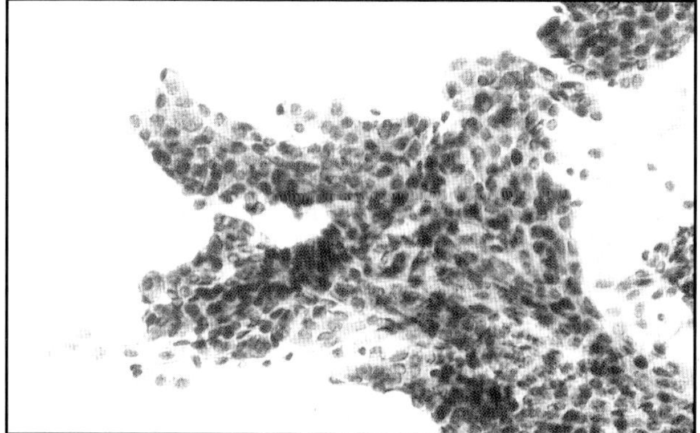

Figure 10.16. Proliferative Breast Disease without Atypia. Cellular smear with clustering of epithelial cells. Papanicolaou stain, magnification 200x.

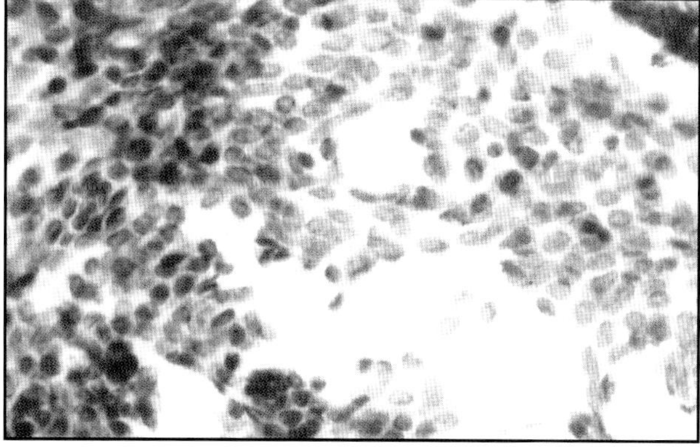

Figure 10.17. Proliferative Breast Disease without Atypia. Crowded epithelial cells with overriding of the nuclei, demonstrating hyperplastic ductal cells and smaller, darker myoepithelial cells. Papanicolaou stain, magnification 200x.

Cytologic differential diagnosis includes low-grade neoplasms, such as noncomedo ductal carcinoma in situ, and lobular and tubular carcinoma. Familiarity of the cytopathologist with the cytomorphology of radial scar may prevent overdiagnosis of malignancy in the stereotactic FNAB specimen. Rare occurrence of carcinoma within a radial scar justifies confirmatory excisional biopsy when, cytologically, the possibility of this diagnosis is entertained.

Atypical Hyperplasia Versus Neoplasia

Atypical hyperplasia presents a diagnostic challenge for cytopathologists. This entity defines a noninfiltrating breast abnormality with some, but not all, of the features of cancer. Thus, atypical hyperplasia occupies an intermediate position between benign and malignant abnormalities. There are already substantial degrees of subjectivity and disagreement in making this diagnosis histologically[51-53]. Therefore, it is reasonable to expect some difficulty in cytologically differentiating this from carcinoma or benign changes without atypia. Such differentiation, however, is important in terms of the different clinical management each of these diagnoses entails.

Using our cytologic grading system, we have been able to prospectively identify 21 out of 23 histologically proven atypical hyperplasia in 100 nonpalpable breast abnormalities (concordance 91%). In a follow-up study challenging our cytologic grading system in 146 cases of palpable breast abnormalities, there were two noncomedo carcinoma in situ, one infiltrating lobular carcinoma, and two infiltrating ductal carcinoma that were misinterpreted as atypical hyperplasia. Thus, difficulty remains in the differentiation between atypical hyperplasia and low-grade neoplasms, such as well-differentiated ductal carcinomas, lobular and tubular carcinoma, and noncomedo ductal cell carcinoma.

Presently, most investigators advocate an intraoperative consultation, or an excisional biopsy, for any case diagnosed as atypical hyperplasia, suspicious, or inconclusive for carcinoma[22,41,42]. Regardless of the experience and the promising reports in the literature defining the cytomorphology, we need to recognize some of the limitations of FNAB in the study of breast disease. This may not necessarily be the result of our inability to recognize different entities. The presence of heterogeneity of individual abnormalities is an important factor to be considered. As an example, in a study conducted by Lennington et al. in 1994[54], the authors reviewed 100 sequentially collected ductal carcinoma in situ cases from a consultation practice. Recognizing the bias of such a series toward exclusion of easily recognizable comedocarcinoma, the authors studied the spectrum of mixed pattern abnormalities to identify variations and common features in the architectural arrangement of the various histologic patterns. Interestingly, atypical ductal hyperplasias were intermixed in 17 cases of ductal carcinoma in situ. Mixed patterns of comedo and noncomedo type ductal carcinoma in situ were seen in 33 cases. In all cases of combined atypical ductal hyperplasia and ductal carcinoma in situ, the more advanced patterns of ductal carcinoma in situ were seen in the central portion of the abnormality, while the atypical ductal hyperplasia components were arranged peripherally. Thus, the presence

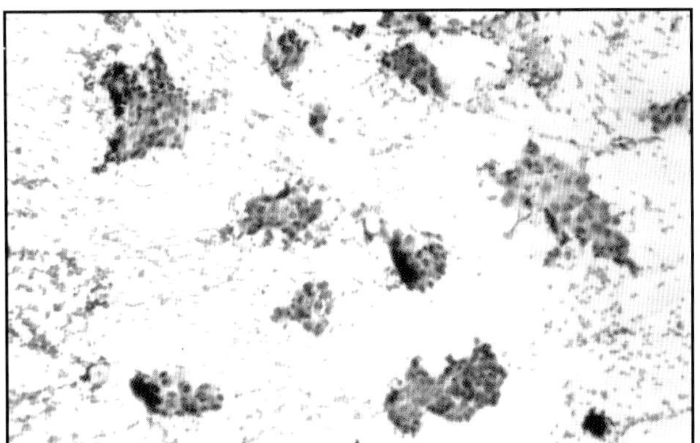

Figure 10.18. Proliferative Breast Disease with Atypia (Atypical Hyperplasia). Cellular smear with crowded clustering epithelial cells. Papanicolaou stain, magnification 100x.

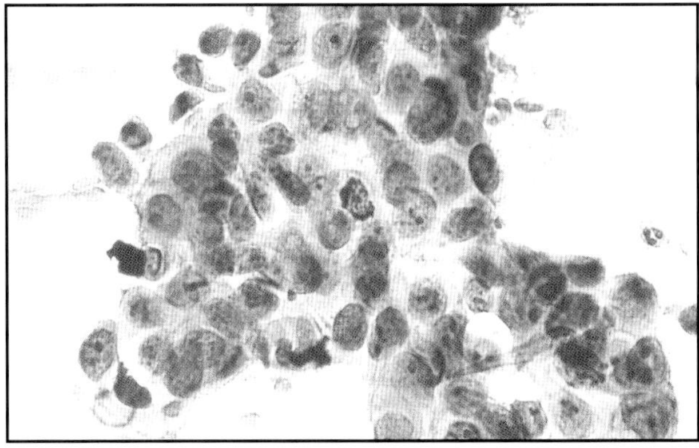

Figure 10.19. Proliferative Breast Disease with Atypia (Atypical Hyperplasia). Cluster of epithelial cells with overriding of the nuclei and cytological atypia. Myoepithelial cells are still seen within the cellular aggregate. Papanicolaou stain, magnification 400x.

of different patterns of ductal carcinoma in situ within individual abnormalities (46 out of 100), and the coexistence of atypical ductal hyperplasia and ductal carcinoma in situ (17 out of 100), strongly support the presence of heterogeneity within an abnormality.

Similarly, if adequately sampled, the spectrum of morphological alterations of fibrocystic change, proliferative breast disease, and atypical hyperplasia are commonly seen in association with carcinoma in situ and/or invasive breast abnormalities. Multiple sampling of a breast abnormality by FNAB may overcome the problem of heterogeneity of individual abnormalities to some extent. However, this remains a limiting factor in interpretation of FNAB and consequently in further management of patients, particularly in palpable breast abnormalities.

Aside from morphology, attempts have been made to utilize ancillary studies to distinguish between atypical hyperplasia and carcinoma in situ. We had already utilized cell image analysis to assess the DNA ploidy pattern of our breast fine needle aspirates to differentiate between atypia and neoplasia. Although the frequency of aneuploidy was higher in carcinoma (59%), the presence of aneuploidy in 28% of the cases of atypical ductal hyperplasia limited the use of this technology. Similar experiences reported by others concluded that DNA analysis and/or nuclear measurements do not provide or substantiate evidence to differentiate between atypical hyperplasia and carcinoma[55-57].

It was also intriguing to speculate that the study of oncogene expression may aid in the differentiation between atypical hyperplasia and carcinoma in situ. We used standard immunocytochemistry to assess the pattern of expression of HER-2/neu oncogene in 65 invasive carcinoma, 36 ductal carcinoma in situ, and 32 atypical ductal hyperplasia. Positive immunostaining for HER-2/neu oncogene was observed in 43% (28/65) of invasive carcinoma, 38% (14/36) of carcinoma in situ, and 12% (4/32) of atypical hyperplasia. Naturally, this finding discourages the use of oncogene study as an adjunct to differentiate hyperplasia from neoplasia[58]. Therefore, based on these observations, morphology still remains an important diagnostic tool.

Aside from the persistence of clustering and cellular cohesion, and the absence of significant numbers of isolated single cells, we believe that the presence of myoepithelial cells within the clusters of atypical cells in a breast aspirate is a significant finding that can separate hyperplasia from neoplasia. We have already demonstrated the value of muscle specific actin (MSA) in differentiation between atypical hyperplasia and carcinoma in situ in surgical cases[59]. In these studies, MSA was found to be a specific marker for detecting myoepithelial cells.

Based on these findings, we have assessed the feasibility of the use of MSA as a marker for myoepithelial cells in aspirated smears and cell block preparations obtained from breast fine needle aspirates[60,61]. The observed staining of myoepithelial cells in benign and high-risk proliferative breast disease can be used as a strong differentiating feature in interpretation of atypical breast fine needle aspirates. This will potentially maximize the diagnostic accuracy of fine needle aspiration biopsies and help to reduce the number of inconclusive cytologic diagnoses.

Reporting and Management

The results of breast fine needle aspirates of nonpalpable breast abnormalities are reported as insufficient, negative, inconclusive (suspicious), or positive for malignancy. The importance of intermediate levels of suspicion beyond simple distinctions of benign and malignancy has been well-demonstrated to improve diagnostic accuracy and reduce false-negative rates[62].

In situations where there is no, or minimal, cellular material, repeat aspiration or excisional biopsy is recommended. The criteria for adequacy of cytologic specimens varies in different institutions. Dowlatshahi et al. recommended the presence of more than six epithelial clusters of more than 10 cells each to be considered sufficient sample[63]. Layfield et al. considered aspirates as sufficient when no less than 25 epithelial cells were present per slide[64].

Smears containing adequate numbers of well-preserved benign cells are reported as negative. Further follow-up of a patient with a nonpalpable breast abnormality and negative FNAB depends on the extent of the mammographic abnormality seen in that patient. Abnormal mammograms depicting either soft tissue masses or microcalcifications may be classified as having a high, intermediate, or low index of suspicion for malignancy. A *highly suspicious abnormality* is usually seen as: a) a solid soft-tissue mass having highly irregular or stellate borders, or b) fine needle-like and linear branching microcalcifications, either clustered or scattered, c) extremely polymorphic clustered microcalcifications, or d) an irregularly marginated solid mass containing suspicious or indeterminate microcalcification. An *intermediate abnormality* is regarded as a solid, soft-tissue mass with partially irregular or obscured borders, or indeterminate microcalcification. A *low suspicious abnor-*

mality is characterized by a 0.5-1.5 cm well-defined mass, a 1-2 cm asymmetric opacity, and a regular and uniform clustered microcalcification[65].

Considering the current increasing liability exposure in the United States, it is advisable to recommend needle localization and open biopsy for mammographically high or intermediate-risk abnormalities, despite a negative fine needle aspiration biopsy result.

An asymptomatic woman whose screening mammogram reveals a low-risk abnormality and whose fine needle aspiration cytology shows no evidence of malignancy may undergo interval mammography within 6-12 months. This strategy is based on the fact that the likelihood of malignancy ranges from 10% in asymmetric parenchymal densities and moderately suspicious microcalcifications to 50-70% for stellate mass and branching microcalcifications[66]. Furthermore, in a well-conducted study in 1991, Sickles[67] reported that patients with a low degree of abnormality in their mammogram may be safely followed with interval mammography. Similarly, Hann et al. suggested that negative cytologic findings in an abnormality with a low suspicion at mammography may be reassuring. In their series, they showed that the predictive value for low-suspicion abnormality with negative cytologic findings was 100%[68].

Breast fine needle aspirates that show cells with significant cytologic atypia, but not conclusive for malignancy, are reported as inconclusive or suspicious. These cases require excisional biopsy and an intraoperative frozen section consultation to establish the final diagnosis.

Aspirates that show conclusive evidence of malignancy are reported as "positive." This diagnosis justifies proceeding directly to definitive therapy without frozen section confirmation, unless the mammographic findings or other clinical factors are not in agreement with the positive FNAB result. In such cases, confirmation of malignancy by an intraoperative consultation diagnosis is recommended prior to definite treatment. It cannot be overemphasized that in management of patients with nonpalpable breast abnormalities, the results of the FNAB procedure should always be complemented by the mammographic findings.

Summary

Fine needle aspiration biopsy can be a potentially effective means of sampling nonpalpable breast abnormalities. Review of the literature with analysis of data on 3,000 cases of FNAB of nonpalpable breast abnormalities with histologic follow-up has demonstrated that the results are comparable to FNAB of palpable breast abnormalities. FNAB of palpable abnormalities has shown a sensitivity of 72-99% (average 87%) for detection of breast cancer. FNAB of nonpalpable abnormalities has shown a sensitivity of 82-100% (average 96%)[69].

The reported false negative rate for FNAB of nonpalpable breast abnormalities ranges from 0-32%[70-72]. This may be due to poor localization technique, small abnormalities (5 mm), and firm masses that may have deflected the needle. Failure due to a missed target, such as a mobile mass or a fibroadenoma, may occasionally occur with SBB.

Sampling error may occur when malignancy is not associated with the abnormality seen on the mammogram. Foci of lobular carcinoma in situ are common incidental findings in tissue adjacent to but not within the abnormality for which the biopsy is performed[38,73-75]. Lobular carcinoma in situ constitutes a major source of false negative cases of FNAB of nonpalpable breast abnormalities, also due to a bland cellular pattern that can be confused with benign breast abnormalities[76]. In situ carcinomas cannot be reliably diagnosed by FNAB in view of the necessity of examining the entire histologic architecture to exclude invasion[76,22,38].

Breast abnormalities may have a complex structure comprising benign as well as malignant components. Aspiration of such an abnormality leads to a cellular yield that may represent the benign part of the abnormality and result in a false negative diagnosis. Thus, the management of patients with nonpalpable breast abnormalities should be based on the combined findings of cytologic study and mammography.

Reported false-positive rates in nonpalpable breast abnormalities varies from 0-6%[25,38,66,68,77-81]. This is usually due to misinterpretation of atypical abnormalities, such as proliferative breast disease, sclerosing adenosis, duct ectasia with inflammation, and intraductal hyperplasia. Naturally, false-positive cases must be minimized by more objective and reproducible interpretation methods, if this technique is to achieve its optimal potential.

Smears from the nonpalpable abnormalities are often of low cellularity[25,68]. This may lead to an impression of benignity or inadequacy and ultimately result in a misdiagnosis. The relatively scant cellularity in occult abnormalities can be related to the size of the abnormality and the aspiration technique. In a large palpable mass, the aspiration needle is easily directed into multiple directions, which leads to obtaining a representative sample. This, however, is more difficult in a small nonpalpable abnormality. The rigid fixation of the aspirating needle will also compound this problem. It is also important to recognize that a certain percentage of cases will always be inadequate, regardless of the type of localizing device. Hann et al.[68] found that 40% of their inadequate cases were from fibrotic and hypocellular abnormalities from which a low cellular yield would be anticipated. The histologic type and the nature of the abnormality also play an important role in a diagnostic yield. Usually, tumors representing medullary, mucinous, and comedocarcinomas are more cellular than infiltrating lobular and scirrhous ductal carcinomas. Benign abnormalities such as sclerosing adenosis and hyalinized fibroadenoma may be associated with a low yield[72].

The rate of insufficient samples in palpable breast abnormalities ranges between 4-13%. In contrast, FNAB of nonpalpable breast abnormalities has shown an insufficient rate of 2-36%. Thus, it appears that FNAB of occult breast abnormalities carries a higher rate of insufficient samples than FNAB of palpable breast abnormalities[45,69]. This limitation has resulted in the increasing use of stereotactic localization and the acquisition of core biopsy specimen with larger (14-gauge) cutting needles[82].

Reports in radiology literature have shown a reduction in the number of insufficient cases by the use of stereotactic core biopsy. However, the superiority of core biopsy versus FNAB in nonpalpable breast abnormalities is not yet established. In a well-designed study, Dowlatshahi et al. suggested that the needle core biopsy and FNAB cytology may complement each other in the diagnosis of nonpalpable breast abnormalities[83]. Others advocate the "long-throw" biopsy gun, using a 14-gauge needle and multiple passes (8-10 samples) as the preferred modality. In one study, the reported diagnostic accuracy between stereotactic core biopsy and surgical biopsy was 96%[84].

Despite these reports, confusion remains in the choice of needle for sampling of occult breast abnormalities. The FNAB procedure suffers from a high rate of insufficient samples, a high false-negative rate, and an inability to distinguish between in situ and infiltrating abnormalities. Core needle biopsy also has important shortcomings. This includes extensive tissue damage by the recommended multiple passes and the use of a 14-gauge needle. There is also a practical limitation to the long-throw mechanized core biopsy needle. It cannot be used in relatively small breasted women with a compressed thickness less than approximately 4 cm, since the needle will hit the opposite skin and film holder and bend. Furthermore, the core needle biopsy is unlikely to allow confirmation of an in situ abnormality. In situ abnormalities diagnosed by means of core needle biopsy may subsequently show invasion at follow-up lumpectomy.

Further well-designed, controlled studies are required to assess the diagnostic value of FNAB and stereotactic core biopsy in nonpalpable breast abnormalities. It should be recognized that the visibility and participation of cytopathologists in multidisciplinary investigations are the key to the success of FNAB techniques. It is important that cytopathologists play an active role in fostering the merits of FNAB. This will only be accomplished by increasing our technical skill and diagnostic ability. We also need to be aware of medicolegal implications and the marketing power of automated stereotactic core biopsy, which naturally influences the practice of medicine in this country.

Overall, to avoid the demise of FNAB in the evolution of nonpalpable breast abnormalities, a concerted effort is necessary among interested cytopathologists to enhance the clinical usefulness of FNAB. Combining the merits and pitfalls of the techniques of FNAB and core needle biopsy may also be an alternative means to increase the overall sensitivity of these procedures and to eliminate the need for surgical biopsy.

References

1. Azavedo, E., Fallenius, A., Svane, G., Auer, G. 1990. Nuclear DNA Content, Histological Grade and Clinical Course in Patients with Nonpalpable Mammographically Detected Breast Adenocarcinoma. *Am J Clin Oncol* 13(1):23-27.

2. Werlheimer, M.D., Castanza, M.E., Dodson, T.F., D'Ars, C., Pastides, H., Zapka, J.G. 1986. Increasing the Effort Toward Breast Cancer Detection. *JAMA* 255:1131-1315.

3. Marrujo, G., Jolly, P.C., Hall, M.H. 1986. Nonpalpable Breast Cancer: Needle Localized Biopsy for Diagnosis and Consideration for Treatment. *Am J Surg* 151:599-602.

4. Hermann, G., Janns, C., Schwartz, I.S., Krivisky, B., Bier, S., Rabinowitz, J.G. 1987. Nonpalpable Breast Lesions. Accuracy of Prebiopsy Mammographic Localization. *Radiology* 165:323-326.

5. Hall, W.C., Aust, J.B., Gaskill, H.V., Polter, J.M., Flournay, J.G., Cruz, A.B. 1986. Evaluation of Nonpalpable Breast Lesions: Experience in a Training Institution. *Am J Surg* 151:467-496.

6. Threatt, B., Appelman, H., Dow, R., O'Rourke, J. 1974. Percutaneous Localization of Clustered Mammary Microcalcifications Prior to Biopsy. *Am J Roentgenol* 121:839-842.

7. Seymour, E.Q., Stanley, J.H. 1985. The Current Status of Breast Imaging. *Am Surg* 51:591-595.

8. Poole, G.V., Chaplin, R.H., Sterch, J.M., Leinbach, L.B., Myers, R.T. 1986. Occult Lesions of the Breast. *Surg Gyn Obstet* 163:107-110.

9. Proudfoot, R.W., Mattingly, S.S., Selling, C.B., Fine, J.G. 1986. Nonpalpable Breast Lesions: Wire Localization and Excisional Biopsy. *Am Surg* 52:117-122.

10. Lefor, A.J., Numann, P.J., Levinsohn, E.M. 1984. Needle Localization of Occult Breast Lesions. *Am J Surg* 148:270-274.

11. Kline, T.S. 1988. Breast In: *Handbook of Fine Needle Aspiration Biopsy Cytology,* 2nd edition New York: Churchill Livingstone 199-252.

12. Frable, W.J. 1984. Needle Aspiration Biopsy of the Breast. *Cancer* 53:671-676.

13. Frable, W.J. 1989. Needle Aspiration Biopsy: Past, Present and Future. *Hum Pathol* 20:504-51.

14. Feldman, P.S., Covell, J.L. 1985. Fine Needle Aspiration Cytology and Its Clinical Applications: Breast and Lung. Chicago: American Society of Clinical Pathologists Press 27-118.

15. Linsk, J.A., Franzen, S. 1983. *Clinical Application Cytology.* Philadelphia: J.B. Lippincott.

16. Rosen, P.P., Braun, D.W., Kinne, D.E. 1980. The Clinical Significance of Preinvasive Breast Carcinoma. *Cancer* 46:919-925.

17. Smart, C.R., Meyers, M.H., Gloeckler, L.A. 1978. Implications from SEER Data on Breast Cancer Management. *Cancer* 41:787-789.

18. Silverstein, M.J., Gamagami, P., Roser, R.J., et al. 1987. Hooked-Wire Directed Breast Biopsy and Overpenetrated Mammography. *Cancer* 59:715-722.

19. Bach, M.M., Barclay, T.H.C., Cutler, S.J., Hankey, B.F., Asive, A.J. 1972. Association of Atypical Characteristics of Benign Breast Lesions with Subsequent Risk of Breast Cancer. *Cancer* 29:338-343.

20. Page, D.L. 1986. Cancer Risk Assessment in Benign Breast Biopsies. *Hum Pathol* 17:871-878.

21. Dupont, W.D., Page, D.L. 1985. Risk Factors for Breast Cancer in Women with Proliferative Breast Disease. *New England Journal of Medicine* 312:136-141.

22. Silverman, J., Masood, S., Ducatman, B.S., Wang, H., Sneige, N. 1993. Can FNA Biopsy Separate Atypical Hyperplasia, Carcinoma In Situ, and Invasive Carcinoma of the Breast? Cytomorphologic Criteria and Limitations in Diagnosis. *Diagn Cytopathol* 9(6):713-728.

23. Wang, H.H., Ducatman, B.S., Eich, D. 1991. Comparative Features of Ductal Carcinoma In Situ and Infiltrating Ductal Carcinoma of the Breast on Fine Needle Aspiration Biopsy. *Am J Clin Pathol* 96:654-659.

24. Dizura, B.R., Bonfiglio, T.A. 1979. Needle Cytology of the Breast. *Acta Cytol* 23:32-340.

25. Bibbo, M., Scheiber, M., Cajulis, R., Keebler, C.M., Wied, G.L., Dowlatshahi, K. 1988. Stereotaxic Fine Needle Aspiration Cytology of Occult Malignant and Premalignant Breast Lesions. *Acta Cytol* 32:193-201.

26. Swain, S.M. 1992. Ductal Carcinoma In Situ. *Cancer Invest* 10:443-454.

27. Bradley, S.J., Weaver, D.W., Bouwman, D.L. 1990. Alternatives in the Surgical Management of In Situ Breast Cancer. A Meta-Analysis of Outcome. *Ann Surg* 56:428-432.

28. Rosen, P.P., Lieberman, P.H., Braun, D.W., Kosloff, M.S., Adair, F. 1978. Lobular Carcinoma In Situ of the Breast. *Am J Surg Pathol* 2:225-250.

29. Anderson, J.A. 1974. Lobular Carcinoma In Situ: A Long Term Follow-up in 52 Cases. *Acta Pathol Microbiol Scan (A)* 82:519.

30. Meyers, J., Kopans, P.E., Stomper, P.C., Lindfors, K.K. 1984. Occult Breast Abnormalities: Percutaneous Preoperative Needle Localization. *Radiology* 150:333-337.

31. Rosenberg, A.L., Schwartz, G.F., Feig, S.A., Patchefsky, A.S. 1987. Clinically Occult Breast Lesions: Localization and Significance. *Radiology* 162:167-170.

32. Kline, T.S., Kline, I.K. 1989. High Risk Lesion In: *Guides to Clinical Aspiration Biopsy.* New York: Igaku-Shoin 235-248.

33. Salhany, K., Page, D.L. 1989. Fine Needle Aspiration of Mammary Lobular Carcinoma In Situ and Atypical Lobular Hyperplasia. *Am J Clin Pathol* 92:22-26.

34. Sneige, N. 1992. Current Issues in Fine Needle Aspiration of the Breast: Cytologic Features of In Situ Lobular and Ductal Carcinomas and Clinical Implications of Nuclear Grading. *Cytopathology Annual,* edited by W. Schmidt 155-171.

35. Azzopardi, J.G. 1983. Benign and Malignant Proliferative Epithelial Lesions of the Breast: A Review. *Eur J Cancer Clin Oncol* 19(2):1717-1720.

36. Wellings, S.R. 1980. Development of Human Breast Cancer. *Adv Cancer Res* 31:287-314.

37. Ashikari, R., Huros, A.G., Snyder, R.E., et al. 1974. A Clinicopathologic Study of Atypical Lesions of the Breast. *Cancer* 33:310-317.

38. Masood, S., Frykberg, E.R., McLellan, G.L., Scalapino, M.C., Mitchum, D.G., Bullard, J.B. 1990. Prospective Evaluation of Radiologically Detected Fine Needle Aspiration Biopsy of Nonpalpable Breast Lesions. *Cancer* 66:1480-1487.

39. Masood, S., Frykberg, E.R., McLellan, G.L., Dee, S., Bullard, J.B. 1991. Cytologic Differentiation Between Proliferative and Nonproliferative Breast Disease in Mammographically Guided Fine Needle Aspirates. *Diagn Cytopathol* 7:581-590.

40. Abendroth, C.S., Wang, H.H., Ducatman, B.S. 1991. Comparative Features of Carcinoma In Situ and Atypical Ductal Hyperplasia of the Breast on Fine Needle Aspiration Biopsy. *Am J Clin Pathol* 96:654-659.

41. Shiels, L.A., Mulford, D., Dawson, A.G. 1993. Cytomorphology of Proliferative Breast Disease. *Acta Cytol* 37(5):768(12)A.

42. Stanley, M.W., Henry-Stanley, M.J., Zera, R. 1991. Prospective Study of High Risk Proliferative Lesions of Breast Duct Epithelium by Fine Needle Aspiration. *Acta Cytol* 35(5):611(36)A .

43. Sneige, N., Staerkel, G.A. 1994. Fine Needle Aspiration Cytology of Ductal Hyperplasia with and without Atypia and Ductal Carcinoma In Situ. *Hum Pathol* 25:485-492.

44. Maygarden, S.J., Novotny, D.B., Johnson, D.E., Frable, W.J. 1994. Subclassification of Benign Breast Disease by Fine Needle Aspiration Cytology: Comparison of Cytologic and Histologic Findings in 265 Palpable Breast Masses. *Acta Cytol* 38:115-129.

45. Masood, S. 1993. Occult Breast Lesions and Aspiration Biopsy: A New Challenge. *Diagn Cytopathol* 9:611-612.

46. Bottles, K., Chan, J.S., Holly, E.A., Chin, S.H., Miller, J.R. 1988. Cytologic Criteria for Fibroadenoma. A Stepwise Logistic Regression Analysis. *Am J Clin Pathol* 89:707-713.

47. Gupta, R.K., Simpson, R.J. 1991. Carcinoma of the Breast in a Fibroadenoma: Diagnosis by Fine Needle Aspiration Cytology. *Diagn Cytol* 7(1):61-62.

48. Fenoglio, C., Lattes, R. 1974. Sclerosing Papillary Proliferations in the Female Breast. A Benign Lesion Often Mistaken for Carcinoma. *Cancer* 33:691-700.

49. Vazquez, M.F., Mitnik, J., Waisman, J., Harris, M.N., Ross, D.F. 1991. Stereotaxic Aspiration of Radial Scars. *Acta Cytol* 35(5):584(A3).

50. Frierson, H.J., Iezzoni, J.C., Covell, J.L. 1993. Stereotaxic Fine Needle Aspiration Cytology of Radial Scars. *Acta Cytol* 37(5):814(A90).

51. Beck, J.S. 1985. Observer Variability in Reporting Breast Lesions. *J Clin Pathol* 38:1358-1365.

52. Rosai, J. 1991. Borderline Epithelial Lesions of the Breast. *Am J Surg Pathol* 15:209-221.

53. Scnitt, S.J., Connolly, J.L., Tavassoli, F.A., Fechner, R.E., Kempson. R.L., Gelman, R., Page, D.L. 1992. Intraobserver Reproducibility in the Diagnosis of Ductal Proliferative Breast Lesions Using Standardized Criteria. *Am J Surg Pathol* 16:1133-1143.

54. Lennington, W.J., Jensen, R.A., Dalton, L.W., Page, D.L. 1994. Ductal Carcinoma In Situ of the Breast: Heterogeneity of Individual Lesions. *Cancer* 73:118-124.

55. Crissman, J.D., Visscher, D.W., Kubus, J. 1990. Image Cytophotometric DNA Analysis of Atypical Hyperplasia and Intraductal Carcinomas of the Breast. *Arch Pathol Lab Med* 114:1249-1253.

56. Teplitz, R.L., Butler, B.B., Tesluk, H., et al. 1990. Quantitative DNA Patterns in Human Preneoplastic Breast Lesions. *Anal Quant Cytol Histol* 12:98-102.

57. Norris, H.J., Bahr, G.F., Mikel, U.V. 1988. A Comparative Morphometric and Cytophotometric Study of Intraductal Hyperplasia and Intraductal Carcinoma of the Breast. *Anal Quant Cytol Histol* 10:1-9.

58. Masood, S. 1991. HER-2/neu Oncogene Expression in Atypical Ductal Hyperplasia, Carcinoma In Situ and Invasive Breast Cancer. *Modern Pathol* 4(1):12A.

59. Masood, S., Sim, S.J., Lu, L. 1992. Immunohistochemical Differentiation of Atypical Hyperplasia Versus Carcinoma In Situ of the Breast. *Cancer Detection and Prevention* 16(4):225-235.

60. Masood, S., Lu, L., Assaf-Munasifi, N., McCaulley, K. 1995. Myoepithelial Cells in Breast Fine Needle Aspirates: Use of Immunostaining for Muscle Specific Actin as Diagnostic Adjunct. *Diagn Cytopath* (In Press).

61. Masood, S. The Value of Muscle Specific Actin Immunostaining in Differentiation Between Atypical Hyperplasia and Carcinoma in Breast Fine Needle Aspirates. Presented at the 1994 42nd Annual American Society of Cytology Meeting, Chicago.

62. Casey, T.T., Rodgers, W.H., Baxter, W.J., Sawyers, J.L., Page, D.L. 1992. Stratified Diagnostic Approach to Fine Needle Aspiration of the Breast. *The American Journal of Surgery* 163:305-311.

63. Dowlatshahi, K., Jokich, P.M., Schmidt, R., Bibbo, M., Dawson, P.J. 1987. Cytologic Diagnosis of Occult Breast Lesions Using Stereotaxic Needle Aspiration. *Arch Surg* 122:1343-1346.

64. Layfield, L., Parkinson, B., Wong, J., Guiliano, A.E., Bassett, L.W. 1991. Mammographically Guided Fine Needle Aspiration Biopsy of Nonpalpable Breast Lesions. Can it Replace Open Biopsy? *Cancer* 68:2007-2011.

65. Dowlatshahi, K., Gent, H.J., Schmidt, R., Jokick, P.M., Bibbo, M., Sprenger, E. 1989. Nonpalpable Breast Tumors: Diagnosis with Stereotaxic Localization and Fine Needle Aspiration. *Radiology* 170:427-433.

66. Ciatto, S., Cataliotti, L., Distante, V. 1987. Nonpalpable Lesions Detected with Mammography: Review of 512 Consecutive Cases. *Radiology* 165:99-102.

67. Sickles, E.A. 1991. Periodic Mammographic Follow-up of Probably Benign Lesion Results in 3,784 Consecutive Cases. *Radiology* 179:463-468.

68. Hann, L., Ducatman, B.S., Wang, H.H., Fein, V., McIntire, J.M. 1989. Nonpalpable Breast Lesions: Evaluation by Means of Fine Needle Aspiration Cytology. *Radiology* 171:373-376.

69. Masood, S. 1994. Fine Needle Aspiration Biopsy of Nonpalpable Breast Lesions. In: *Cytopathology Annual* 1993, edited by W. Schmidt, Baltimore: Williams and Wilkins Publications.

70. Lofgren, M., Andersson, I., Bondenson, L., Lindholm, K. 1988. X-ray Guided Fine Needle Aspiration for the Cytologic Diagnosis of Nonpalpable Breast Lesions. *Cancer* 61:1032-1037.

71. Svane, G., Silfversward, C. 1983. Stereotaxic Needle Biopsy of Nonpalpable Breast Besions: Cytologic and Histologic Findings. *Acta Radial* [Diagn](Stockh) 24:283-288.

72. Hall, F.M., Sotrella, J.M., Silverstone, D.Z., Wyshak, G. 1988. Nonpalpable Breast Lesions: Recommendation for Biopsy Based on Suspicion of Carcinoma at Mammography. *Radiology* 167:252-258.

73. Schwartz, G.F., Feig, S.A., Patchefsky, A.S. 1988. Significance and Staging of Nonpalpable Carcinomas of the Breast. *Surg Gynecol Obstet* 166:6-10.

74. Fisher, E.R., Fisher, B. 1988. Lobular Carcinoma of the Breast: An Overview. *Am Surg* 185:377-385.

75. Gent, H.J., Sprenger, E., Dowlatshahi, K. 1986. Stereotaxic Needle Localization and Cytological Diagnosis of Occult Breast Lesions. *Ann Surg* 204:580-584.

76. Sneige, N., Fornage, B., Salch, G. 1994. Ultrasound Guided Fine Needle Aspiration of Nonpalpable Breast Lesions. Cytologic and Histologic Findings. *Am J Clin Pathol* 102:98-101.

77. Helvie, M.A., Baker, D.E., Adler, D.D., Anderson, I., Naylor, B., Backwalter, K.A. 1990. Radiographically Guided Fine Needle Aspiration of Nonpalpable Breast Lesions. *Radiology* 174:657-61.

78. Arishita, G.I., Cruz, B.K., Harding, C.L., Arbiutina, D.R. 1991. Mammogram-Directed Fine Needle Aspiration of Nonpalpable Breast Lesions. *Journal of Surgical Oncology* 48:153-157.

79. Dent, D.M., Kirkpatrick, A.E., McGoogan, E., Chetty, U.,

Anderson, T. 1989. Stereotaxic Localization and Aspiration Cytology in Nonpalpable Breast Lesions. *Clin Radiol* 40:380-382.

80. Lofgren, M., Anderson, J., Lindholm, K. 1990. Stereotaxic Fine Needle Aspiration for Cytologic Diagnosis of Nonpalpable Breast Lesions. *AJR* 154:1191-1195.

81. Fajardo, L.L., Davis, J.R., Weins, J.L., Trego, D.C. 1990. Mammography Guided Stereotactic Fine Needle Aspiration Cytology of Nonpalpable Breast Lesions: Prospective Comparison with Surgical Biopsy Results. *AJR* 155:977-981.

82. Dowlatshahi, K., Yaremko, N.L., Kluskens, L.F., Jokich, P.M. 1991. Nonpalpable Breast Lesions: Findings of Stereotaxic Needle Core Biopsy and Fine Needle Aspiration Cytology. *Radiology* 181(3):745-750.

83. Jackson, V.P., Reynolds, H.E. 1991. Stereotaxic Needle-Core Biopsy and Fine Needle Aspiration Cytologic Evaluation of Nonpalpable Breast Lesions. *Radiology* 188:633-634.

84. Parker, S.H., Lovin, J.D.F., Jobe, W.E., Burke, N.J., Hopper, K.D., Yakes, W.F. 1991. Nonpalpable Breast Lesions: Stereotactic Automated Large Core Biopsies. *Radiology* 180:403-407.

Risk of Breast Cancer Assessed by Histopathology

David L. Page, M.D.
Roy A. Jensen, M.D.

11

Introduction

When specifically defined, certain histologic patterns in otherwise benign biopsies of breast indicate a medically relevant risk of breast cancer development. Four to five percent of women undergoing surgical biopsy without an abnormality recognized as cancer will have these histologic abnormalities. The clinically relevant group is largely confined to elevated risk levels of at least 4 times that of similar women, that is, of the same age, geographic background, and at risk for the same length of time. The length of projected risk used for clinical management decisions is best limited to 10-15 years. This restriction is further explained below, but is largely because our reliably validated evidence does not extend further in time. These anatomic risk indicators are recognized by specific combined cytologic and histologic pattern criteria.

Histologic and cytologic epithelial alterations presage the development of carcinomas in many body sites. In the breast, as elsewhere, premalignancy or the borderline between benignancy and malignancy has engendered many forms of inquiry. Current knowledge supports risk assessment as an acceptable approach to stratification and definition in this area. Thus, specifically defined risk indicators or associations are tested and, for simplification, may be found to fall within one or another of the following categories (**Figure 11.1** and **Figure 11.2**):

1) Unassociated with an increased cancer risk (or risk magnitude less than 50% elevated).

2) Associated with increased risk approaching double (1.5-2 times, which is greater than 50% elevated and not greater than 100% increased) that of the comparable group (slight).

3) Associated with a risk of 4-5 times (moderate).

4) Associated with a risk of 9-11 times (high).

This arrangement of histologic groups into varied levels of subsequent risk of invasive breast cancer has gained wide acceptance in the last 10 years and corroboration from various studies, detailed below. Since the 1985 Consensus Conference[1], few changes have been made in general approach, except for the placement of well-developed examples of sclerosing adenosis [2, 3] within the slightly increased risk category. There may still be some question about where this change actually belongs, but as this discussion will indicate, the slightly increased risk category has no great clinical importance. In any case, women with only slight risk are not women who should be treated greatly different than the general population.

Somewhat fewer than 5% of women in a premammographic series[4, 5] had specific histopathologic patterns of atypical hyperplasia (AH) that approached the patterns of carcinoma in situ (CIS: LCIS or DCIS, lobular or ductal). The women with AH had a risk of cancer 4-5 times that of the general population, or about one half the risk associated with microscopic carcinoma in situ (LCIS or small, noncomedo DCIS untreated after biopsy). When cases with original diagnoses (derived from a large number of different pathologists) were utilized in a similarly designed cohort study, AH still elevated risk[6], but only to about 3 times. Presumably, this lowering of risk was a result of the pathologists using less stringent criteria for making the diagnosis of AH, thereby including cases with lesser inherent risks.

This study strongly supports the use of more stringently defined histologic criteria to identify higher risk. Several recent studies support the utility and predictability of specifically defined AH[7-9]. Comparable follow-up studies involving women with mammographically detected abnormalities

		Site of Cancer Risk	
		Local Risk	**General Risk (Both Breasts)**
Magnitude of Risk	**Moderate (4-5x)**	None recognized	ALH, ADH
	High (9-11x)	Noncomedo DCIS	LCIS
	Very High	Comedo DCIS	None recognized

Figure 11.1 Stratification of Premalignant Abnormalities by Magnitude and Site of Cancer Risk. Note that while some abnormalities indicate a generalized increased risk of invasive breast cancer and therefore are best thought of as marker abnormalities, DCIS predicts with a high degree of certainty the development of breast cancer at a specific site. Therefore, DCIS should be considered a determinant or true precursor abnormality.

Relative Risk for Invasive Breast Carcinoma

No increased risk

Women with any abnormality specified below in a biopsy specimen are at no greater risk for invasive breast carcinoma than are comparable women who have had no breast cancer.

- Adenosis
- Apocrine metaplasia
- Cysts, macro and/or micro†
- Hyperplasia (mild, more than 2 but not more than 4 epithelial cells in depth)
- Duct ectasia
- Fibroadenoma††
- Fibrosis
- Mastitis (inflammation)
- Periductal mastitis

Slightly Increased Risk (1.5-2 times)

Women with any abnormality specified below in a biopsy specimen are at slightly increased risk for invasive breast carcinoma relative to comparable women who have had no breast biopsy.

- Hyperplasia, moderate or florid, solid or papillary
- Papilloma with fibrovascular core
- Sclerosing adenosis, well-developed

Moderately Increased Risk (4-5 times)

Women with an abnormality specified below in a biopsy specimen are at moderately increased risk for invasive breast carcinoma relative to comparable women who have had no breast biopsy.

- Atypical hyperplasia (borderline abnormality)
- Specific patterns of atypical ductal hyperplasia
- Specific patterns of atypical lobular hyperplasia

Figure 11.2. Relative Risk for Invasion Breast Carcinoma Based on Pathologic Examination of Benign Breast Tissue.
†,†† See notes on next page.

Notes for Figure 11.2:

† Cysts were placed in this category in 1985 [1] and probably should remain there, although there is some interest in analyzing special subsets of cysts identified biochemically or by apocrine cytology. These studies are in progress. There is a suggestion that women with a family history and cysts (presumably large and palpable) have a slightly greater risk than the risk identified by their family history alone, but the effect does not as much as double the familial indicator, and has not been controlled for the simultaneous presence of hyperplastic abnormalities.

†† There is a suggestion from large epidemiologic studies that women with fibroadenomas (FA) have a slightly increased risk of later carcinoma, by about 1.7 times. This is "slight," less than double that of comparable women. Note that the absolute risk of cancer for these young women is not greatly changed, that is, women under age 40 in North America have less than a 0.1% incidence of breast cancer per year.

are not available. However, it is clear that the incidence of AH is higher in mammographically directed biopsies[10].

Further studies have indicated an appreciable interaction between atypical hyperplasia and other nonanatomic risk factors, particularly a family history of breast cancer[8]. Also, lower dosage estrogen replacement (specifically, conjugated preparation) after menopause does not appear to further affect risk in any histologically defined group[11].

Clinical Implications of Increased Cancer Risk

Patients are only considered at a medically meaningful elevated risk for the development of carcinoma if the risk is reliably determined to approach double that of the general population. Lesser magnitudes of risk may be important in nonclinical settings but are not considered here. Even a doubling of risk may not be of direct clinical relevance. This is because the practical impact is minimal. Elevated breast cancer risk is unquestionably clinically important when its magnitude approaches 5 times the general population.

Note that comments on the magnitude of relative risks are inherently confusing without an immediate reference group. This reference or comparison group is usually the general population of women without the risk factor.

The age of a patient, as well as the number of years at risk are of great importance when evaluating the impact of risk statements in a clinical setting. Thus, in the clinical setting relating to a single patient, absolute risk statements are more relevant. However, these statements, rendered as a single fraction or percentage, must be known to have relevance to comparable women over a similar period of time.

It is important not to extrapolate such risks to time intervals that are longer than those documented by follow-up studies in the literature. In particular, projecting risk over the entire lifetime of an individual patient is misleading, and usually overstates the magnitude of the patient's absolute risk[12,13].

Relative risk (RR) always compares one group with another and therefore is of less direct relevance than determining the experience of comparable women and relaying the information in a more direct way, as with absolute risk (AR). For example, a 10% likelihood of developing invasive carcinoma in 10-15 years is an AR statement. A specific period of time is necessary in the statement.

Generally, we do not feel that prediction of breast cancer risk should be extended beyond 10-15 years[13] because the stability of risk with time is unproven. It is our experience, particularly with older women, that these elevated risks will fall (at least in relative terms) 10-15 years after detection[13]. Thus, AR should be used preferentially with an individual patient, and should be carefully sculpted to the clinical setting.

AR may be derived from RR[12]. However, overestimates of AR will occur even if the relative risk is assumed to be constant for a full 20 years when, in fact, RR falls with time after biopsy. This is precisely what happens for proliferative disease[13]. Thus, AR is the most useful in the clinical setting[14]. However, AR must be derived with care for each individual patient, assessing the relevance of published figures to the specific patient being advised. For example, few women less than 30 and more than 60 years of age were present in any follow-up studies. Risk figures for atypical abnormalities must be understood to be less certain for women in younger and older age groups[14,15].

The diagnostic phrase *proliferative breast disease* (PBD or PD) indicates that there are proliferative alterations noted by histology, and that they indicate a disease by their demonstrated link to an increased risk of subsequent carcinoma development[16]. This term may be used to connect the histologic and risk statements for slight and greater risk abnormalities (Figure 11.2). The greatest utility of the diagnostic phrase is in the clinical use of the negative phrase "negative for PBD" or "no PBD." These phrases are used to indicate that abnormalities with cancer risk implications have been sought but not found.

Slightly Increased Risk (PBD without Atypia, PBDWA)

The magnitude of risk elevation in this slightly elevated group is recognized as slight because it is not proven to be as high as doubled. However, breast cancer risk is reliably increased to more than 50% that of women of similar age from the general population. The risk of developing invasive carcinoma does not reliably attain the magnitude of 100% greater or double that of the reference population. This range of risk may be recorded as 1.5-2 times that of the general population, and emphasizes that risk assessment of assignment is not precise but is rather probabilistic and should be understood to include a range of values. The magnitude of the relative risk has varied little with different populations used for comparison. Thus, we found a risk elevation of 1.6 times when the general population was used as a comparison group, and 1.9 when women from our study with only mild or no hyperplasia were the comparison population[4].

The major histologic patterns and categories contained in this slight elevation of risk category are more developed, usual, or common types of epithelial hyperplasia. The terms "papillomatosis" and "epitheliosis" have been used for these changes[17]. These terms will still find utility but have caused confusion and are inconsistently applied in different countries. The term "usual" refers to commonly found patterns of cytology and cell relationships that are seen when cell numbers are increased within the basement membrane-bound spaces in the breast. These alterations are most common in the immediate premenopausal ages. The 1985 Consensus Conference[1] defined this histologic pattern as having a more extensive degree of epithelial proliferation than 4 cells above a basement membrane. This is largely true, and serves as a good rule of thumb in separating mild hyperplasia (epithelial lining or 2-4 cells deep with no increased cancer risk) from abnormalities with slight cancer risk implications.

Sclerosing adenosis had not been repeatedly demonstrated as an indicator of increased risk in 1985, and was not independently linked to increased risk. Since that time, we have completed an analysis of sclerosing adenosis and its various associations. When rigorously defined histologically, sclerosing adenosis is an indicator of slightly increased risk of subsequent breast carcinoma apart from its association with other risk indicators[2]. McDivitt and associates have also found sclerosing adenosis to be an indicator of increased risk in the magnitude of double that of the general population[3].

Fibroadenomas have recently been evaluated with regard to their implications for subsequent breast cancer risk. In several studies, these characteristic abnormalities of young women have been found to indicate an increased risk of subsequent breast carcinoma development in the range of 1.6 or 1.7 times that of the general population. A recent study recognized the same magnitude of risk in an entire group of women with fibroadenoma in a large cohort, which was followed up for over 20 years and was 90% successful in follow-up[18]. The important outcome of this study was to indicate that there were three additional discernible risk factors in addition to fibroadenoma. Despite having a fibroadenoma, women without any of these additional risk factors had the same risk as the general population. These three factors were: a slight family history of breast cancer (at least one first degree relative); proliferative breast disease in the surrounding parenchyma outside the fibroadenoma; or a "complex" fibroadenoma histology. This latter feature was recognized by any combination of cyst formation, sclerosing adenosis, epithelial related calcification, or papillary apocrine change. This finding is unexpected and needs validation. These four alterations had no compelling relevance to breast cancer risk elevation when found in the breast parenchyma. One of the most interesting observations about the risk associated with fibroadenoma is that it may not decrease 5 or 10 years after identification. In contrast, the risk of the indicators of ordinary hyperplasia or atypical hyperplasia in the breast parenchyma does decrease subsequently.

Moderately Increased Risk

This term was originally chosen by the Consensus Conference[1] to place these abnormalities in a category between those noted above and microscopic examples of in situ carcinoma. Microscopic appearances are similar to analogous CIS abnormalities (**Figure 11.3**) and reach a high degree of consensus when histologic criteria are applied[19,20]. The relative risk for subsequent invasive carcinoma attributable to atypical hyperplasias is 4-5 times that of the general population. In absolute terms, this risk averages 8-10% over 10-15 years after biopsy (**Figure 11.4**) and applies to each breast. This is approximately half the risk experienced by women after biopsy only with microscopic in situ carcinoma (Figure 11.1), specifically LCIS (generalized to both breasts)[21] and microscopic DCIS of noncomedo variety[16] (local, regional risk).

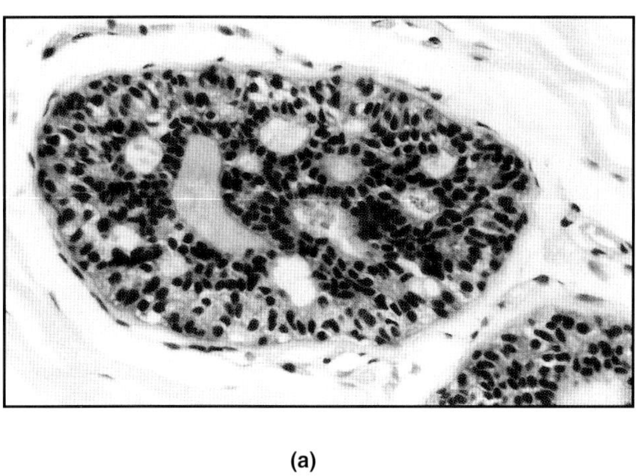

(a)

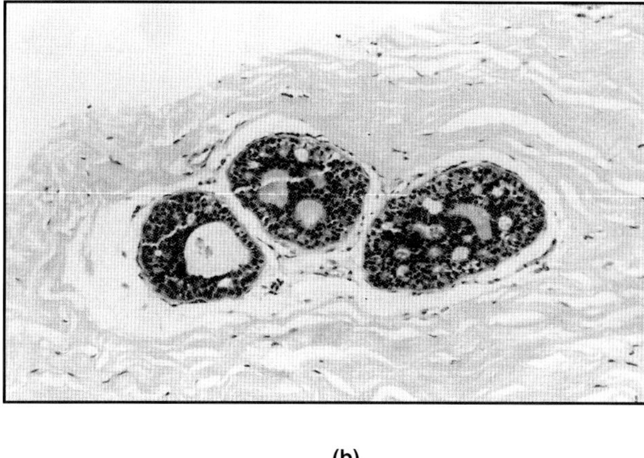

(b)

Figure 11.3. Atypical Ductal Hyperplasia. High **(a)** and low **(b)** magnification photographs of a focus of atypical ductal hyperplasia (ADH). The involved area (three basement membrane-bound spaces) is less than 2 mm in overall diameter. The restricted nature of these changes (small size) is a usual factor in their presentation and definition. Similar changes, when present in foci over 3 to 4 mm in size, are regularly regarded as low-grade ductal carcinoma in situ.

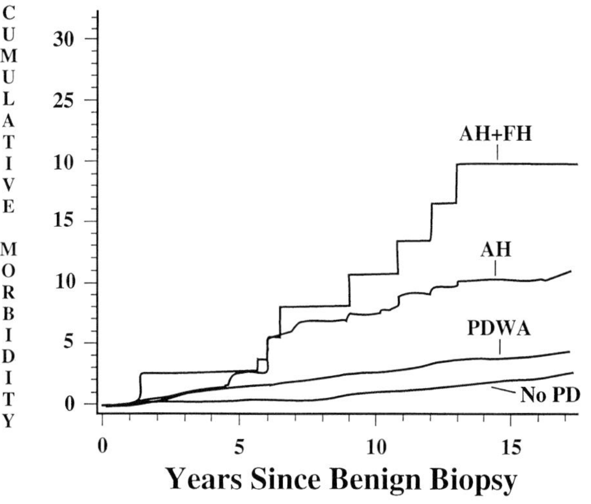

Figure 11.4. Incidence of Invasive Breast Cancer After Biopsy. Cumulative morbidity graph of the incidence of invasive breast cancer for women with different diagnoses recognized at time of breast biopsy (modified from Dupont and Page, 1985[4]). Note that this is an average experience for all women in the study, and would be recognized as a lower risk for women younger than 45 and a high risk for women over 55, at least for the atypical ductal series abnormalities. There is evidence that the risk for women with ALH is less after 55 or 50.

There is such a strong interaction with family history and AH that it is relevant to consider women with atypical hyperplasia, who have a positive family history (FH) of breast cancer, separately from those who do not. The defin ition of a positive FH in these studies was at least a first degree relative (mother, daughter, sister) with proven breast cancer. The absolute risk of breast cancer development in women with atypical hyperplasia without a family history was 8% in 10 years, whereas those with a positive family history experienced a risk of about 20-25% at 15 years[4,5]. This interaction with family history has been supported in a recent study[7,8]. The magnitude of risk for women with AH and FH is closely analogous to that accorded lobular carcinoma in situ[21-25].

Several confirming studies link more complex and "atypical" abnormalities to future risk of breast cancer[26]. Most recently, London et al.[8] have used the original histologic criteria [5,19] and found the same risks for atypical hyperplasia in a very large cohort, primarily from the 1970s and 1980s. This extends the relevance of AH because the initial studies[4,5] involved a cohort biopsied in the 1950s and 1960s. Also, Tavassoli and Norris have documented the experience of a reference center with atypical hyperplasia[9]. Using criteria similar to those of Page et al.[5,19] but including a criterion of abnormality size (up to 2-3 mm in greatest dimension), they found similar risks for later carcinoma development as previously recorded for AH, based on specific histologic criteria.

Clinical Management

Mammographic surveillance is widely accepted as a clinical alternative over extirpative surgery for most women with increased risk. The logic of this decision rests largely in the knowledge that: 1) mastectomy would remove many more breasts than ever would develop cancer, 2) the patient's breast cancer risk will more closely approximate that of slightly elevated risk if she remains free of cancer for 10 years after biopsy, indicating moderate risk[13], and 3) the current era of mammography should only improve the good prognosis after treatment of later developing breast cancer in women with moderate and high risk, followed closely by palpation[27].

It is abundantly clear that many factors will affect the clinical management of women with high risk attending AH and family history. Although indications for biopsy (surgical or needle) will remain the same as for other women, it is also clear that biopsies will be performed more frequently in this group, based on less certain indications. If frequent biopsies are performed, then preventive surgical strategies, such as subcutaneous mastectomy, should be more seriously considered[28]. Preventive surgery will certainly be more frequently considered in women with a 20% risk of invasive carcinoma in the next 15 years, especially if they have emotional trauma from the death of family members with breast cancer. In any case, even bilateral mastectomy need not be an urgent action. A 6-month delay in decision making is not likely to place a patient at risk.

Mammography Correlation

Few studies have rigorously sought correlates between histopathology and mammography[29, 30]. It appears that the degree of nodularity and density combine to produce some degree of increased risk indication, apart from a proven link to histology[31, 32]. This may be more important in some age groups than in others, as indirect correlates with high risk histopathology are more common in older age groups where the less dense and fatty mammographic pattern is most frequent[30]. However, this may not be the age group in which AH has its greatest clinical importance. The correlation of invasive cancer and some types of in situ carcinoma with mammographic findings is well-documented, but the correlates with atypical hyperplasia are not well-defined. This is largely because considerable overlap exists in the mammographic findings of atypical hyperplasia and usual hyperplasia (irregular densities)[33].

A positive association also exists between the presence of benign patterns of calcification detectable by mammography and the presence of atypical hyperplasia. These calcifications may be in benign lobular units unaffected by atypical hyperplasia. Two studies have shown that the co-occurrence of benign calcifications and hyperplastic abnormalities elevates breast cancer risk higher than when either is present alone[4, 34]. However, this is not of sufficient magnitude to be of clinical importance.

Fine Needle Aspiration

The utilization of fine needle aspiration cytology for the evaluation of proliferative, premalignant, or high risk abnormalities is an important consideration. This is an area of current controversy in which some people use the classic cytologic criteria for atypia and assume that this has intrinsic meaning. Recently, Stanley et al.[35] and Sneige and Staerkel[36] have demonstrated that the specific criteria for atypical hyperplasia derived from histology cannot be readily transferred into fine needle aspiration specimens. Furthermore, the rarity and sparsity of the abnormalities add to the difficulties. Stanley et al. documented a large series of breast FNA. Using classical cytology criteria, they were not able to identify cases that had histologically identified atypical hyperplasia on subsequent tissue biopsies. However, Sneige and Staerkel have demonstrated that, occasionally, the elements of atypical ductal hyperplasia may be present at fine needle aspiration, which has also been commented upon by Abendroth et al[37].

The features of lobular cytology, when seen by fine needle aspiration, may indicate atypical lobular hyperplasia, or lobular carcinoma in situ[38], or even more advanced abnormalities. Obviously, when they are identified, a biopsy is mandated. Care must be taken, then, about interpretation of fine needle aspiration cytology reports (just as in histology reports) that the term atypical hyperplasia has more than a general meaning as somewhat abnormal or unusual presentation, or is linked by epidemiologic studies to a larger increased risk as identified by AH.

Molecular Markers

Protein markers, growth factors, receptors, and various indices of proliferation, etc. have not yet found clear clinical relevance in premalignant abnormalities and breast cancer risk predictability. We have suggested that if there is any sharp divide within noninvasive proliferative abnormalities, it would be between comedo DCIS and lesser examples of in situ disease[39]. This is supported by oncogene studies noted below, as well as by the few studies of DNA content (ploidy)[40] that show aneuploidy largely confined to comedo DCIS.

Many studies of the c-erB-2 protein in noninvasive proliferative diseases have shown remarkable uniformity of overexpression in comedo DCIS, up to 80% in some series, and a lack of expression in LCIS and noncomedo examples of DCIS[41-43]. Apparently, the mechanism for this is most often gene amplification[44]. Most of these studies have been done searching for the protein product by immunohistochemistry. Some more recent studies examining mRNA expression have found overexpression in an even higher percentage of cases[45].

There have been few studies of the presence of estrogen or progesterone receptors in the in situ proliferative diseases[46]. Although there is no known clinical or therapeutic correlate of the demonstration that estrogen receptor protein is present in most AH and CIS abnormalities, the demonstration certainly would support the current interest in preventive trials using antiestrogens.

Another interesting approach to this study of a basic molecular biological understanding of these premalignant abnormalities is by Guidi et al.[47] in which microvessel density was evaluated adjacent to DCIS abnormalities. This study showed that neovascularization was not limited to the comedo-type DCIS, but that lower grade noncomedo abnormalities also increased neovascularization, occasionally. Clearly, the understanding and cataloging of molecular events in premalignant abnormalities may lead to improved ways of stratifying, prognosticating, and guiding novel therapeutic approaches.

Conclusion

Women with histologically determined slightly increased risk abnormalities should be encouraged to follow a regular (yearly) program of mammographic surveillance. These women, in practical terms, are not regarded as different from other women of similar age. Women with abnormalities associated with moderately increased risk (AH) should follow a yearly program without fail, probably by age 40. Atypical hyperplasia is rare, occurring in only 4% of breast biopsy specimens, prior to the mammography era. However, this incidence is currently higher in mammographically directed biopsies. Other considerations such as mammographic density, family history, and high anxiety will impinge on clinical management decisions. AH of either lobular or ductal pattern interacts with slight family history data (cancer in any first degree relative) to produce a further doubling of risk to 9-10 times. The absolute magnitude of this combined risk of AH and FH for a woman in her forties and early fifties is 15-20% in 10-15 years. The high risks attending membership in densely hereditary breast cancer, such as BRCA1 families, do not have known anatomic precursors.

Efforts to understand the molecular basis of the varied patterns of ductal carcinoma in situ, the related abnormalities of lobular carcinoma in situ, and the specifically defined atypical hyperplasias are ongoing, but as yet have no known clinical role in premalignancy.

References

1. Hutter, R.V.P. 1986. Consensus Meeting. Is "Fibrocystic Disease" of the Breast Precancerous? *Arch Path Lab Med* 110:171-173.

2. Jensen, R.A., Page, D.L., Dupont, W.D. and Rogers, L.W. 1989. Invasive Breast Cancer Risk in Women with Sclerosing Adenosis. *Cancer* 64:1977-1983.

3. McDivitt, R.W., Stevens, J.A., Lee, N.C., et al. 1992. Histologic Types of Benign Breast Disease and the Risk for Breast Cancer. *Cancer* 69:1408-1414.

4. Dupont, W.D. and Page, D.L. 1985. Risk Factors for Breast Cancer in Women with Proliferative Breast Disease. *New England Journal of Medicine* 312:146-151.

5. Page, D.L., Dupont, W.D., Rogers, L.W. and Rados, M.S. 1985. Atypical Hyperplastic Lesions of the Female Breast. A Long-Term Follow-up Study. *Cancer* 55:2698-2708.

6. Dupont, W.D. and Page, D.L. 1987. Breast Cancer Risk Associated with Proliferative Disease, Age at First Birth, and a Family History of Breast Cancer. *Am. J. Epidemiol.* 125:769-779.

7. Dupont, W.D., Parl, F.F., Hartmann, W.H., et al. 1993. Breast Cancer Risk Associated with Proliferative Breast Disease and Atypical Hyperplasia. *Cancer* 71:1258-1265.

8. London, S.J., Connolly, J.L., Schnitt, S.J. and Colditz, G.A. 1992. A Prospective Study of Benign Breast Disease and Risk of Breast Cancer. *JAMA* 267:941-944.

9. Tavassoli, F.A. and Norris, H.J. 1990. A Comparison of the Results of Long-Term Follow-up for Atypical Intraductal Hyperplasia and Intraductal Hyperplasia of the Breast. *Cancer* 65:518-529.

10. Rubin, E., Alexander, R.W., Visscher, D.W., Urist, M.M. and Maddox, W.A. 1988. Proliferative Disease and Atypia in Biopsies Performed for Mammographically Detected Nonpalpable Lesions. *Cancer* 61:2077-2082.

11. Dupont, W.D., Page, D.L., Rogers, L.W. and Parl, F.F. 1989. Influence of Exogenous Estrogens, Proliferative Breast Disease, and Other Variables on Breast Cancer Risk. *Cancer* 63:948-957.

12. Dupont, W.D. 1989. Converting Relative Risks to Absolute Risks: A Graphical Approach. *Stat Med* 8:641-651.

13. Dupont, W.D. and Page, D.L. 1989. Relative Risk of Breast Cancer Varies with Time Since Diagnosis of Atypical Hyperplasia. *Hum Pathol* 20:723-725.

14. Page, D.L. and Dupont, W.D. 1988. Histopathologic Risk Factors for Breast Cancer in Women with Benign Breast Disease. *Sem Surg Onc* 4:213-217.

15. Dupont, W.D. and Page, D.L. 1991. Risks Factors for Breast Carcinoma in Women with Proliferative Breast Disease. In: *The Breast,* edited by Bland, K.I. and Copeland, E.M. Philadelphia: W. B. Saunders, 292-298.

16. Page, D.L. and Dupont, W.D. 1990. Anatomic Markers of Human Premalignancy and Risk of Breast Cancer. *Cancer* 66:1326-1335.

17. Azzopardi, J. 1979. Nomenclature of the Microanatomy of the Breast: Parts Affected in Different Diseases: Normal Structure and Involution. In: *Problems in Breast Pathology,* London: Saunders, 11-16.

18. Dupont, W.D., Page, D.L., Parl, F.F., et al. 1994. Long-Term Risk of Breast Cancer in Women with Fibroadenoma. *New England Journal of Medicine* 331:10-15.

19. Page, D.L. and Rogers, L.W. 1992. Combined Histologic and Cytologic Criteria for the Diagnosis of Mammary Atypical Ductal Hyperplasia. *Hum Pathol* 23:1095-1097.

20. Schnitt, S.J., Connolly, J.L., Tavassoli, F.A., et al. 1992. Interobserver Reproducibility in the Diagnosis of Ductal Proliferative Breast Lesions Using Standardized Criteria. *Am J Surg Pathol* 16:1133-1143.

21. Page, D.L., Kidd, T.E., Dupont, W.D., Simpson, J.F. and Rogers, L.W. 1991. Lobular Neoplasia of the Breast: Higher Risk for Subsequent Invasive Cancer Predicted by More Extensive Disease. *Hum Pathol* 22:1232-1239.

22. Frykberg, E.R., Santiago, F., Betsill, W.L. and O'Brien, P.H. 1987. Lobular Carcinoma In Situ of the Breast. *Surg Gynecol Obstet* 164:285-301.

23. Gump, F. E. 1990. Lobular Carcinoma In Situ: Pathology and Treatment. *Surg Clin N A* 70:873-883.

24. Hutter, R.V.P. 1984. The Management of Patients with Lobular Carcinoma In Situ of the Breast. *Cancer* 53:798-802.

25. Wapnir, I.L. Rabinowitz, B. and Greco, R.S. 1990. A Reappraisal of Prophylactic Mastectomy. *Surg Gynecol Obstet* 171:171-184.

26. Palli, D., Rosselli del Turco, M., Simoncini, R. and Bianchi, S. 1991. Benign Breast Disease and Breast Cancer: A Case-Control Study in a Cohort in Italy. *Int. J. Cancer* 47:703-706.

27. Haagensen, C.D., Lane, N., Lattes, R. and Bodian, C. 1978. Lobular Neoplasia (So-Called Lobular Carcinoma In Situ) of the Breast. *Cancer* 42:737-769.

28. Shack, R.B. and Page, D.L. 1988. The Patient at Risk for Breast Cancer: Pathologic and Surgical Considerations. *Perspectives in Plast Surg* 2:43-62.

29. Arthur, J.E., Ellis, I.O., Flowers, C., Roebuck, E., Elston, C.W. and Blamey, R.W. 1990. The Relationship of "High Risk" Mammographic Patterns to Histological Risk Factors for Development of Cancer in the Human Breast. *Br J Radiol* 63:845-849.

30. Bartow, S.A., Pathak, D.R. and Mettler, F.A. 1990. Radiographic Microcalcification and Parenchymal Pattern as Indicators of Histologic "High-Risk" Benign Breast Disease. *Cancer* 66:1721-1725.

31. Goodwin, Pamela J. and Boyd, Norman F. 1988. Mammographic Parenchymal Pattern and Breast Cancer Risk: A Critical Appraisal of the Evidence. *Am J Epidemiology* 127:1097-1108 .

32. Saftlas, A.F., Hoover, R.N., Brinton, L.A., et al. 1991. Mammographic Densities and Risk of Breast Cancer. *Cancer* 67:2833-2838.

33. Oza, A.M. and Boyd, N.F. 1993. Mammographic Parenchymal Patterns: A Marker of Breast Cancer Risk. *Epidemiol Rev* 15:196-208.

34. Hutchinson, W.B., Thomas, D.B., Hamlin, W.B., Roth, G.J., Peterson, A.V. and Williams, B. 1994. Risk of Breast Cancer in Women with Benign Breast Disease. *JNCI* 65:13-20.

35. Stanley, M.W., Henry-Stanley, M.J. and Zera, R. 1993. Atypia in Breast Fine-Needle Aspiration Smears Correlates Poorly with the Presence of a Prognostically Significant Proliferative Lesion of Ductal Epithelium. *Hum Pathol* 24:630-635.

36. Sneige, N. and Staerkel, G.A. 1994. Fine-Needle Aspiration Cytology of Ductal Hyperplasia with and without Atypia and Ductal Carcinoma In Situ. *Hum Pathol* 25:485-492.

37. Abendroth, C.S., Wang, H.H. and Ducatman, B.S. 1991. Comparative Features of Carcinoma In Situ and Atypical Ductal Hyperplasia of the Breast on Fine-Needle Aspiration Biopsy Specimens. *Am J Clin Pathol* 96:654-659.

38. Salhany, K.E. and Page, D.L. 1989. Fine-Needle Aspiration of Mammary Lobular Carcinoma In Situ and Atypical Lobular Hyperplasia. *Am J Clin Pathol* 92:22-26.

39. Page, D.L. and Dupont, W.D. 1990. Anatomic Markers of Human Premalignancy and Risk of Breast Cancer. *Cancer* 66:1326-1335.

40. Norris, H.J., Bahr, G.F. and Mikel, U.V. 1987. A Comparative Morphometric and Cytophotometric Study of Intraductal Hyperplasia and Intraductal Carcinoma of the Breast. *Analytical and Quantitative Cytol Histol* 10:1-9.

41. Bartkova, J., Barnes, D.M., Millis, R.R. and Gullick, W.J. 1990. Immunohistochemical Demonstration of c-erbB-2 Protein in Mammary Ductal Carcinoma In Situ. *Hum Pathol* 21:1164-1167.

42. Lodato, R.F., Maguire, H.C., Greene, M.I., Weiner, D.B. and LiVolsi, V.A. 1990. Immunohistochemical Evaluation of c-erbB-2 Oncogene Expression in Ductal Carcinoma In Situ and Atypical Ductal Hyperplasia of the Breast. *Modern Pathol* 3:449-454.

43. VanDeVijver, M.J., Peterse, J.L., Mooi, W.J., et al. 1988. Neu-protein Overexpression in Breast Cancer: Association with Comedo-Type Ductal Carcinoma In Situ and Limited Prognostic Value in Stage II Breast Cancer. *New England Journal of Medicine* 319:1239-1245.

44. Iglehart, J.D., Kraus, M.H., Langton, B.C., Huper, G., Kerns, B.J. and Marks, J.R. 1990. Increased erbB-2 Gene Copies and Expression in Multiple Stages of Breast Cancer. *Cancer Res* 50:6701-6707.

45. Hubbard, A.L., Doris, C.P., Thompson, A.M., Chetty, U. and Anderson, T.J. 1994. Critical Determination of the Frequency of c-erbB-2 Amplication in Breast Cancer. *Br J Cancer* 70:434-439.

46. Barnes, R. and Masood, S. 1990. Potential Value of Hormone Receptor Assay in Carcinoma In Situ of Breast. *Am J Clin Pathol* 94:533-537.

47. Guidi, A.J., Fischer, L., Harris, J.R. and Schnitt, S.J. 1994. Microvessel Density and Distribution in Ductal Carcinoma In Situ of the Breast. *J Natl Cancer Inst* 86:614-619.

Quality Assurance: The Mammography Practice Audit

Laurie L. Fajardo, M.D.
Gia A. DeAngelis, M.D.
Jennifer A. Harvey, M.D.

12

Introduction

A comprehensive quality assurance (QA) program for a mammography practice involves not only evaluations of equipment, image processing, and image quality but also an assessment of image interpretation accuracy and the appropriateness of recommendations for subsequent patient management. This chapter will outline and summarize currently recommended approaches to auditing a mammography practice. With minor modifications, the following concepts can be applied to evaluate a screening mammography practice, a screening and/or diagnostic practice, or a practice situation involving primarily imaging guided percutaneous breast needle biopsy.

A Mammography Practice Audit

A mammography practice audit is an evaluation of the appropriateness and accuracy of mammographic image interpretation. A properly performed audit also provides a facility or practice with insight regarding the appropriateness of recommendations for surgical consultation, surgical biopsy, or imaging guided needle biopsy made by the interpreting radiologists. To be useful, an audit must be properly planned, executed, and interpreted and the outcomes used to improve the operation of the practice.

How to Collect Data

The volume of data required for analysis depends on the depth of analysis desired, and can sometimes present an imposing challenge. Certainly, the data can be gleaned manually, however, many facilities recommend and have even created specially designed computer software programs to perform such tasks. Such computer data collection programs can also be incorporated as part of a complete mammography reporting system.

What Data to Collect

The first step in conducting an audit involves deciding which data to collect. Attempts at achieving completeness, although commendable, must be tempered by the realization that some data has relatively little importance, other data is essentially impossible to acquire, and the gathering of each additional data item increases time and expense.

Proponents of the mammography practice audit advocate two formats: the *Basic (or minimal) Audit* and the *Comprehensive (or detailed) Audit.* **Figure 12.1** provides detailed approaches to both formats, including definitions for the core information and data to be collected, and the mathematical equations for calculating the outcome statistics. The term raw data refers to the actual data collected, whereas the term derived data refers to the statistical metrics that are subsequently calculated from the raw data.

Derived Data—Calculating Audit Statistics

After a mechanism is established for collecting the raw data for either a basic (minimal) or comprehensive audit, a facility can calculate its audit statistics (or derived data) based on the definitions and equations presented in this chapter under the heading *Definitions and Methods for Calculating Statistics.* **Figure 12.2** outlines the derived data obtainable from the raw data (Figure 12.1) for each audit.

Raw Data Required for Audits	
Basic Audit	**Comprehensive Audit**
1. Dates of audit period (6 mo., 12 mo.)	1. Dates of audit period (6 mo., 12 mo.)
2. Total no. of examinations performed* a. no. of screening exams b. no. of diagnostic exams	2. Total no. of examinations performed* a. no. of screening exams b. no. of diagnostic exams
3. Risk factors a. age at time of exam	3. Risk factors a. age at time of examination b. personal history — breast Ca (especially premenopausal cancer in first degree relative) c. family history — breast Ca **d. hormonal replacement therapy **e. previous diagnosis of LCIS† or atypia
4. N/A	4. Type of exam: screening vs. diagnostic
5. N/A	5. First-time or repeat exam
6. N/A	6. Mammographic interpretation a. negative, benign, probably benign
7. Mammographic recommendation a. routine follow-up (negative exam) b. early follow-up (that is, 6 mo.) c. further imaging evaluation (recall) d. biopsy or surgical consultation	7. Mammographic recommendation a. routine follow-up (negative exam) b. early follow-up (that is, 6 mo.) c. further imaging evaluation (recall) d. biopsy or surgical consultation (suspicious, malignant)
8. Biopsy results a. benign, malignant b. lymph node status	8. Biopsy results (separate data collection for FNA/core vs. surgical biopsy) a. benign/malignant
9. N/A	9. Cancer/staging data: a. Mammographic findings — mass, microcalcifications b. Clinical breast exam findings (palpable vs. nonpalpable tumor) c. Pathologic tumor staging - tumor size, in situ vs. invasive, nodal status, tumor grade, distant metastases

* Separate statistics are recommended for symptomatic vs. asymptomatic women.
** Optional data points.
†NOTE: LCIS should not be considered a breast cancer.

Figure 12.1. Raw Data Table. This table presents the raw data needed for basic and comprehensive audits.

Derived Data	
Derived Data for Basic Audit	Derived Data for Comprehensive Audit
1. N/A	1. Population risk factors and frequency by age
2. N/A	2. Population characteristics by type of examination (asymptomatic vs. symptomatic)
3. N/A	3. Prevalent vs. incident cancers
4. True positive and false positive rates	4. True positive and false positive rates
5. Recall rate (overall frequency and frequency by age)	5. Recall rate (overall frequency and frequency by age)
6. Estimate of sensitivity* [TP / TP + FN] (However, true FN rate will not be known.)	6. Sensitivity* [TP / TP + FN] (Accuracy will depend on FN rate tracking.)
7. N/A	7. False negative rate (not always practical)
8. Positive Predictive Value PPV_3 (easiest) or PPV_2	8. Positive Predictive Value: PPV_1, PPV_2, or PPV_3, depending on how rigorous all abnormal mammogram readings are tracked
9. N/A	9. Specificity: [TN / FP + TN] requires follow-up of all negatives
10. N/A	10. Accuracy of interpretation
11. Cancer detection rate: a. overall cancer detection rate (per 1,000 examinees screened)	11. Cancer detection rates: a. overall cancer detection rate (per 1,000 examinees screened) b. prevalent vs. incident cancer rates c. cancer detection rates in screening vs. diagnostic exams d. cancer detection rates by age
* Sensitivity can be estimated from the benign or probably benign mammographic diagnoses that develop interval changes, prompting biopsy that reveals cancer. For most accurate determination, false negative cancers (interval cancer occurrences) must also be tracked.	

Figure 12.2. Derived Data Table. This table presents the derived data, that is the statistics calculated from the raw data for basic and comprehensive audits.

Expected Outcome Measures of Mammography Practice Audit

There are several valid reasons for conducting periodic audits of mammography or imaging guided breast needle biopsy practices. A well-designed audit can demonstrate a practice's success to patients and to referring physicians. Routine audits assist a group in determining whether individuals and the group as a whole are finding a high percentage of the cancers that exist within a specific population (that is, by calculating sensitivity and the number of cancers found per 1,000 women screened) **(Figure 12.3)**. The group can also evaluate whether cancers are being found within an acceptable level of total biopsies (by evaluating the *positive predictive value* for the group and for individual group members). Successful outcomes data can be beneficial in building a referral base and in demonstrating an acceptable level of performance to third party payors and managed care organizations. Other positive aspects of performing regular mammography and needle biopsy practice audits are listed in **Figure 12.4**.

Definitions and Methods for Calculating Statistics

True Positive (TP) Mammographic Examination—Cancer is diagnosed within one year after biopsy recommendation based on *abnormal* mammogram.

True Negative (TN) Mammographic Examination—No known breast cancer diagnosis within one year of *normal* mammogram. Note: some authorities recommend using a two or three-year period.

False Negative (FN) Mammographic Examination—Cancer is diagnosed within one year of a *normal* mammogram. Note: some authorities recommend using a two or three-year period. The specific type of false negative examination can be further categorized as:
a. interpreter false negative - a mammographic abnormality is detected on second blind reading or in retrospect.
b. technical false negative - positioning or imaging factors are primarily responsible for the nondetection of a significant mammographic abnormality, rather than an error of interpretation.

Analysis of Mammography Practice Audit Data—Desirable Goals

Derived Statistic	Desirable Goal
Positive Predictive Value	
Based on abnormal screening exam	5-10%
Based on recommendation for biopsy (surgical, core, or fine needle)	25-40%
Cancers detected - Stage 0 or Stage 1	>50%
Minimal cancer detection rate*	>30%
Lymph node positivity	<25%
Cancers detected per 1,000 women screened	2-10
Prevalent cancers detected per 1,000 women having first screening examination	6-10
Incident cancers detected per 1,000 women having repeat screening examinations	2-4
Recall rate	<10%
Sensitivity (if measurable)	>85%

* Minimal cancer = invasive cancer $\leq$ 1 cm, or in situ ductal carcinoma.

Figure 12.3.

Expected Outcomes of a Mammography Audit

1. Evaluation of a mammography program's success or failure to detect occult cancers at the expected rate.
2. Provide interpreting radiologists with feedback on their individual performances and on the performance of the group as a whole.
3. Analysis of trends in clinical performance that may indicate less than optimal care and suggest the need for corrective action.
4. Positive outcomes data will indicate acceptable levels of technology performance to third party payors and government agencies.
5. Timely audits of abnormal mammograms can assure optimal follow-up of individual patients as part of risk management programs.
6. Positive outcomes data can improve compliance of referring physicians and women with screening guidelines.
7. Programs can ultimately assist with monitoring population outcomes related to effectiveness of screening programs (national mammography registry).

Figure 12.4. Positive Aspects of Performing Regular Mammography and Needle Biopsy Practice Audits.

False Positive (FP) Mammographic Examination—Three separate definitions of a false positive mammographic examination are found in the literature:
a. No known cancer is diagnosed within one year of a *non-negative screening mammogram* (that is, mammographic interpretation of suspicious or malignant abnormality). (FP_1)
b. No known cancer is diagnosed within one year after a biopsy recommendation based on *abnormal* mammogram. (FP_2)
c. Benign disease (no cancer) is found at biopsy following a recommendation for biopsy or surgical consultation based on *abnormal* mammogram. (FP_3)

Figure 12.5 provides a visual summary of derived data categories.

Derived Data Catagories

Ca	No Ca
TP abnormal mammo	FP (abnormal mammo, no Ca) • abnormal mammo (non-neg.) • abnormal mammo • (benign) abnormal mammo
FN normal mammo	TN normal mammo

Figure 12.5. A Visual Summary of Derived Data Catagories.

Sensitivity—The probability of detecting a cancer when a cancer exists, or the percent of all patients found to have cancer within one year of screening, who were correctly diagnosed as having breast cancer at screening:

$$\text{Sensitivity} = \frac{TP}{TP + FN}$$

Specificity—The probability of a normal mammogram report when no cancer exists, or the percent of all patients who remain free of breast cancer within one year of screening, correctly identified as normal at time of screening (note: some authorities recommend using a two or three-year period):

$$\text{Specificity} = \frac{TN}{FP + TN}$$

The major difficulty in collecting data to calculate the specificity of a mammography practice is tracking all negative screening examinations. However, follow-up tracking of patients having negative stereotactic needle biopsy is more easily accomplished because the total number of patients is significantly less.

Positive Predictive Value—Three definitions for positive predictive value are found in the literature, depending on how a false positive examination is defined and on the method chosen for tracking true and false positive examinations (that is, mammographic interpretations of probably benign, suspicious, or malignant abnormalities).

a. The percent of all non-negative screening exams that result in a diagnosis of cancer:

$$PPV_1 = \frac{TP}{\text{no. non-negative screening exams}}$$

This definition is based on the careful tracking of any non-negative screening mammographic interpretation and is the only option for calculation of positive predictive value for a facility that performs only screening mammography. It is the least practical and most difficult approach to tracking patient outcomes due to the large numbers of women who must be followed.

b. The percent of all cases recommended for biopsy as a result of screening that resulted in a diagnosis of cancer (that is, follow-up of recommendation for biopsy having/not having biopsy):

$$PPV_2 = \frac{TP}{\text{no. recommended for biopsy}}$$

This definition is based on tracking all recommendations for biopsy or surgical consultation.

c. The percent of all biopsies done as a result of screening that resulted in diagnosis of cancer or positive biopsy rate:

$$PPV_3 = \frac{TP}{TP + FP} \quad \text{or} \quad \frac{TP}{\text{no. of biopsies}}$$

This definition is based on the results of surgical pathology and requires tracking only those patients having surgical biopsy. It is the least difficult approach for collecting data to calculate the positive predictive value of a mammography practice or a breast needle biopsy database.

Overall Cancer Detection Rate—The overall cancer detection rate is defined as the number of cancers detected by mammography at a facility within a year per 1,000 women screened.

Minimal Cancer—A minimal cancer is generally defined as an invasive carcinoma less than or equal to one centimeter in size with *negative* lymph nodes. The percentage of minimal invasive cancers is the number of minimal cancers diagnosed among all cancers as a result of mammography:

% minimal cancer = [(no. minimal cancers detected by mammography)/ (all breast cancers detected by mammography)] x 100

Percentage of Ductal Carcinoma In Situ (DCIS)—The percent of DCIS is calculated as follows:

% DCIS = [(the no. of women diagnosed with DCIS by mammography) / (the total no. of breast cancers detected as a result of mammography)] x 100

Prevalent Cancer—Prevalent cancers are those detected in women undergoing their first screening examination.

Incident Cancer—Incident cancers are those detected in women undergoing a repeat screening examination.

Interval Cancer—Interval cancers are those (clinically) diagnosed between routine screening examinations. These cases should be reviewed by a facility when evaluating *potential* false negative mammograms.

References

1. Kopans, D. 1992. The Positive Predictive Value of Mammography. *American Journal of Radiology* 158:512-26.

2. Linver, M.N., Paster, S., and Rosenberg, R., et al. 1992. Improvement in Mammography Interpretation Skills in a Community Radiology Practice After Dedicated Teaching Courses: 2-Year Medical Audit of 38,633 Cases. *Radiology* 184:39-43.

3. Monticciolo, D.L., and Sickles, E.A. 1990. Computerized Follow-up of Abnormalities Detected at Mammography Screening. *American Journal of Radiology* 155:751-3.

4. Moskowitz M. 1988. Predictive Value, Sensitivity and Specificity in Breast Cancer Screening. *Radiology* 167:576-8.

5. Sickles, E.A. Ominsky S.H., and Sollitto, R.A., et al. 1990. Medical Audit of a Rapid-Throughput Mammography Screening Practice: Methodology and Results of 27,114 Examinations. *Radiology* 175(2):323-7.

6. Spring, D.B. and Kimbrell-Wilmot, K. 1987. Evaluating the Success of Mammography at the Local Level: How to Conduct an Audit of Your Practice. *Radiol Clin North Am* 25:983-92.

Acceptance Testing, Quality Control, and the Medical Physicist's Role

13

Robert J. Pizzutiello

Introduction

At this time, no formal protocols exist for acceptance testing or quality control of dedicated stereotactic breast biopsy (SBB) systems. However, experience with medical physics evaluations of SBB systems has continued to evolve over the last few years. Our group has developed a procedure for testing these units based on communications with representatives of LORAD® and Fischer Imaging Corporation, a recent medical physics publication[1], and numerous personal communications with other medical physicists, radiologic technologists, and service engineers experienced with SBB.

This chapter contains a description of the procedures we use during the acceptance testing process, as well as sample test results. These procedures address image quality and other technical factors that are essential to a successful SBB procedure. Acceptance testing of any x-ray producing equipment, whether a diagnostic mammography unit or a fluoroscopically guided lithotripsy unit, should evaluate all functions of the system that relate to x-ray production image quality, as well as other key performance parameters unique to the specific functions of the system.

An individual who did not install the unit, and who is qualified to evaluate the performance of the system should perform the acceptance testing. Independent acceptance testing by a qualified third party provides a "fresh look" at equipment performance and an objective evaluation of patient and operator safety. A medical physicist who is qualified to perform acceptance testing on diagnostic mammography units should acquire additional preparation before undertaking acceptance testing of an SBB system. A medical physicist may prepare further by consulting with more experienced colleagues (medical physicists, technologists, or manufacturers' representatives), referring to technical publications, and attending seminars. This additional preparation assures that the medical physicist understands the unique performance features of SBB systems. Attempts to bypass this important step may compromise the value of the acceptance testing process and potentially jeopardize the safety of the patient, personnel, and the equipment. With the proper background, the medical physicist should use his or her knowledge of x-ray imaging, three-dimensional coordinate systems, and radiation safety principles to devise and perform an acceptance test that assures proper performance of the SBB system and the safety of patients and operators.

After an SBB system has been in operation for some time, a medical physicist should perform periodic medical physics surveys to verify that acceptable system performance is maintained. Modeled after the annual medical physics survey for diagnostic mammography systems, our annual medical physics survey for SBB systems includes a minimum protocol to verify that all critical performance and safety parameters associated with the system are being met. Our annual surveys include the full acceptance testing protocol on the SBB equipment. Of course, the radiation protection survey is only performed once (upon acceptance testing), unless machine configuration, workload, or other facility changes mandate a repeat survey. A medical physics survey is also useful, in whole or in part, when troubleshooting any subtle performance degradation of the system.

At the time of this writing, the *Interim Final Regulations* (21 CFR 900), implementing the *Mammography Quality Standards Act*, does not include SBB systems in the Federal regulation[2]. For each facility, the acceptance testing and ongoing quality control (QC) program must comply with the local, state, and federal regulations that apply to SBB systems. A qualified medical physicist should be able to clarify these criteria. Furthermore, as the state of the art in SBB systems advances, further technical publications will likely appear in the literature. Acceptance testing and QC programs should also keep current with these developments.

This chapter addresses the following parameters of image quality, system performance, and the dose and safety aspects included in acceptance testing and quality control of dedicated SBB systems:

Assembly Evaluation
Output Calibration
Phantom Imaging
Focal Spot Measurement
Line-Pair Resolution
Grid Artifact Evaluation
Targeting Accuracy QC
Average Glandular Dose
Radiation Protection Survey

Acceptance testing of nondedicated SBB systems requires only those tests that are *not* included in the annual medical physics survey of the mammography unit. For nondedicated screen-film imaging systems, only assembly evaluation and positioning accuracy QC are required during acceptance testing on the SBB apparatus. For nondedicated digital imaging systems, beam limitation (to the digital image receptor), image quality, and resolution tests should be performed in addition to those for nondedicated screen-film systems.

As with all performance evaluations, test results should be compared with manufacturers' specifications. Acceptable tolerances should be determined by a qualified medical physicist, who should consider clinically acceptable tolerances and the effect of any variations in performance introduced by the field testing protocol.

General

Stereotactic breast biopsy (SBB) units are very different from diagnostic mammography machines. Both systems use similar x-ray tubes and image receptors. However, the purpose of an SBB unit is primarily *biopsy*, with x-ray imaging used for localization and guidance. As a result, imaging is a means to an end, not an end in itself.

For dedicated SBB systems, the prone patient configuration (and the horizontal x-ray beam direction) makes positioning test equipment much more difficult than with upright systems. Some dedicated units do not have x-ray field lights, further complicating the positioning of test equipment. Once proper positioning of test equipment has been determined, we have found it useful to document these positions with sketches denoting the exact placement of test equipment with respect to the breast support device (BSD), SID, etc. Sketches speed positioning of test equipment, minimize unnecessary multiple exposures while repositioning test equipment, and expedite future evaluations.

Acceptance Testing Procedures

This section provides a detailed description of our acceptance testing procedures.

Assembly Evaluation

1. Verify that all motorized and manual controls, locks, detents, biopsy illuminating lights, and controls are operating smoothly. Check to see that all cables are safely routed to avoid injury and have not been spliced or damaged between the digital acquisition unit and the monitor.

2. If the unit has a light field, verify that the light field-to-x-ray field coincidence is acceptable, using a procedure similar to that for evaluating diagnostic mammography units. Position a loaded cassette between the image receptor and the compression paddle. Hold the cassette in place using a compression paddle. Tape four coins to a cassette, positioning each coin within the light field and tangent to each edge of the light field. Tape an additional coin (of a different denomination) to the chest-wall edge of the compression-paddle wall. Make an exposure and evaluate the image on the test film, as described in the *ACR Mammography Quality Control Manual*[3]. The light field-to-x-ray field coincidence should be within +/- 2% of the SID.

3. Assess x-ray beam limitation in both screen-film and digital imaging modes.

a) Evaluate screen-film beam limitation by using the procedure in item 2 above, placing an additional cassette in the image receptor holder. In the absence of performance standards specifically for SBB equipment, it is reasonable to apply the standards for diagnostic mammography units to this evaluation. The measured x-ray beam size should be completely within the 18 x 24 cm image receptor holder assembly, except for the edge of the beam at the chest wall. Beam limitation should be evaluated as described in the *ACR Mammography Quality Control Manual*[3].

b) Beam limitation in the digital imaging mode is evaluated with the digital image receptor and appropriate x-ray aperture in place. Place a loaded cassette in contact with the BSD. Use the "cut-out" compression device to hold the cassette in place. Use tape to position four coins to delineate the edges of the opening in the compression device, corresponding to the digital image receptor area. Make an x-ray exposure using the digital mode. Compare the resultant digital and screen-film images. The measured x-ray beam size should be within the digital image receptor size, as described in the *ACR Mammography Quality Control Manual*[3].

Output Calibration

The medical physicist can verify the output and calibration of the unit using the following modified procedures for testing a standard diagnostic mammography unit.

1. Position an ion chamber or appropriate noninvasive test device in front of the BSD. Use an inexpensive lab jack and BR-12 slabs to provide a stand with the variable height necessary to position test equipment **(Figure 13.1)**.

2. Unlike a diagnostic mammography unit, the BSD on some units can be moved along the tube-image receptor axis. Keep the BSD at the 0 position, or any other preferred consistent position. Document the position of the BSD in the report.

3. The steep target angle makes positioning in the anode-cathode axis critical for output and kVp measurements. We have found that the most easily reproducible position of the test instrument is where the chamber is exposed to the maximum mR/mAs output at a clinically used kVp. That is, the chamber is positioned where the active volume of the chamber is centered (left to right) and nearest to the chest-wall edge of the x-ray beam, while being fully exposed. Verify that the chamber is positioned to measure the maximum output by making repeated exposures, adjusting the position of the chamber slightly until the maximum mR/mAs (at a clinically used kVp) reading is achieved. Collect data using the ion chamber in the position that produces the maximum mR/mAs.

4. Use the largest aperture in the slot at the x-ray tube port, that is, an 18 x 24 cm screen-film aperture.

5. We do not use the 5 x 5 cm compression paddle (for digital imaging) for QC measurements because the field of view is too small to obtain consistent results with our noninvasive meter. We also avoid the perforated paddle used for needle localization because the attenuation differences from the holes in the paddle may affect the output and noninvasive kVp measurements. We prefer to use the large, open

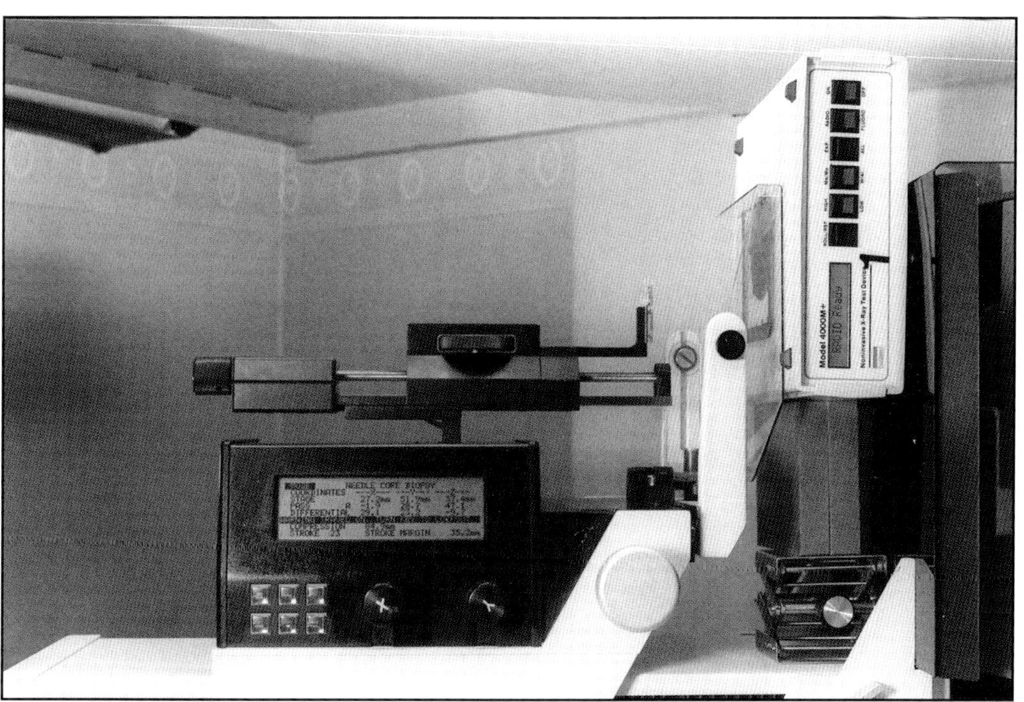

Figure 13.1. Experimental Setup of Test Equipment. This setup utilizes a lab jack and BR-12 slabs to adjust the position of the multifunction meter.

compression device. This is clinically relevant because during breast biopsy, the area of interest is *never* compressed by the compression paddle surface. The area of interest must be open and accessible to the needle. Note that this differs from a diagnostic mammography unit, where nearly all patient exposures take place through the compression paddle.

6. Use noninvasive multifunction test instrument(s) to measure mR/mAs, kVp, and timer accuracy. The test instrument should be calibrated for use at mammographic energies. If the SBB unit has a digital imaging capability, we find the digital mode to be more time-efficient than using the screen-film mode.

7. Evaluate kVp accuracy/reproducibility and beam quality (HVL), using the established procedures for evaluating diagnostic mammography generators[3]. We modify our standard mammography test protocol so that most exposures are performed at 28 kVp, the preferred kVp for digital imaging. We also measure kVp accuracy at 26 and 30 kVp.

Because SBB units are frequently used without Automatic Exposure Control, we also document mR/mAs for each exposure. The mR/mAs may be used to determine Average Glandular Dose.

Phantom Imaging

1. The field of view for digital imaging is about 50 x 50 mm, requiring multiple exposures to image the critical details of the standard ACR Accreditation Phantom.

2. On dedicated prone biopsy units, positioning the ACR Accreditation Phantom with the **nipple indentation up** will produce phantom images that appear in the familar orientation seen on the CRT screen. However, imaging the phantom with the **nipple indentation down** better simulates the geometry and heel effect of phantom imaging with conventional mammography units. We now image the phantom in this way.

3. Obtain screen-film images of the phantom. For systems that are not equipped with AEC, use estimated conventional techniques from the facility technique chart. Typical techniques are 26 kVp at 100 mAs for a 100-speed system.

4. Digital imaging on the LORAD® SBB system is accomplished without AEC. A pixel value histogram is available when in the window/level mode of the distal imaging system. LORAD reports that optimal imaging occurs when many pixels have values near 2k. This prevents over or undersaturating the CCD camera and the analog-to-digital converter. We have found typical good imaging techniques to be 28 kVp at 96 mAs (512 x 512) images, and 28 kVp at 192 mAs (1024 x 1024).

5. Visualizing all objects in the phantom requires four digital images. Three images will visualize all critical areas of the phantom. Position the phantom using the lab jack and additional spacer blocks as needed. It may be useful to document the positions of the phantom with a sketch or to create a template. This will save time in positioning the phantom during future testing. New phantoms have recently become available that provide the critical objects from the ACR Accreditation Phantom in a 66 x 66 x 42 mm slab, suitable for imaging with a single exposure **(Figure 13.2)**.

6. For each phantom position, acquire a digital (512 x 512) image. Adjust window and level controls for maximum object visibility. The INVERT, MAG, and ZOOM software functions may improve the visibility of speck groups.

7. Repeat step 6 for a 1024 x 1024 matrix size. Images are automatically annotated with matrix size, kVp, and mAs. Evaluate image scores and record the results based on viewing the image from the CRT display. See the sample score sheet in **Figure 13.3**. Note that screen resolution, brightness, and contrast may or may not be optimized, which can introduce a significant variable.

8. If desired, evaluate additional images using the MAG function, which acts like a small magnifying loupe, or enlarge the entire image to full screen size using the ZOOM mode.

9. Repeat steps 6-8 for each phantom position. If possible, also score phantom images from a hard copy output device and summarize the results. Note that many hard copy devices degrade image quality. However, digital imaging systems are used clinically with images evaluated from the CRT, with hard copy imaging used primarily for documen-

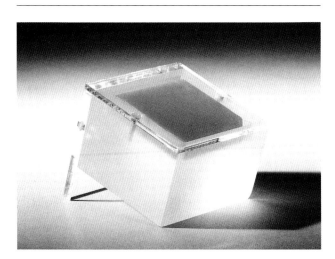

Figure 13.2. Mammography Phantom Designed for Use with Digital SBB Units. Photo, courtesy of Nuclear Associates, Carle Place, New York.

Phantom Imaging Score Sheet					
	Digital 512	Digital 1024	Digital 512	Digital 1024	Screen-Film
Viewing Mode	CRT	CRT	Film	Film	Film
AEC Mode	Manual	Manual	Manual	Manual	Manual
kVp	28	28	28	28	25
mAs	96	192	96	192	136
Fibers	5.0	5.0	5.0	5.0	5.0
Specks	4.0	4.0	3.5	4.0	3.0
Masses	4.0	4.0	4.0	4.0	3.5
Artifacts	None	None	None	None	None

Figure 13.3. Sample Score Sheet for Phantom Imaging.

tation purposes. It may also be useful to evaluate the image quality as affected by the hard copy output device.

Focal Spot Measurement

The horizontal x-ray beam configuration makes it impossible to use the standard test stand to hold the slit camera in a perfectly vertical, centered position. LORAD® has built a limited number of special jigs to hold the slit camera (**Figure 13.4**). The test jig can also be used to position a star pattern. It is preferable to evaluate the focal spot using the slit camera, if the physicist can properly position the camera. A star pattern† may be used, making positioning somewhat less critical. Line-pair resolution may be evaluated instead of focal spot size measurement, if the special jig is unavailable, and for all subsequent quality control measurements. Once the physicist properly positions the test device, he or she may use the established procedures for evaluating focal spot size[3].

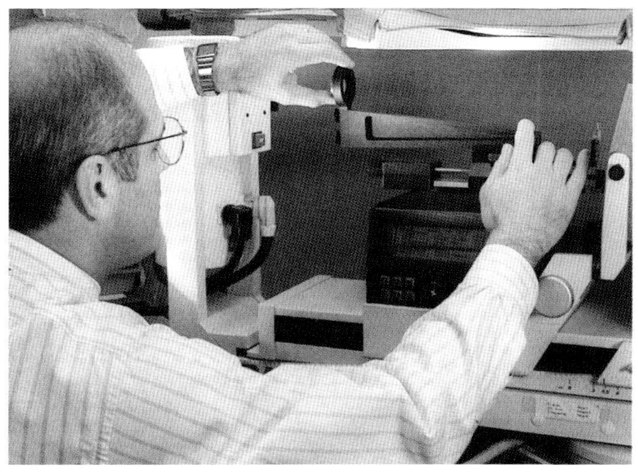

(a)

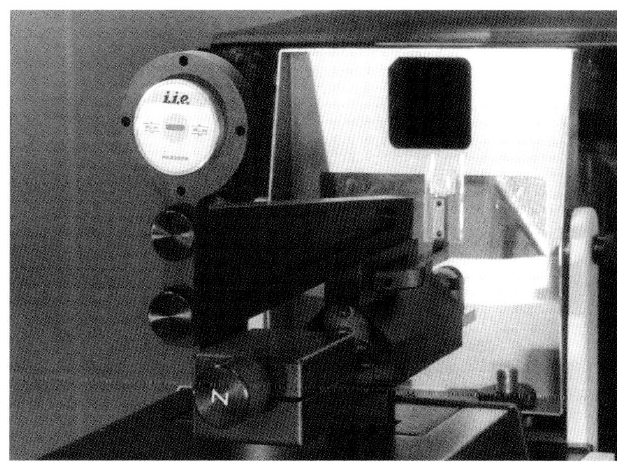

(b)

Figure 13.4 a and b. Focal Spot Measurement. Positioning the slit camera in a test jig, specially designed by LORAD ® **(a)**. A near "beam's eye-view" showing the slit camera, test jig, and compression device **(b)**.

† Manufactured by Siemens Corporation.

Line-Pair Resolution

1. Perform this test using screen-film and digital modes, as recommended in the *Mammography Quality Control Manual*[3].

2. Tape the LP test pattern to the 50 mm window of the steel-lined compression paddle with the lines of the LP test pattern positioned parallel to the anode-cathode axis. Position the compression paddle with the LP test pattern at a distance of 4.5 cm from the BSD. There is no need to use additional scattering material. Note that there is some additional magnification in the LORAD® unit due to the distance between the BSD and the image receptor.

3. Image the LP test pattern in 512 x 512 and 1024 x 1024 matrix modes to determine the effect of the digital imaging system, CRT, and hard copy unit on high-contrast resolution. Evaluate resolution on both CRT and hard copy images. Record results on an LP Score Sheet; a sample appears in **Figure 13.5**.

4. Repeat step 3 with the lines of the LP test pattern positioned perpendicular to the anode-cathode axis. Record results on the LP Score Sheet.

5. Obtain LP test pattern images using the screen-film image receptor to evaluate the inherent high-contrast resolution, limited by focal spot size and imaging geometry. Place the cassette in the Bucky and obtain images with both test pattern orientations: lines parallel and perpendicular to the anode-cathode axis. Record results on the LP Score Sheet.

6. At this time, no suggested criteria for evaluating *digital* LP resolution have been published. Screen-film imaging by its nature will always provide higher LP resolution than digital imaging modes. For the screen-film images, the physicist may wish to use the suggested performance criteria from the *ACR Mammography Quality Control Manual*[3] to evaluate LP resolution, which are ≥13 lp/mm (bars parallel to the anode-cathode axis) and ≥11 lp/mm (bars perpendicular to the anode-cathode axis).

Grid Artifact Evaluation

1. Using the largest screen-film x-ray aperture, obtain screen-film images of a 2 cm slab of clear acrylic to evaluate grid artifacts. Depending on the model of the SBB system, it may be possible to disable the Bucky motion. (Unplugging the grid motion cable on some systems is interpreted by the software as selecting the digital imaging mode, which requires the digital image receptor.) Evaluate the image for grid uniformity. Note that the heel effect is severe over the field of view due to the steep target angle.

2. Report any significant grid nonuniformities.

Targeting Accuracy QC

1. Manufacturers recommend that the technologist perform this test each day before the first SBB procedure. This test is a closed-loop evaluation of the needle position, stereo position calculations, and the user interface. The procedure and performance criteria are described in the SBB unit *User's Guide*, and should be performed at acceptance testing.

2. Sample results appear in **Figure 13.6**

Average Glandular Dose (AGD)

For the digital imaging mode, it may be helpful to use the mR/mAs output data in conjunction with the phantom imaging technique (kVp and mAs) to determine the Entrance Skin Exposure (ESE). Average Glandular Dose may be determined for screen-film and digital imaging

Line-Pair Resolution Results					
	Digital 512	**Digital 1024**	**Digital 512**	**Digital 1024**	**Screen-Film**
Viewing Mode	CRT	CRT	Film	Film	
Limiting Resolution (lines parallel to tube axis)	5	6	5	6	14
Limiting Resolution (lines perpendicular to tube axis)	7	10	7	10	17

Figure 13.5. Sample Report Table Showing Line-pair Resolution Results for all Modes of an SBB System.

Targeting Accuracy			
	X	Y (Angle 1)	Z (Angle 2)
Coordinates of needle tip	9.4	19.8	29.9
Calculated coordinates	10.0	20.0	30.0
Evaluation		**Acceptable**	

Figure 13.6. A Sample Report Table Showing Results of Targeting Accuracy Test.

modes using the method described in the *ACR Mammography Quality Control Manual*[3]. Using typical mammography screen-film systems and film processing, SBB equipment should be capable of delivering Average Glandular Doses comparable to diagnostic mammography units. For digital imaging during SBB, the dose versus image quality comparison is not resolved at this time. Furthermore, the risk/benefit trade-off for SBB patients may be different than that for diagnostic and screening mammography patients. The medical physicist should exercise caution in interpreting Average Glandular Dose results, particularly for digital imaging systems, until these issues are better understood.

Radiation Protection Survey

1. A qualified medical physicist should determine the adequacy of radiation protection using the standard measurement techniques for radiation protection surveys of diagnostic mammography equipment. Be sure to consider the range of orientations of the x-ray beam with respect to the table, taking advantage of left to right symmetry to reduce the number of measurements required.

2. When calculating exposure levels to personnel in the vicinity of the x-ray room, use realistic exposure and workload estimates. Obtain estimates from the facility, if possible.

Summary

Summarize the results of each of these tests in a simple table or executive summary. Results should indicate the parameters upon which acceptable or unacceptable performance was judged. Highlight any items that require further or corrective action.

Acceptance testing of SBB systems provides the user with baseline performance data to evaluate the installation. Results from subsequent surveys should be compared with acceptance testing results if image quality degradation is suspected after major service that could affect image quality, or when follow-up medical physics survey tests are performed.

At this time, quality control for SBB systems is in a nascent stage, particularly when compared with diagnostic mammography. As the professional community addresses this issue, testing protocols and evaluation criteria will become more standardized.

References

1. Kimme-Smith, C. and Solberg, T. 1994. Acceptance Testing Prone Stereotactic Breast Biopsy Units. *Medical Physics* 21(7) 1197-1201.

2. Federal Register, Part VII, Department of Health and Human Services—Food and Drug Administration, 21CFR Part 900, Mammography Facilities—Requirements for Accrediting Bodies and Quality Standards and Certification Requirements; Interim Rules, Dec. 21, 1993.

3. American College of Radiology (ACR), *Mammography Quality Control Manual*. Committee on Quality Assurance in Mammography. Revised edition 1994.

Cost-Effectiveness of Stereotactic Breast Biopsy

Laurie L. Fajardo, M.D.

14

Carrying out cost-effectiveness analyses has become increasingly popular in economic evaluations of health care technologies. Scientifically valid evaluations of technologies are crucial for medicine, hospitals, insurers, policy makers and the public, if decisions concerning technologies are to be made on a rational basis. Currently, such decisions are made in the context of a wide array of expensive medical technologies and increasing and unrelenting budget pressures. In an environment of fierce competition among providers and payors, decision makers face demands to lower health care costs, while health care providers and patients demand the latest technologies.

Within the field of medical technology assessment, the process of technology assessment has been defined as the careful evaluation of a medical technology with relation to safety, efficacy, cost, cost-effectiveness, and ethical and legal considerations—both in absolute terms and in comparison with competing technologies[1, 2]. Technology assessment also relates to quality of life and to patient preferences [3, 4] and, ideally, is a comprehensive form of policy research that examines short- and long-term social consequences of the application of technologies[5]. The "language" of medical technology assessment is often not readily understood. Some of the common terms and basic concepts are defined in **Figure 14.1**.

For diagnostic imaging examinations and procedures, efficacy studies provide a way of understanding and comparing alternative modalities. Validation of the value of diagnostic imaging requires that researches show benefits related to improving the quality of life. However, the efficacy of diagnostic imaging is complicated by the fact that imaging is one step in a larger process of patient management. Furthermore, distinguishing between cost-benefit analysis and cost-effectiveness analysis is difficult for many health care providers and researchers. The distinction is subtle, but important.

In cost-benefit analysis, the costs and benefits are expressed in the same units. Thus, one can use cost-benefit analysis to determine whether benefits exceed costs and for deciding whether a program is worth undertaking. Cost-benefit analysis evaluates whether the improved outcomes are worth the cost by measuring both in the same units. Net benefit or net cost savings is calculated by subtracting costs from benefits. The comparison may also be achieved by calculating the ratio of benefits to costs for two competing technologies or diagnostic modalities, where

$$\frac{\mathrm{Cost}_A - \mathrm{Cost}_B}{\mathrm{Benefit}_A - \mathrm{Benefit}_B} = \frac{\Delta\ \mathrm{Cost}}{\Delta\ \mathrm{Benefit}}$$

Cost-effectiveness analysis is a method for comparing two or more strategies whose benefits can be measured in the same terms. Cost-effectiveness analysis considers both cost and effect by measuring the net cost of providing a service (that is, expenditures minus savings), as well as the outcomes obtained. Cost-effectiveness analysis is used primarily to evaluate improved outcomes in exchange for the use of more resources.

Implicitly, cost-effectiveness research acknowledges that there are insufficient resources for health care, and seeks to provide the information necessary for society to prioritize the available funds. The intent of cost-effectiveness is not to guide health care providers with regard to patient care decisions, but to guide rationing decisions on a more reasonable

Medical Technology Assessment: Common Terminology

Cost-benefit analysis: Comparison of management (or diagnostic) strategies, for which the costs and benefits are expressed in the same terms.

Cost-effectiveness analysis: Comparison of management (or diagnostic) strategies in terms of the cost per unit of output, where output is an outcome such as additional years of life, utility, or additional cases of newly detected disease.

Incremental cost: The additional resources required for a new therapy, beyond the cost of usual care for similar patients.

Incremental benefit: The additional benefit obtained by changing from one therapeutic option to another.

Perspective: The point of view (that is, society, third party payor, hospital, or patient) for a cost-effectiveness analysis that affects the types of costs that are included in the study.

Quality adjusted life year (QALY): Analysts use the cost per additional life expectancy produced by an intervention when comparing alternative treatment choices. They also recognize that the purpose of health care should include not only improvement in life expectancy but also in quality of life. The QALY incorporates changes in survival and morbidity into a single measure that reflects the trade-offs between costs and outcomes. The QALY has become the desired unit of comparison for economic analyses because it allows results of widely differing therapies and programs to be compared and for evaluations to be made over time.

Sensitivity: The proportion of patients with disease who have a positive test result.

Specificity: The proportion of patients without disease who have a negative test result.

Sensitivity analysis: The recalculation of study results using alternative values for some of the variables to determine whether different sets of inputs produce different conclusions. These analyses are particularly important if specific data points critical to economic analysis have not been reported with other data from a clinical trial.

Figure 14.1. Some Common Terms and Basic Concepts of Medical Technology Assessment.

basis than the current method of awarding scarce resources to those most able to pay for them. When an application of a technology is more effective and less costly (that is, Technology 1 in **Figure 14.2**), it almost certainly is cost-effective. In contrast, when a technology is both less effective and more costly than the alternative, we generally would think that it is not cost-effective. For technologies that are both more effective and costly (that is, Technology 2 in Figure 14.2), we must consider questions related to "value." That is, how much additional cost are we willing to accept for how much additional benefit?

Another outcome category that has been addressed by other countries operating under national health care plans, but less so in the United States, is that illustrated by Technology 3 (Figure 14.2). Increasingly, health care providers may be offered technologies that are significantly less costly, but perhaps slightly less effective than the competing alternative. Although practiced with near comparability to surgical excisional biopsy under ideal practice conditions, under general radiologic practice, stereotactic breast needle biopsy may fall into this category. Here the pertinent query becomes: "How much less efficacy will we accept to reduce our costs by a certain amount?" Or, "If one is willing to save X number of dollars per delayed diagnosis (or missed breast cancer), then the most cost-effective strategy is..." Proponents of stereotactic biopsy over excisional biopsy for nonpalpable breast abnormalities will likely find it necessary to address the concept of decremental cost-effectiveness analysis.

These examples point to societal decisions that are considerably influenced by such considerations as: (1) who bears the costs; (2) who derives the benefit; and (3) what are the opportunities that must be foregone if resources are allocated to employing one technology rather than another?

Cost and Efficacy Trade-offs of Surgical Biopsy Versus Stereotactic Biopsy in Women with Nonpalpable Mammographically Detected Abnormalities

During the last 20 years, a recurring pattern of new imaging technologies disseminating rapidly into routine use without controlled scientific studies has occurred. The use of stereotactic breast needle biopsy (SBNB) to replace the surgical excision biopsy (SEB) is a recent example of this phenomenon.

Considered in isolation, the performance of SEB over time has been generally excellent, with specificity and sensitivity approaching 90-100% (that is, no false positive and very few false negative histologic outcomes)[6-8]. Unfortunately, the decision to evaluate nonpalpable breast abnormalities is driven by mammography, a technology with lower sensitivity. Thus, the outcome of a majority of SEBs

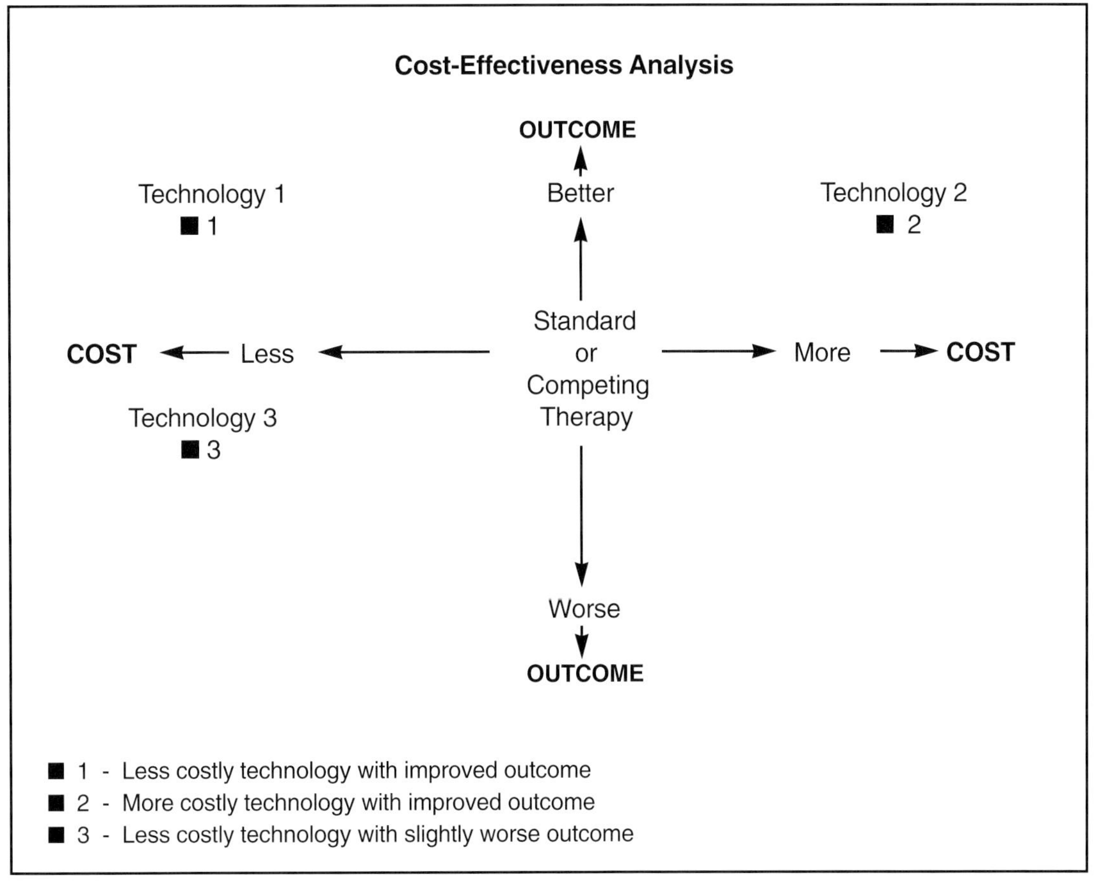

Figure 14.2.

(70-90%) is negative[9-12] and the issue of "unnecessary breast surgery" has arisen. Because SBNB can be performed less expensively, less invasively, with local anesthesia only, and with better cosmesis, it has undergone increasing utilization over the last five years. However, the comparisons reported to date can be criticized because the majority have evaluated fewer than 100 patients[13-23]. Studies reporting larger populations have been where most patients do not undergo surgical biopsy to confirm pathologic findings and, for those not undergoing surgery, sufficient mammographic follow-up (that is, at least two years) has not been performed[24-28].

Discussed here are the results for a study group comprising 400 patients evaluated by SBNB. The specific aims for this trial were to evaluate the efficacy of SBNB for primary management of nonpalpable breast abnormalities and to determine whether SBNB is a cost-effective substitute for SEB. This study was supported by NIH Grant CA56073 and by a General Electric Radiology Research Academic Fellowship.

Methods and Patients

Four hundred patients with nonpalpable (mammographic) breast abnormalities were enrolled prospectively into the study. For each abnormality, a mammographic characterization was made, according to the ACR lexicon, and a mammographic suspicion was assigned[19].

For each abnormality, at least five stereotactic core needle (14-gauge) biopsies were performed using either the Bard or Manan automated biopsy devices. All procedures were performed on a LORAD DSM® prone stereotactic biopsy system equipped with digital imaging capability.

Core biopsy material was routinely processed and evaluated using the following determinants: (1) insufficient sample; (2) negative (or nonspecific benign abnormality such as hyperplasia without atypia) or specific benign abnormality (such as fibroadenoma); (3) hyperplasia with atypia (or other "premalignant" abnormality); (4) ductal carcinoma in situ (DCIS); and (5) invasive carcinoma.

The results of core needle biopsy were correlated with the prebiopsy mammographic characterization. Patients were managed by the following protocol:

1. Patients with probably benign or indeterminate mammographic abnormalities, whose core biopsy results showed negative, specific benign, or benign abnormalities without atypia, comprised the nonsurgical group. These patients underwent mammographic follow-up at 6, 12 and 24 months following the negative SBNB. On follow-up mammography, the study abnormality was classified as: (a) no longer visible on the mammogram; (b) decreased in size; (c) stable, without significant change in size, number of microcalcifications, or character; or (d) increased in size, number of microcalcifications, or mammographic suspicion. Any patient in the latter group underwent subsequent evaluation either with SBNB or SEB, according to the preferences of the patient and her health care provider.

2. Patients with any mammographic diagnosis having insufficient or inadequate core biopsy material underwent immediate repeat evaluation, either by SBNB or SEB.

3. Likewise, patients with suspicious or malignant-appearing abnormalities by mammography, having a negative or nonspecific benign SBNB result, underwent immediate re-evaluation by either repeat SBNB or SEB.

4. Patients with any mammographic diagnosis having DCIS on SBNB underwent an outpatient lumpectomy under local anesthesia with intravenous sedation. If the surgical specimens demonstrated evidence of invasive carcinoma, a second surgical procedure was performed to stage the axillary lymph nodes.

5. Patients having invasive carcinoma on SBNB were managed with the definitive therapeutic procedure of choice, either mastectomy or lumpectomy, with axillary lymph node dissection.

Management Outcomes and Results

A total of 129 patients underwent surgical procedures; 94 of these were cancer and 35 were benign. The overall positive predictive value for the group undergoing SEB following SBNB was 24%.

Twelve patients with indeterminate or suspicious mammography findings had immediate re-evaluations following inadequate SBNB or negative nonspecific benign SBNB results. Five of the 12 patients had repeat SBNB; three showed cancer, while the other two had benign results. The latter two patients were subsequently managed in the follow-up and showed no change on mammography for a follow-up period of two years. Seven of the 12 patients were re-evaluated by SEB; two surgical specimens were malignant and five were benign.

Two hundred seventy-one patients comprised the follow-up group. Compliance with the protocol for follow-up mammography after negative SBNB is shown in **Figure 14.3**. One hundred ninety-one patients underwent all three recommended follow-up mammographic examinations; 13 patients had none of the recommended follow-up studies. **Figure**

Compliance with Follow-Up Mammography

6, 12, 24-month follow-up mammogram	Number of patients	Number of patients with no 24 month follow-up mammogram
Number of patients having all 3 follow-up exams	191	N/A
Number of patients having 2 of 3 follow-up exams	48	6
Number of patients having 1 of 3 follow-up exams	19	11
No follow-up	13	13
TOTAL	271	30

Figure 14.3. Compliance with the Protocol for Follow-up Mammography After Negative SBNB.

Mammographic Findings at Two Years

Stable, NSC	162
Decrease in size or number	39
Abnormality no longer visible	29
Increase in size or number	11
"Noncompliant" *	30
TOTAL number of patients	271

*Patients who did not return for a 24-month mammogram are considered "noncompliant."

Figure 14.4. Mammographic Findings at Two Years Following a Negative Stereotactic Breast Needle Biopsy.

14.4 provides the findings on follow-up mammography for the 271 patients in the follow-up arm. The 30 patients not having a 24-month examination are designated as "noncompliant."

Eleven abnormalities, previously diagnosed as negative by SBNB, demonstrated interval changes (that is, increase in size, number of microcalcifications, or mammographic suspicion) on follow-up mammograms. Four of these were identified on the 6-month follow-up examination and 7 were identified on the 12-month follow-up mammogram. No worrisome interval changes were detected on the 24-month follow-up studies. When the 11 abnormalities were re-evaluated by SEB or SBNB, 8 were benign and 3 were malignant. The 8 benign abnormalties included 4 fibroadenomas that grew, 3 benign groups of microcalcifications (without atypia) that increased in number and 1 nonspecific benign mass (apocrine metaplasia). All 3 of the malignant abnormalities were Stage I ductal carcinomas and had negative lymph nodes. Two of the abnormalties were less than 1 cm in size and the third was 1.8 cm in size. The malignant diagnoses were made at 6, 8, and 13 months following negative SBNB.

Figure 14.5 demonstrates two methods for calculating the sensitivity and specificity for SBNB that have appeared in the literature. The first method considers false negative SBNB outcomes only when a delay in diagnosis results. The second method considers cases where immediate rebiopsy was performed for inadequate SBNB sampling, or for discordance with mammographic findings as false negative and false positive results for SBNB, in addition to those where a delay in diagnosis occurred. The latter method more accurately reflects the performance of SBNB and the patient outcomes to be expected.

Cost-Efficacy Analysis

For the cost-efficacy analysis, a societal perspective was assumed and the following endpoints examined: (1) disease

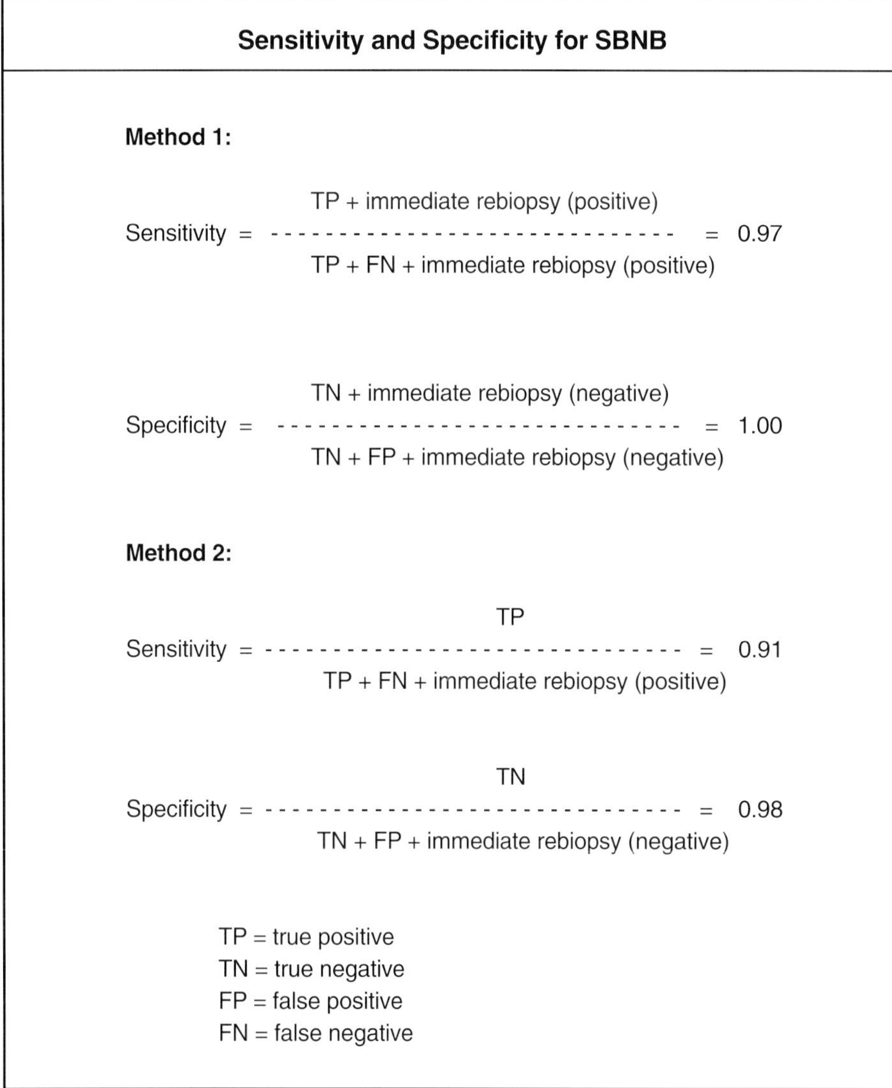

Sensitivity and Specificity for SBNB

Method 1:

$$\text{Sensitivity} = \frac{\text{TP + immediate rebiopsy (positive)}}{\text{TP + FN + immediate rebiopsy (positive)}} = 0.97$$

$$\text{Specificity} = \frac{\text{TN + immediate rebiopsy (negative)}}{\text{TN + FP + immediate rebiopsy (negative)}} = 1.00$$

Method 2:

$$\text{Sensitivity} = \frac{\text{TP}}{\text{TP + FN + immediate rebiopsy (positive)}} = 0.91$$

$$\text{Specificity} = \frac{\text{TN}}{\text{TN + FP + immediate rebiopsy (negative)}} = 0.98$$

TP = true positive
TN = true negative
FP = false positive
FN = false negative

Figure 14.5. This table demonstrates two methods for calculating the sensitivity and specificity for SBNB that have appeared in the literature. Method 2 more accurately reflects the performance of SBNB and the patient outcomes to be expected.

diagnosed by SBNB (DCIS or invasive breast cancer); (2) missed diagnosis; (3) cost; (4) "unnecessary" (negative SEBs). We assumed a base case probability of cancer for patients undergoing SBNB to be 10% for both DCIS and invasive cancer. Furthermore, we used cost-to-charge ratios for a single institution (University of Virginia) to determine that the average cost of SBNB and mammographic follow-up for patients with negative SBNB results to be 40% of the cost for SEB. The cost of outpatient SEB was calculated at $1,500. When calculating the cost for patients requiring a second SBNB or SEB for inadequate initial biopsies for discordance with the mammographic findings (that is, suspicious mammogram with negative or nonspecific benign SBNB), we used the cost of SEB for all cases. We further assumed that outpatient SEB would suffice as a definitive lumpectomy for patients having DCIS (that is, the SEB would have negative surgical margins and re-excision would not be necessary). These assumptions are conservative and are biased in favor of SEB. A further assumption was that if delayed diagnoses by SBNB were Stage 1 with negative lymph nodes, then treatment costs for cancers diagnosed by SBNB versus SEB would not differ. If this holds true uni-

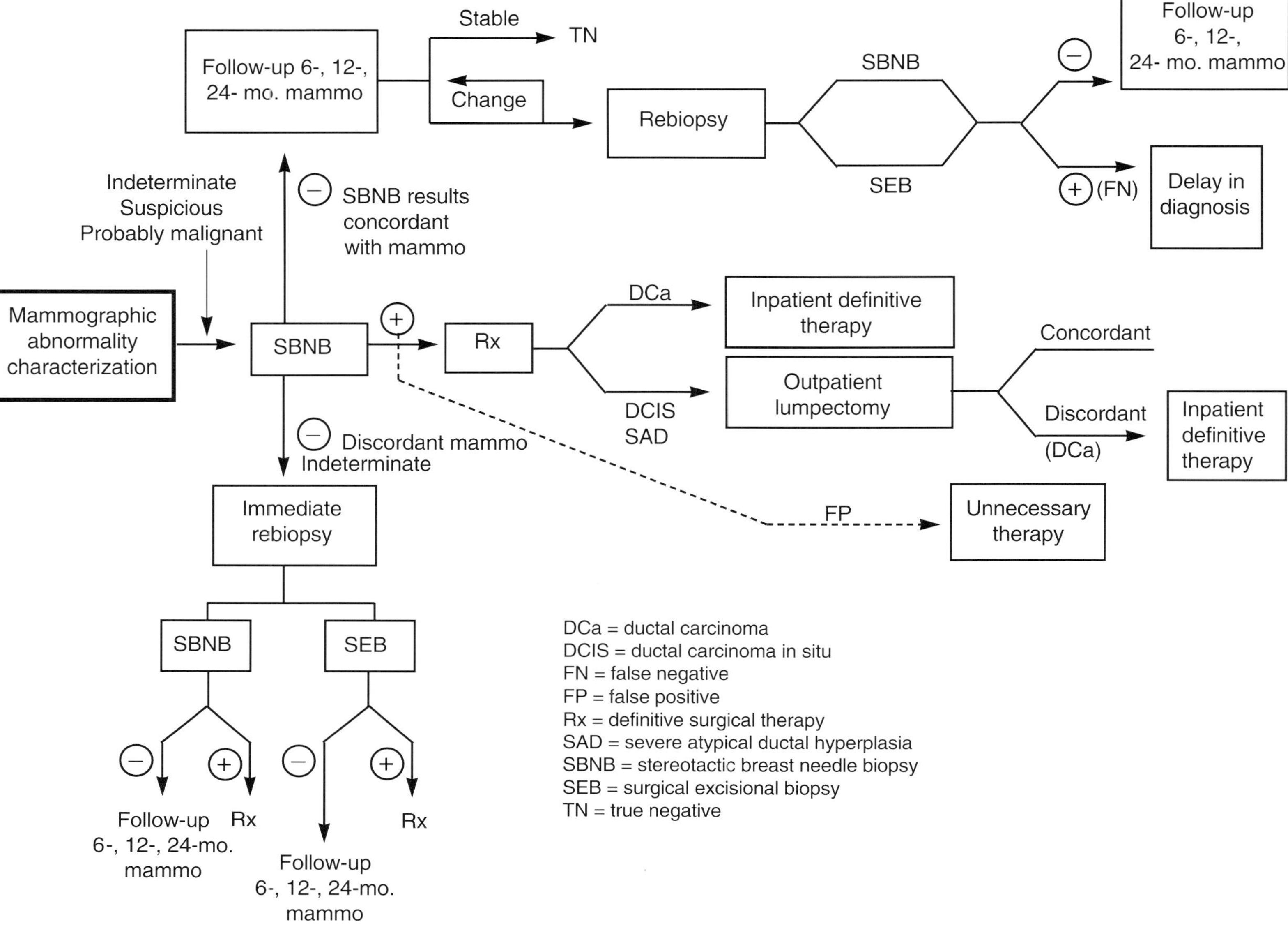

Figure 14.6. Decision Tree for Cost-Effectiveness Analysis

versally, subsequent treatment costs can be ignored. If not, the incremental cost of a delayed diagnosis versus immediate treatment becomes relevant. The decision tree for the cost-analysis is shown in **Figure 14.6**.

Using the assumptions described above, we found the following financial trade-offs for SBNB versus SEB:

1. SEB costs on average $645 more per patient.
2. SEB costs an additional $86,000 per additional Stage 1 invasive cancer detected. (Stated otherwise, SBNB saves $86,000 per delayed breast cancer diagnosis).

Limitations and uncertainties in the analysis include: (1) the uncertainty related to the exact probability of DCIS and invasive carcinoma in a broad population, who would be considered eligible for diagnosis using SBNB; (2) limited controlled trial data on the test characteristics of SBNB; (3) limitations in deriving true costs for SEB and SBNB; and (4) uncertainty related to the prognostic significance of a 6-12 month delay in diagnosis of an early breast cancer.

A randomized trial, the Radiologic Diagnostic Oncology Group-5 (breast RDOG 5) Trial is in progress. This study will randomize 3,600 women to undergo breast needle biopsy by either fine versus core needle, and with stereotactic versus sonographic imaging guidance. Until this randomized-controlled trial is completed to better define the test characteristics for SBNB, this work provides dimension to the patient and financial trade-offs in using SBNB in lieu of surgical biopsy.

Summary

While cost-efficacy/benefit/effectiveness analyses can prove the potential advantages of a diagnostic imaging procedure or intervention for a particular medical indication, the larger goal should be to establish rational public policy in the 1990s when health care resources are limited. The percentage of our GNP and health care dollars that will be available for cancer care will have some limit. Similar to reductions in the ordering of diagnostic imaging procedures, reducing unnecessary breast surgery could preserve scarce resources and save millions of health care dollars.

References

1. Perry, S. Technology Assessment in Health Care: The U.S. Perspective. *Health Policy* 9:317-324.

2. Hillman, B.J. 1994. Outcomes Research and Cost Effectiveness Analysis for Diagnostic Imaging. *Radiology* 193:307-310.

3. Banta, H.D., Luce, B.R. 1993. Health Care Technology and Its Assessment: An International Perspective. Oxford: Oxford University Press.

4. Rettig, R.A. 1991. Technology Assessment—An Update. *Investigative Radiology* 27:165-173.

5. Office of Technology Assessment. 1976. Development of Medical Technology: Opportunities for Assessment. Washington, D.C.: Office of Technology Assessment. Publication OTA-H-34.

6. Norton, L.W., Pearlman, N.W. 1988. Needle Localization Breast Biopsy: Accuracy Versus Cost. *Am J Surg* 156(2):13-15.

7. Gallagher, W.J. Cardenosa, G., Rubens, J.R., McCarthy, K.A. 1989. Minimal-Volume Excision of Nonpalpable Breast Lesions. *AJR* 153:957-961.

8. Landercasper, J., Gunderson, S.B., Gunderson, A.L., Cogbill, T.H. Travelli, R. 1987. Needle Localization and Biopsy of Nonpalpable Lesions of the Breast. *Surg Gynecol Obstet* 164(5): 399-403.

9. Schwartz, G., Feig, S., Patchefsky. 1988. Significance and Staging on Nonpalpable Carcinomas of the Breast. *Surg Gynecol Obstet* 16:6-10.

10. Skinner, M.A., Swain, M., Simmons, R., et al. 1988. Nonpalpable Breast Lesions at Biopsy. A Detailed Analysis of Radiographic Features. *Ann Surg* 208 (2): 203-208.

11. Wright, C. 1986. Breast Cancer Screening. *Surgery* 100 (4): 594-598.

12. U.S. Preventative Services Task Force. 1989. Guide to Clinical Preventive Services: An Assessment of the Effectiveness of 169 Interventions. Baltimore: Williams & Wilkins. Ch. 6. 39-62.

13. Dowlatshahi, K., Yaremko, M.L., Kluskens, L.F., Jokich, P.M. 1991. Nonpalpable Breast Lesions: Findings of Stereotaxic Needle-Core Biopsy and Fine-Needle Aspiration Cytology. *Radiology* 181:745-750.

14. Schmidt, R., Morrow, M., Bibbo, M., Cox, S. 1992. Benefits of Stereotactic Aspiration Cytology. *Administrative Radiology* 9:35-42.

15. Parker, S.H., Lovin, J.D., Jobe, W.E., Luethke, J., Hopper, K., et al. 1990. Stereotactic Breast Biopsy with a Biopsy Gun. *Radiology* 176:741-747.

16. Evans, W.P., Cade, S.H. 1989. Needle Localization and Fine-Needle Aspiration Biopsy of Nonpalpable Breast Lesions with Use of Standard and Stereotactic Equipment. *Radiology* 173:53-56.

17. Dowlatshahi, K., Gent, H., Schmidt, R., Jokich, P., Bibbo, M., Sprenger, E. 1989. Nonpalpable Breast Tumor: Diagnosis with Stereotactic Localization and Fine-Needle Aspiration. *Radiology* 170:427-433.

18. Fajardo, L.L., Davis, J.R., Wiens, J.L., Trego, D.C. 1990. Mammography-Guided Stereotactic Fine-Needle Aspiration Cytology of Nonpalpable Breast Lesions: Prospective Comparison with Surgical Biopsy Results. *AJR* 155:977-981.

19. Bibbo, M., Scheiber, M., Cajulis, R., Keebler, C., Wied, G., Dowlatshahi, K. 1988. Stereotactic Fine-Needle Aspiration. *Acta Cytologica* 32(2):193-201.

20. Dronkers, D. 1992. Stereotactic Core Biopsy of Breast Lesions. *Radiology* 183:631-634.

21. Jackson, VP., Reynolds, H.E. 1991. Stereotaxic Needle-Core Biopsy and Fine-Needle Aspiration Cytologic Evaluation of Nonpalpable Breast Lesions. *Radiology* 181:633-634.

22. Elliot, R.L., Haynes, A.E., Bolin, J.A. Boagni, E.M., Head, J.F. 1992. Stereotactic Needle Localization and Biopsy of Occult Breast Lesions: First Year's Experience. *Am J Surg* 58:126-131.

23. Hann, L., Ducatman, B.S., Wang, H.H., et al. 1989. Nonpalpable Breast Lesions: Evaluation by Means of Fine Needle Aspiration Cytology. *Radiology* 171(2):373-376.

24. Parker, S.H., Burbank, F., Jackman, R.J., Aucreman, C.J., Cardenosa, G., et al. 1994. Percutaneous Large-Core Breast Biopsy: A Multi-Institutional Study. *Radiology* 193:359-364.

25. Kopans, D.B. 1994. Caution on Core. *Radiology* 193:325.

26. Parker, S.H. 1994. Response to 'Caution on Core'. *Radiology* 193:326.

27. Kopans, D.B. 1994. Reply. *Radiology* 193:327.

28. Parker, S.H. 1994. Final Reply. *Radiology* 193:328.

Future Innovations in Breast Imaging

Laurie L. Fajardo, M.D.
Mark B. Williams, Ph.D.
Jennifer A. Harvey, M.D.

15

Digital Acquisition

This chapter discusses image acquisition and transmission technology for digital mammography. The majority of the text focuses on the most important technical requirements and features of digital detectors for both spot mammography and full breast imaging. The remainder of the chapter reviews the status of telemammography and its potential benefit to clinicians and other health care providers.

Digital imaging systems provide advantages over conventional screen-film radiography in image processing, display, transmission, and archiving. Electronic image detectors provide increased x-ray detection efficiency and scatter reduction. However, mammography is among the most challenging of imaging tasks. Detection of irregularly shaped masses must be performed in the presence of an intricate background structure of fibroglandular breast tissue. Since the x-ray attenuation characteristics of the surrounding breast tissue are similar to those of a mass, excellent detector contrast resolution is required for digital mammography[1]. In addition, detection of microcalcifications demands very high spatial resolution (50-100 microns) over areas up to 24 cm x 30 cm.

The simultaneous requirements of high spatial resolution and large area necessitate detectors with 13 to 30 million usable pixels (usable means the resolution must be comparable to the pixel size), and a very low fraction of unusable pixels. Furthermore, the image must be acquired with minimum x-ray dose (<3.0 mGy to a 4.5 cm thick, 50/50 glandular/adipose breast) to the patient[2]. To achieve these goals, a detector for mammography must have the following properties: (1) good modulation transfer function (MTF); (2) good contrast resolution over a large dynamic range; and (3) high detective quantum efficiency (DQE).

Imaging Requirements for Digital Mammography Detectors

High Spatial Resolution/MTF

The MTF measures the spatial-resolving power of an imaging system as a function of spatial frequency. Screen-film systems have high MTFs, limited primarily by light spreading in the phosphor screen. Under optimum conditions, high resolution mammographic screen-film systems can have MTFs of up to 20% at 10 cycles/mm, and limiting resolutions of 20-21 cycles/mm (at MTF=0.05)[3]. However, because of the effects of film granularity, the resolving power of screen-film systems at high frequency is not limited by the MTF, but by the signal-to-noise ratio (SNR)[4, 5].

Based on receiver operating characteristic curve (ROC) studies of radiologists' observations of microcalcifications in mammographic films and digitized film images, Karssemeijer et al. state that "...even under the most optimal circumstances, isolated spherical calcifications with diameters smaller than 0.13 mm are not detectable with film-screen mammography, despite its resolution limit of 15 lp/mm[6]." Other studies have suggested that this minimum detectable size may be as large as 0.20 mm[7].

The limiting resolution of digital systems is set by the pixel-to-pixel spacing, p, and the Nyquist condition, and is given in lp/mm by 1/(2p), where p is in millimeters. However, the MTF may be very low at this frequency because of blurring effects, such as light scatter, electron drift, or defocusing by optical components.

Each of the commercially available small area digital detectors for stereotactic needle biopsy exhibit significantly different MTFs[8]. The MTF of a prototype scanned-slot digital mammographic system at the University of Toronto was reported as 0.2, 0.07, and 0.02 at 5, 8, and 10 lp/mm, respectively, in the slot direction, with values approximately half of those in the scan direction[9, 10]. Even with that relatively limited resolution, the scanned-slot system displays 4 masses, 3 speck groups, and 5 fibers in the ACR Accreditation Phantom. This result compares favorably with the mean scores of 3.6 masses, 3.4 speck groups, and 4.4 fibrils found for screen-film images with mammographic grids in applications for ACR accreditation[11]. *Thus, the superior contrast resolution and SNR of well-designed digital systems are able to compensate for their relatively poorer spatial resolution.*

Good Contrast Resolution Over a Wide Dynamic Range

Dynamic range is the ratio of the maximum and minimum signals that can be accurately measured by a detector. The response of screen-film systems as a function of integrated photon flux at the phosphor surface is linear over only a small portion of the relatively limited dynamic range. Outside of this range, the gradient of the film's characteristic curve is insufficient to allow visualization of low-contrast objects, such as a mass with superimposed fibroglandular tissue. In fact, even relatively high-contrast objects such as microcalcifications can be rendered invisible because of poor contrast resolution[12], especially when imaging radiodense breasts and dense regions near the chest wall.

Screen-film imaging in these situations can result in the utilization of the "toe" or "shoulder" region of the sigmoidal characteristic curve for film. The ratio of maximum and minimum exposures at which the film gradient is appreciable is on the order of 40 or less, whereas the ratio of maximum and minimum x-ray fluxes at the exit surface of the breast can be several hundred, particularly for thicker breasts[5, 12]. Attempts to increase the dynamic range for film inevitably result in further degradation of contrast resolution.

The dynamic range of CCD-based devices is set at the low signal end by the intrinsic detector noise (primarily thermal and read noise) and at the high signal end by the pixel full well capacity. The full well capacity depends on factors including pixel size, the manner in which the CCD is biased, and whether techniques to reduce dark noise (that is, multi-pinned-phase operation) are used. A typical full well capacity for a pixel size of 15 microns is 160,000 e-, with higher values for larger pixels. The minimum possible CCD noise is set by the read noise generated by the on-chip amplifier. The effect of this amplifier noise is determined by the required bandwidth of the CCD signal processor, increasing approximately as the square root of the bandwidth. For read-out times of ~ 1μs per pixel, read noise floors of less than 5 e-rms can be achieved, with values as low as 1.5 e-rms reported. Thermal noise is equal to the square root of the dark current, which is an exponential function of temperature and can be reduced to less than 20 e-/pix/sec at -20°C.

Because of their low dark current and large full well capacities, CCD-based systems typically exhibit linear responses as a function of the integrated signal per pixel over a dynamic range of several thousand[10, 13], thereby maintaining good contrast characteristics over a much wider latitude than that of screen-film systems. In theory, the latitude of a digital system can be made arbitrarily large through integration in digital memory.

High Detective Quantum Efficiency (DQE)

The ability to discern small or low-contrast objects in an image is determined by the image contrast and signal-to-noise ratio (SNR)[14]. The DQE of an imaging system is a measure of how well the SNR, present in the image at the system input, is preserved in the process of converting, amplifying, and displaying the image. All real imaging systems do this in an imperfect way as a result of finite sensitivity, limited spatial resolution, or the addition of noise. The DQE is defined as the square of the ratio of output and input signal-to-noise ratios (SNRs):

$$\mathrm{DQE} = \frac{[\mathrm{SNR}_{out}]^2}{[\mathrm{SNR}_{in}]^2}$$

A perfect detector has a DQE of unity. Primary factors determining the DQE are: (1) the absorption efficiency of the x-ray absorber; (2) the statistical noise associated with the x ray-to-light conversion process; (3) the efficiency with which signal is coupled from one stage to another (for example, for detectors utilizing phosphors or scintillators, the efficiency with which visible photons are coupled to the light-sensing portion of the detector); (4) the efficiency of the sensor, and (5) the amount of noise added by detector components (for example, thermal noise in solid state detectors, or film granularity noise in film-based systems).

For a Poisson distributed x-ray input, such as is encountered in mammography, the input SNR is proportional to the square root of the number of incident x-ray photons. Thus, the above equation indicates that for a given minimum acceptable signal-to-noise ratio present in the output image, *the required dose is inversely proportional to the DQE*[15, 16]. Therefore, increasing the DQE of mammographic detectors is a prerequisite to achieving a lower glandular dose.

The maximum DQE of current screen-film systems is

slightly more than 20% at low spatial frequencies ($< 1\ mm^{-1}$), and falls to less than 1% at higher frequencies (8-12 mm^{-1})[3,17,18]. The loss of DQE is due primarily to film granularity noise, which contributes nearly half of the total noise at low frequency (~ 1 mm^{-1}) and up to 75% at higher frequencies (5 mm^{-1})[17-19]. Furthermore, because of the limited useful exposure range of film, this relatively low DQE is available over only a narrow range of exposures. This narrow range of usable exposure means that screen-film systems may result in unnecessarily high dose in some cases (for example, when imaging high contrast objects such as microcalcifications in fatty breasts), or render clinically important objects invisible (for example, low contrast or small objects).

The low noise characteristics and high sensitivity of current solid state devices such as CCDs result in DQEs of >50% for low frequency systems, when combined with rare earth oxysulfide phosphors or alkali halide scintillators[8,20,21]. The rate of decrement in DQE with increasing frequency is determined by the decreasing system MTF, and the shape of the noise power spectrum (NPS). The latter is determined in large part by the statistical noise of the optical photons incident upon the CCD[8,9,20].

Other Properties, Advantages and Disadvantages of Mammographic Detectors

Scatter Rejection—Detectors for mammography may be usefully categorized as area detectors and scanned-slot devices. Area detectors offer the advantages of rapid acquisition and low mechanical complexity, disadvantages include poor scatter rejection and high cost. Scanned-slot detectors provide excellent scatter rejection and potential cost savings, but may result in excessive tube loading and motion artifacts because of long acquisition times.

Newer digital detectors being developed for whole breast mammographic imaging are hybrids of these two types. Some utilize an array of small area detectors (6.1 cm x 6.1 cm), which are translated to four discrete locations to acquire an image. Unlike scanned-slot detectors, there is no data acquisition during translation, during which time the x-ray beam is turned off and the detectors are read out in parallel. During any given acquisition period, detectors occupy 25% of the image area. Thus, the acquisition time is between that of a single-area detector and a scanned-slot detector.

Similarly, the scatter rejection of a discontiguous array of small area detectors falls between that of full-area detectors and slot-shaped detectors. Using Monte Carlo simulations, Andre et al. have shown that with a 4 cm air gap between the detector and the exit surface of the breast, scatter into the center of a 5 cm x 5 cm detector is similar to that for a standard-sized area detector using a 5:1 grid[22]. This is a very encouraging result, since it means that small area detectors can achieve good scatter rejection without the long acquisition times of scanned-slot devices, or the higher radiation dose associated with grids.

Separation of Acquisition and Display—One of the main advantages of digital imaging is the ability to optimize the inherent signal-to-noise ratio of an input image by separating image acquisition from image display. With screen-film systems, the exposure technique and film optical density must be optimized for the human visual response when viewing film on a light box. This viewing constraint limits the range of useful exposures and may result in improperly exposed images. Even if the desired optical density is obtained, only by coincidence will this exposure be that which results in an acceptable image signal-to-noise ratio at a minimum dose. In digital systems, the dose that provides the desired signal-to-noise ratio is used, and the resulting range of pixel intensities is spread over the full range of the display.

Post-Acquisition Image Processing and Handling—Other advantages of digital mammography over conventional film-based mammography include: compatibility with Picture Archiving and Communication Systems (PACS) for image transmission and storage; the ability to transmit images between remote locations and large health centers; the ability to enhance images with digital filtering, feature extraction, zooming, windowing and leveling; and the potential to use Computer Aided Diagnosis (CAD) algorithms for abnormality detection and classification.

Digital Systems Under Investigation for Full Breast Imaging

Area Detectors

Photostimulable Phosphor Plates—Photostimulable storage phosphor plates have been applied successfully to some areas of radiography for more than a decade[23]. The storage phosphor plate consists of a flexible substrate covered by a layer of BaFBr:Eu2+ crystals in an organic binder. When exposed to x rays, the plates develop a latent image of metastable "f-centers," which is stable for hours afterward. The f-centers de-excite when the plates are scanned by a He-Ne laser beam, producing visible photons that are sensed by a photomultiplier tube.

The dynamic range of storage phosphor plates is higher than that of film by several orders of magnitude[24] . However, due to light scattering in the phosphor layer, the spatial resolution is poorer, with an MTF of less than 5% at 8 lp/mm[25]. Thus, the true resolution is worse than the limiting resolution as determined by the pixel size. For this reason, the use of photostimulable phosphor plates has been limited to imaging tasks with less stringent resolution requirements than those of mammography.

Amorphous Silicon Arrays—Amorphous silicon (a-Si:H) array technology has undergone vigorous development, primarily because of the commercial interest in flat panel displays. Amorphous silicon offers a distinct advantage over crystalline silicon because it can be fabricated in large sheets; arrays of up to 23 cm x 25 cm have been constructed with 512 x 560 pixels[26]. Typical pixel sizes are 100-200 microns and the active (sensing) portion is less than 100% of the pixel. The active fraction (fill factor) decreases with decreasing pixel size, and is currently only 35% for a pixel size of 127 microns[27]. In contrast, the fill factor for CCDs is 100%, independent of pixel size. Because of this fill factor constraint and because current technology limits the minimum feature size of a-Si:H arrays to be larger than that of crystalline Si devices, pixel sizes of less than 100 microns appear impractical in the near future.

Amorphous Selenium (a-Se) Arrays—Amorphous selenium sensors store a latent charge image that is read out by either a scanning electrometer or by a laser[28]. Although selenium-based detectors have been used in a slot-scanning format with electrometer readout[29], the development of larger a-Se plates is still in its early stages. Initial results are promising, however, the application to digital mammography is likely to be several years away.

Slot-Scanning Detectors

Detection schemes utilizing narrow fan-shaped beams that are scanned over the breast simultaneously with a slot-shaped detector can significantly reduce the amount of scatter in the image, because many of the photons scattered in the breast are not intercepted by the detector[30]. This scatter reduction leads to greatly improved contrast without additional radiation dose (roughly by a factor of two [31]),which occurs when grids are used. Unfortunately, any given location on the patient is exposed to x rays for a fraction of the total scan time equal to the ratio of the slot width to the size of the imaged area in the scan direction. Therefore, the acquisition time for a scanned-slot system is longer than that for an area detector of the same size and DQE by the ratio of the scan distance to the slot width. Since typical slot widths are less than 1 cm, this ratio can be significant. Any reduction in this scan time requires an increase in x-ray flux. In all cases, heat dissipation from the target of the rotating anode tube becomes a limiting factor. Even with increased flux through the use of a modified tungsten target angiographic tube, a 7.8 s scan is required to achieve an exposure of about 200 mR at the breast entrance[10]. In addition, to preserve adequate spatial resolution, the scan velocity for systems using x-ray phosphors or scintillators is limited by the phosphor or scintillator decay time.

Time Delay Integrated (TDI) CCD Schemes

TDI-CCD detectors that use phosphors coupled by fiber optic tapers to slot-shaped CCDs are being utilized in full breast imagers under development at the University of Toronto[10, 32]. By setting the scan velocity equal and opposite to the vertical shift velocity of the CCD, the pixel charge corresponding to a given spot on the patient remains approximately stationary in the patient's reference frame, and is integrated during the entire time (slot width/scan velocity) the spot is exposed.

A prototype unit, utilizing a Gd_2O_2S:Tb phosphor screen and 2:1 fiber optic tapers exhibits reasonable sensitivity (about half of the incident x rays from a tungsten target at 40 kVp are absorbed, with 6 electrons per absorbed x ray)[6] and adequate resolution (MTF of 1% in both dimensions at 10 cycles/mm)[10]. For slot-scanning devices, tungsten targets are favored over molybdenum targets because of their higher loading capability and greater flux. Thicker phosphors would improve absorption at the expense of poorer resolution. Currently, resolution in the scan direction is limited by the decay time of the phosphor[33].

A particularly promising variation on the TDI-CCD approach utilizes direct absorption of the incoming x rays in crystalline silicon that is indium-bonded to a CCD array[34]. To form the mammographic image, slightly overlapping rows of the hybrid detectors are scanned over the field of view. Electrons generated in the silicon by the absorption of an x-ray photon are collected in the CCD pixels in a TDI fashion. The absorbing layer must be thick (~1.5 mm) to ensure a high absorption probability in the silicon. Therefore, individual detectors are set with their perpendicular bisectors intersecting the x-ray focal spot to reduce parallax. Preliminary tests made on individual detectors have demonstrated high DQE and high resolution, with an MTF of 40% at 10 lp/mm[34].

Telemammography

Currently, there are active research and industrial efforts for developing clinically useful telemammography systems. The usefulness and cost of a telemammography system depend on the wide area network links available and their interface into radiology department infrastructures. Terrestrial networks are rated by data rates such as the following: (a) DS-0 (56/64 kbits-per-second); (b) DS-1 or T-1 (1.544 Mbps); (c) DS-3 or T-3 (45 Mbps); and (d) ATM (155 Mbps). Higher rates of digital service are possible but not available for most of the country. Clinics and hospitals with mammography service programs would benefit by interfacing to other sites using telemammography. However, except for urban areas, these terrestrial networks are expensive.

The potential significance of the application of satellite communications to telemammography is the connection of remote, rural, or small medical facilities with experts located at large medical complexes. Within urban areas, fiber optic networks can handle the requirements for transmission of mammographic images; they are available now, or will become available in the near future. However, in areas of smaller population and in remote areas, fiber optic connections may be years or decades away. Therefore, satellite transmission is a practical alternative. A successful telemammography system using an integrated satellite and/or terrestrial communication link would provide several benefits to breast screening programs, as listed below.

Expert Consultation

Telemammography offers the ability to provide mammography consultations to underserved and remote areas. If telemammography systems can achieve the mammographic image quality necessary for primary diagnosis, expert opinion outreach programs can be established to enhance breast cancer detection and improve patient care.

Group Practice Distributed Over Multiple Sites

As awareness of the role of mammography in early detection of breast cancer increases, so does the need for access to low-cost screening. Many practices are responding to the increasing needs for mammography services by establishing mobile mammography and/or satellite sites. Telemammography would enable a group with a limited number of expert mammographers to handle multiple off-site practices. In addition, if appropriate for the practice, the radiologist could supervise screening mammograms offsite while determining the need for any additional views "online," rather than having the patient return for further imaging. Image quality could also be supervised offsite via telemammography. Due to efficiencies of scale, mammography interpretation costs could be lowered by avoiding the need for an on-site radiologist.

Overreading Mammographic Images

There is increasing emphasis on the interpretive skills of radiologists who read mammograms by the regulations mandated by the *Mammography Quality Standards Act*. Residency programs now offer more formal training time in mammography, and there are formal, standardized training programs underway for radiology residents and mammography technologists through the American College of Radiology-Center for Disease Control cooperative agreement. Nonetheless, the impact of accreditation guidelines and training programs will not be immediate, and the need remains for expert mammography interpretation in many practices. With telemammography, a small number of expert mammographers could provide consultation services or second readings of mammograms for a large number of general radiologists to improve the quality of care.

Interdisciplinary Consultation

Using telemammography capabilities, primary care physicians and clinicians can readily review images and plan patient care. On a broader scale, the utilization of telemammography at multiple radiology practices in a referral region can provide improved access to a patient's prior examinations.

The importance of such transmission would be multifold: original films would not have to be mailed, risking their loss; the cost of making copy films could be avoided; and the facility interpreting the current study would have faster access to prior exams, thereby improving the accuracy and timeliness of reporting or results. Prior mammograms are particularly critical when an equivocal breast abnormality is identified, so that the need for early follow-up versus immediate intervention can be determined.

Regional Breast Cancer Outcomes Databases

A national database for breast cancer screening does not exist and regional databases are extremely limited. Telemammography, along with transmission of clinical information, would enable the development of electronic databases that could be interfaced for regional or national systems. Clinicians could monitor biopsy rates for various types of abnormalities, histopathology results, breast cancer incidence, stage, management, etc. Access to such information would also be particularly helpful for auditing breast imaging practices.

Summary

Although active work in the area of full breast digital imaging is ongoing, screen-film systems will remain the primary technology used in mammography imaging for the next several years[16-18]. It is generally accepted that replacement of screen-film mammography by digital systems will reduce costs, enhance reliability, and permit broader interpretation of mammograms by trained subspecialists. Telemammography and PACS infrastructures will enable clinicians and other health care providers to further exploit the availability of digital image data and the advantages of digital mammography.

References

1. Johns, P.C. and Yaffe, M.J. 1987. X-ray Characterization of Normal and Neoplastic Breast Tissues. *Phys Med Biol* 32-675-695.

2. *21 CFR Part 900,* 1993. FDA Requirements for Mammographic Facilities, December 21.

3. Haus, A.G. 1994. Screen-Film Image Receptors and Film Processing, in Syllabus: A Categorical Course in Physics, Technical Aspects of Breast Imaging, eds. Haus, A.G. and Yaffe, M.J. *Radiological Society of North America.* Oak Brook, IL 85-101.

4. Yaffe, M.J. 1994. Digital Mammography, in Syllabus: A Categorical Course in Physics, Technical Aspects of Breast Imaging, eds. Haus, A.G. and Yaffe, M.J. *Radiological Society of North America.* Oak Brook, IL 275-286.

5. Nishikawa, R.R., Mawdsley, G.E., Fenster, A., and Yaffe, M.J. 1987. Scanned-Projection Digital Mammography. *Med Phys* 14(5):717-729.

6. Karssemeijer, N., Frieling, J.T.M., and Hendriks, J.H.C.L. 1993. Spatial Resolution in Digital Mammography. *Invest Radiol* 28(5):413-419.

7. Kimme-Smith, C., Bassett, L.W., Gold, R.H., Zheutlin, J., and Gornbein, J.A. 1990. New Mammographic Screen/Film Combinations: Imaging Characteristics and Radiation Dose. *AJR* 154:713-719.

8. Roehrig, H., Fajardo, L.L., Yu, T., and Schempp, W.S. 1993. Signal, Noise, and Detective Quantum Efficiency in CCD Based X-ray Imaging Systems for Use in Mammography. *Proc. SPIE* 2163:320-332.

9. Nishikawa, R.M. and Yaffe, M.J. 1990. Model of the Spatial-Frequency-Dependent Detective Quantum Efficiency of Phosphor Screens. *Med Phys* 17(5):894-904.

10. Maidment, A.D.A., Yaffe, M.J., Plews, D.B., Mawdsley, G.E., Soutar, I.A., and Starkoski, B.G. 1993. Imaging Performance of a Prototype Scanned-Slot Digital Mammography System. *Proc. SPIE* 1896:92-103.

11. Barnes, G.T. and Hendrick, R.E. 1994. Mammography Accreditation and Equipment Performance. *Radiographics* 14:129-138.

12. Nishikawa, R.M. and Yaffe, M.J. 1983. An Investigation of Digital Mammographic Imaging. *Proc. SPIE* 419:192-200.

13. Strauss, M.G., Westbrook, E.M., Naday, I., Coleman, T.A., Westbrook, M.L., Travis, D.F., Sweet, R.M., Pflugrath, J.W., and Stanton, M. 1990. CCD-Based Detector for Protein Crystallography with Synchrotron X-rays. *Nucl Instrum Meth Phys Res* A 297:275-295.

14. Rose, A. 1973. Vision, Human and Electronic. New York: Plenum Press.

15. Gruner, S.M., Milch, J.R., and Reynolds, G.T. 1978. Evaluation of Area Photon Detectors by a Method Based on Detective Quantum Efficiency (DQE). *IEEE Trans Nucl Sci* NS-25(1):562-565.

16. Rose, A. 1946. A Unified Approach to the Performance of Photographic Film, Television Pick-up Tubes, and the Human Eye. *J Soc Motion Picture & Telev Engrs* 47:273.

17. Nishikawa, R.M. and Yaffe, M.J. 1985. Signal-to-Noise Properties of Mammographic Film-Screen Systems. *Med Phys* 12(1):32-39.

18. Bunch, P.C., Huff, K.E., and Van Metter, R. 1987. Analysis of the Detective Quantum Efficiency of a Radiographic Screen-Film Combination. *J Opt Soc Am A* 4(5): 902-909.

19. Bunch, P.C., Huff, K.E., and Van Metter, R. 1986. *Proc. SPIE* 626-63.

20. Maidment, A.D.A. and Yaffe, M.J. 1994. Analysis of the Spatial-Frequency-Dependent DQE of Optically Coupled Digital Mammography Detectors. *Med Phys* 21(6):721-729.

21. Standon, M., Phillips, W., Li, Y., and Kalata, K. 1992. The Detective Quantum Efficiency of CCD and Vidicon-Based Detectors for X-ray Crystallographic Applications. *J Appl Cryst* 25:638-645.

22. Andre, M.P., Rudzevich, B.L., Stoller, M., and Tran, J. 1994. Scatter Reduction and Contrast Improvement with Air Gaps for Full-View Digital Mammography. *Radiology* 193 (P) suppl. :360.

23. Minoru, S., Masao, T., Miyahara, J., and Hisatoyo, K. 1983. *Radiology* 148 833-838.

24. Amemiya, Y., Nakagawa, A., Kishimoto, S., Matsushita, T., Ando, M., Chikawa, J., and Miyahara, J. 1989. *Proc. SPIE* 1140: 167-173.

25. Sanada, S., Doi, K., Xu, X., Yin, F., Giger, M.L., and Macmahon, H. 1991. *Med Phys* 18(3):414-420.

26. Antonuk, L.E., Yorkston, J., Huang, W., Boudry, J., Morton, E.J., and Street, R.A. 1993. Large Area, Flat-Panel a-Si:H Array for X-ray Imaging. *Proc. SPIE* 1896:18-29.

27. Antonuk, L.E., Boudry, J.M., El-Mohri, Y., Huang, W., Siewderden, J., and Yorkston, J. 1994. High-Resolution, Flat-Panel, Digital Imager for Diagnostic Radiography and Fluoroscopy. *Radiology* 193 (P) suppl.:940 (abstract).

28. Rowlands, J.A., Hunter, D.M. and Araj, N. 1991. X-ray Imaging Using Amorphous Selenium: A Photoinduced Discharge Readout Method for Digital Mammography. *Med Phys* 18(3):421-431.

29. Hillen, W., Schiebel, U., and Zaengel, T. 1988. *Proc. SPIE* 914:253-261.

30. Barnes, G.T., Cleare, H.M., and Brezovich, I.A. 1976. Reduction of Scatter in Diagnostic Radiology by Means of a Scanning Multiple Slit Assembly. *Radiology* 120:691-694.

31. Barnes, G.T. 1991. Contrast and Scatter in X-ray Imaging. *Radiographics* 11:307-323.

32. Maidment, A.D.A. and Yaffe, M.J. 1990. Scanned-Slot Digital Mammography. *Proc. SPIE* 1231:316-326.

33. Yaffe, M.J., Plewes, D.B., Maidment, A.D., Lewkow, R., Mawdsley, G.E., and Starkoski, B.G. 1994. Clinical Digital Mammography System: Initial Results. *Radiology* 193(P) suppl: 361.

34. Roehrig, H., Yu, T., Gaalema, S., Minteer, J.A., Sharma, S.D., and York, W.E. 1994. Slot Scanner for Mammography: Application of Hybrid Detector Technology. *Radiology* 193 (P) suppl. :36.

Appendix A
Quality Control Visual Checklist

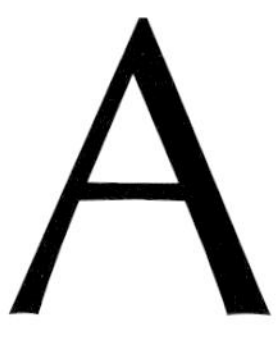

Pass = P
Fail = F
Not applicable = N/A

Technologist ____________________

Date																							
Generator																							
Key pads																							
X-ray key																							
X-ray key light																							
Screen visibility																							
Table Unit																							
Integrity and cleanliness of table covering																							
Leg extensions move freely																							
C-arm Controls																							
Control indicators visible																							
Table movement–up/down																							
C-arm movement–up/down																							
Table/c-arm movement–simultaneous																							
Rotational control through 180°																							
Panning control																							
Compression controls–finger switch																							
Compression controls–foot switch																							
Lamp rheostat																							
Control lock-out																							

C-arm

C-arm detents into +/- 15°																							
Apertures slide in and fix easily																							
Halogen lamps operation																							
Emergency switch operation																							
Digital camera slide																							
Digital camera centering detent																							
Camera connectoins to table																							
Wire connections to digital camera																							

Breast Support

Number markings																							
Moves easily between detented positions																							
Integrity of support																							
Drip pan																							

Compression Arm

Manual control																							
Biopsy/compression plate detents center																							
Biopsy/compression plate–integrity																							
Cam lever lock																							
Scout paddle–integrity, readable scale																							

Stage

Markings evident and clear																							
X, Y, Z–manual controls																							
Stage coordinates change accurately along full range of scale, with knob movements																							
Integrity and cleanliness of Z axis																							
Anterior needle guide mount moves easily along axis																							
Posterior needle guide placement																							
Biopsy instrument holder–set screw																							

Motorized Movement

Occurs only when "enable" key depressed																							
Moves to 0 position																							
Moves to "target" or "pass"																							
Warning display occurs with incomplete movement																							

LCD Display (Check both numeric and graphic screens.)

All lines functioning																							
Changes between windows (core, FNA, wire loc, 0 preset)																							
Cursor key moves cursor																							
Enter key changes line-LCD display																							
Stroke margin and compression numbers change with detented breast tray positions																							
Zero preset functions and disengages when 0 set manually																							
Coordinate transmission																							
Negative stroke margin indicators: audible tone and highlighted stroke margin line																							

Workstation

Markings clear on CPU																							
Optical disk drive																							
Integrity and cleanliness of monitors																							
Keyboard functional																							
Trackball moves easily (remove ball and check rollers)																							
Buttons on trackball functional																							
On-screen cursor functional with trackball																							

Appendix B
Suggested Sterile Tray Setup

B

Basic

- Sterile drape for tray
- Biopsy instrument (not sterile)
- Desired biopsy needle (core, localization, FNA)
- Needle guides
- Gauze (4x4)
- Povidone-iodine solution or similar wash - swabs work best for easier access.
- Sterile water - for swabbing needle in between specimen samples and for cleaning the breast postprocedure; also may be used in a syringe to "push"specimen out of sample notch. Avoid sterile saline as this can corrode the biopsy instrument.
- Sterile container - for sterile water
- Syringes:
  - 3 cc - for anesthesia
  - 5 cc - for "pushing" specimen off needle (optional)
- Needles:
  - 18-gauge for drawing up anesthesia
  - 25-gauge or similar for infusion of anesthesia
- Anesthesia:
  - Lidocaine hydrochloride, 1% or 2%
  - Optional:
    - Sodium bicarbonate - may be mixed with anesthesia to reduce burning just prior to biopsy. Ratio 1:10 sodium bicarbonate to lidocaine (or similar).
    - Epinepherine - may be used to reduce bleeding; purchase premixed with anesthesia or separately. Ratio 1:100,000 epinepherine to lidocaine hydrochloride.
- Scalpel/blade # 11 - long handle provides better access
- Sterile 6" swabs for swabbing incision prior to needle insertion
- Steristrips for incision closure
- Specimen collector/holder for samples

Other Needs

- Sterile and unsterile gloves
- Dressings
- Topical antibiotic ointment in single-use packets
- Instant (or other) ice packets

Index

Note: Figures are represented by *f* following their page number.

A

B

Note: Figures are represented by *f* following their page number.

C

Note: Figures are represented by *f* following their page number.

D

Note: Figures are represented by *f* following their page number.

E

F

G

H

Note: Figures are represented by *f* following their page number.

Note: Figures are represented by *f* following their page number.

N

O

P

Note: Figures are represented by *f* following their page number.

Q

Note: Figures are represented by *f* following their page number.

Note: Figures are represented by *f* following their page number.

T

Note: Figures are represented by *f* following their page number.

Note: Figures are represented by *f* following their page number.